HOW
Can I
HELP?

A Week in My Life as a Psychiatrist

David Goldbloom, M.D.,
and
Pier Bryden, M.D.

Published by Simon and Schuster
New York London Toronto Sydney New Delhi

SIMON &
SCHUSTER
CANADA

Simon & Schuster Canada
A Division of Simon & Schuster, Inc.
166 King Street East, Suite 300
Toronto, Ontario M5A 1J3

This Simon & Schuster Canada edition February 2016

SIMON & SCHUSTER CANADA and colophon are registered
trademarks of Simon & Schuster, Inc.

For information about special discounts for bulk purchases,
please contact Simon & Schuster Special Sales at 1-800-268-3216
or CustomerService@simonandschuster.ca.

Library and Archives Canada Cataloguing in Publication
Goldbloom, David S., author
How can I help? : a week in my life as a psychiatrist /
David Goldbloom, M.D. and Pier Bryden, M.D.
Includes bibliographical references and index.
Issued in print and electronic formats.
ISBN 978-1-4767-0678-8 (bound).—ISBN 978-1-4767-0680-1 (ebook)
1. Goldbloom, David S. 2. Mentally ill—Care—Ontario—Toronto.
3. Centre for Addiction and Mental Health. 4. Psychiatry. 5. Physician
and patient. 6. Psychiatrists—Ontario—Toronto—Biography.
I. Bryden, Pier, 1964–, author II. Title.
RC438.6.G64A3 2016   616.890092   C2015-905066-9
C2015-905067-7

Interior design by Lewelin Polanco

Manufactured in the United States of America

3 5 7 9 10 8 6 4 2

ISBN 978-1-4767-0678-8
ISBN 978-1-4767-0680-1 (ebook)

For people with mental illnesses and their families

Contents

Introduction

Almost thirty years ago, a patient on the psychiatry inpatient unit where I had just started working approached me as if we were lifelong friends. He was tall, skinny, unshaven, dressed in threadbare jeans and a pale blue hospital pajama shirt. His hair was long and matted, and it was clearly some time since he had bathed. I assumed my best psychiatrist manner – unthreatening, warm but not familiar, and firm – and prepared to tell him that I was not actually his doctor, that we had never met, and that my colleague Dr. Buckingham would be looking after him.

He started speaking before I could deliver my blurb.

"David Goldbloom! I heard you had gone to medical school. How amazing to see you here. Do you remember me?"

There was something about the man's deep, slow voice, with an Ottawa valley drawl, that was familiar. But I couldn't recognize or place him.

"It's Andrew. Andrew Balkos. We played squash together at university."

His voice, height, and smile coalesced immediately into an older, gaunt phantom of the muscular twenty-something squash player who had won a healthy number of games off me during round-robins in university. We had been part of a group of young men who played sports and socialized before we all headed off to further education or our first serious jobs. We were a confident bunch in those days, encouraged by our education, our youth, and our health to think we would attain whatever life goals we set ourselves. I hadn't known him particularly well, but I now recalled that he had dropped out of school – no one said why – and that I was short a squash partner as a result.

Usually when I run into old school friends, we discuss work, family, travel. Andrew told me that he had been admitted from the emergency room the previous night. He explained that he had been struggling with mental illness for years, and this was not the first time he had been hospitalized.

I made the right noises about Dr. Buckingham being a good psychiatrist and about the treatments available in the hospital, but my brain was in overdrive. It was hard to reconcile this emaciated, unkempt individual who looked easily fifteen years older than me with the virile young man with whom I had competed for corner drop shots ten years earlier.

It was clear from our discussion that whatever psychiatric disorder Andrew was suffering from had completely changed his life course. He told me that he was estranged from his family and had never married. He had dropped out of school and done odd jobs, but within a few years he started to experience the paranoia and hallucinations that continued to haunt him, despite his intermittent efforts to quiet them with medication and talk therapy. Currently he was living in a rooming house a few blocks away, surviving on public assistance. His only social contact was with the other inhabitants of the rooming house and a social worker assigned to him after his most recent hospitalization.

I told him how sorry I was to hear about his illness and wished him well in his treatment. I couldn't think of what else to say. What I didn't tell him was how sorry I was that a decade earlier I had not been attuned to whatever struggle he was having, that I was oblivious. Back then, I knew nothing about mental illness.

Andrew told me that knowing I worked in the hospital as a psychiatrist would help him to trust Dr. Buckingham and his recommendations for treatment, something that had been difficult for him during past hospitalizations. I didn't comment at the time but have wondered in retrospect why our meeting – our first in more than ten years – had this impact on him. I know that he stayed until Dr. Buckingham thought he was ready for discharge and accepted both medication and referrals for outpatient therapy.

My hypothesis, looking back, is that his knowledge of me as a person rather than simply as a psychiatrist helped him to trust me and to think differently about psychiatrists in general, including Dr. Buckingham. I also believe the fact that I had known him before his illness made a difference. I hadn't known him well, just in the way young men know each other when they share similar backgrounds, goals, and an enjoyment of sports. We had been equals once in terms of our potential, and he knew that to me he was more than just a patient with a psychiatric disorder. I wonder if his experience of knowing and being known by me in a way not limited to his illness spread to his relationships with his doctor, nurses, and social worker, allowing him to trust.

Andrew left the hospital two weeks later, and I have neither seen nor heard from him since. But that brief encounter at the beginning of my clinical career would be an enduring reminder that "they" are "us."

WHEN I BEGAN A career in psychiatry in 1982, five years after Andrew and I had played squash together, I was naïve about what my choice would mean. I didn't realize then that I was entering the most misunderstood – and mistrusted – specialty in medicine. Coming from a family of physicians and inspired by my father-in-law, who was a psychiatrist, I assumed that everyone saw psychiatry the way I did: as the branch of medicine that offered its most complex diagnoses, its most profound relationships with patients, and its most dazzling frontiers for scientific discovery. Given my youth and relative inexperience, it was arguably a natural mistake.

My early passion for psychiatry has not changed over the intervening decades, even if my view and understanding of it has: psychiatry remains for me medicine's most intellectually challenging, eclectic, and diverse specialty. It is also the most open to considering different theories of illness, examining explanatory models that bring together the contributions of biology, psychology, culture, and society into a coherent whole. I tell my residents that all their prior education – whether in the sciences, social sciences, or humanities – will be relevant to their work in psychiatry, and that they will need to read voraciously in all those disciplines to keep up in a field where knowledge is constantly expanding and intellectual paradigms evolving.

More selfishly, as a natural extrovert who is incurably curious, I revel in the opportunity that psychiatry gives me to meet new people almost every day of my working life, to hear their stories, and to try to help them. I also love the variety inherent in my work: seeing patients with a range of psychiatric disorders in different settings, teaching students, working with colleagues from various disciplines, participating in research, and speaking publicly about mental illness and its treatment. I am too restless and easily bored to do the same thing every day.

But thirty years later, my naïveté in believing that my passion for psychiatry would be shared uniformly by others is long gone. I now recognize that powerful forces (both inside and outside my specialty) dog public perceptions of psychiatry and psychiatrists, and converge to create an environment of mistrust and skepticism regarding our potential to help people struggling with mental illness.

Some of the damage to public trust, of course, has been perpetrated by psychiatrists themselves. It would be disingenuous not to acknowledge the role that psychiatry's own history – its fads, therapeutic dead ends, and ethical breaches and abuses – has played in creating its persistently negative image, amplified by the popular culture of movies and television where both patients and psychiatrists are either mocked or vilified. It is also unarguable that modern psychiatry's close relationship with the pharmaceutical industry – a partnership that some characterize as a pact with the devil – has done great harm to the perceived integrity of the research that lends our treatments credibility. No psychiatrist I know wants to return to the era before the 1950s, when there were no effective medications for anxiety, depression, psychosis, and mania; it would be like being nostalgic for the pre-antibiotic era of infections. But as good as the current medications are, they are still not good enough. We need to find new paths for drug development and clinical evaluation where the legitimacy of the results is not compromised by conflict of interest. At the same time, we need more research on the effectiveness of nondrug interventions – psychotherapy, of course, but also interventions relating to housing, employment, income support, and social engagement.

Some of society's ambivalence toward psychiatry stems from its historically and legally assigned ability and responsibility to detain individuals in the hospital against their will, and in certain cases to force treatment upon them. It's not a simple equation, however, between those powers and public fear and mistrust because in most jurisdictions, including my own, the Canadian province of Ontario, all doctors – not only psychiatrists – have those powers, at least for certain periods of time and under certain carefully and legally prescribed circumstances. It fascinates me that a family physician, an obstetrician, or a surgeon can hold patients for up to seventy-two hours in a hospital to allow for psychiatric assessment and decide that a patient is not able to make treatment decisions for himself or herself without prompting any of the public debate or protest that psychiatrists exerting the same powers evoke.

I think that superimposed on people's philosophical concerns over depriving someone of fundamental civil liberties is the fear of the kind of illness that at times warrants some such action. There is no greater threat to our sense of personal integrity and identity than mental ill-ness. If you break your leg, you're still you. If your brain is broken, are you still you?

Psychiatrists can't win on this one. Some critics argue that psychi-atrists don't use their power to detain and treat patients often enough, allowing acutely ill patients to fall through the cracks by waiting until their disorders bring them to the brink of disaster or beyond. Oth-ers argue that psychiatrists are simply agents of social control, treat-ing nonconformity and alternative ways of being as illnesses requiring forceful intervention.

Most societies have a long tradition of isolating, shunning, and victimizing people with mental illness. Although this has improved substantially in the last century, it is still acceptable to lampoon them in popular culture, in ways that would no longer be politically correct for any other form of disability.

Even within the health-care community, I have been exposed to far too many professionals who regard psychiatric patients, and to a lesser extent those of us who work in the mental health field, with suspicion and even contempt. And my personal experience is sadly reinforced by studies that report health-care professionals, and even some mental health professionals, hold biased and negative perceptions of psychiat-ric patients.[1]

The most sweeping and potentially powerful force undermining the public's trust in psychiatry derives from the accumulation of mis-information, myths, bias, and stigma about psychiatric disorders and the people who suffer from them (not to mention the people who treat them) propagated by mainstream media. It is easy to recall a nega-tive portrayal of a psychiatric patient or a psychiatrist from film or television (*One Flew Over the Cuckoo's Nest* being the defining image for many generations) but harder to pull out a memory of a positive one. And the positive ones have their own issues. Patients' symptoms are frequently romanticized and minimized in order to elicit the audi-ence's sympathy. The mental health professionals who are viewed with relative approval are most often nonmedical psychotherapists (in contrast to pill-pushing or sinister psychiatrists), or if they are psychiatrists, they demonstrate their caring for patients by crossing long-established professional boundaries.

The popular media's emphasis on recent razzle-dazzle neuroscience advances in brain imaging and genetics has been a double-edged sword. It reflects the excitement of discovery, but at the expense of spotlighting more mundane interventions that currently have far greater potential for significant and immediate impact on the quality of life and prospects of people with mental illness: housing, employment, social network, and the right level of clinical care available when needed.

The most dangerous consequence of all these forces – those that serve to stigmatize individuals suffering from psychiatric disorders and the health professionals who look after them, and which characterize psychiatric disorders as not real diseases, and psychiatry therefore as not real medicine – is that many people who are suffering are too frightened to see a psychiatrist and to try psychiatric treatments. They are more scared of taking medication, entering psychotherapy, or considering a hospital admission than they are of their own symptoms: the suicidal thoughts, the voices in their heads telling them they are being followed and spied upon, or the fear that the recurrent cardiac palpitations and shortness of breath represent a heart attack rather than a panic attack. By the time they are referred to a psychiatrist, patients may have seen doctors or health-care practitioners who have told them that their struggles are beyond conventional medicine's ability to help them. Or they have been told by relatives and friends, similarly wary, that a psychiatrist is simply a pill pusher, and that they should lean on friends, go to church, go for a run, volunteer – anything other than see a specialist doctor with knowledge of psychiatric disorders.

It is the admittedly ambitious goal of this book to combat this fear and to reassure patients and their families that if they need to see a psychiatrist and pursue treatment, they will be met by a doctor who has had years of training and supervision; who has been taught to take care of his or her own well-being, and to be aware of professional and personal biases and judgments in order not to inflict these, even inadvertently, on patients. Psychiatrists trained today are taught not only about psychiatry's historical abuses of patients with the goal that they will not be blind to the risks that can characterize patients' and psychiatrists' desperate search for better treatments, but also about the conflicts of interests that have marred and continue to exist within psychiatric research.

This book is not meant to whitewash or oversimplify the state of contemporary psychiatry, which deals with difficult and sometimes frightening disorders and faces problems that need to be confronted. It is meant to provide an honest, informed, and ultimately personal account of both psychiatric disorders and the problems psychiatrists encounter in trying to help sufferers, while also describing the specialty's numerous successes and strengths. In doing so, we hope it will provide prospective patients, their families and friends, and the health professionals who refer them to us with the opportunity to know who psychiatrists are, how we are trained, how we practice, how we cope with the tragedies and horror that are part of all physicians' work, as well as the nature of the scientific evidence that supports our diagnoses and treatment recommendations.

I have been extraordinarily lucky to have as my coauthor Dr. Pier Bryden. We met twenty years ago when Pier was a second-year psychiatry resident and I was a staff psychiatrist providing her with occasional supervision during her training. In the course of writing this book together, Pier and I returned over and over to the centrality of different types of trust: between patient and physician, between psychiatry and society, between researchers and their subjects, and between us and our readers. We agreed that to build trust with our readers, it would be important for me to acknowledge my own biases and judgments about psychiatry, given our shared perception that the traditional image of the therapist/psychiatrist as omniscient but neutral has not served our profession well, portraying us as uncaring, arrogant, and at some level inhuman.

I am, as you will read, anything but neutral in my professional and personal lives. I am intermittently insensitive, arrogant, impatient, and an incorrigible performer and teller of tasteless jokes. As you will see, I am very much part of my family in my professional inclinations and behavior. But I hope as a result of what was – at least to my family and friends – an unpredictable career choice that I am a better person, physician, and teacher than I otherwise would have been. It is a choice that has not only satisfied my natural extroversion and curiosity about people but also compelled me to understand better the experiences of individuals suffering from psychiatric disorders and their families. It has also helped me understand myself better, despite my default style of nonreflection. And it has humbled me, forcing me to recognize the limitations of what I am likely to achieve, and what psychiatry as a specialty can achieve, during my professional lifetime.

Over the course of writing this book, events in my own life occurred that changed my thinking about psychiatry and the rest of medicine – and changed me. After much thought and discussion, Pier and I decided to include those events to emphasize the intersection between the lives of psychiatrists and their patients. Introspection on the part of psychiatrists keeps us honest and helps us build trust with our patients. More than any other aspect of the doctor-patient relationship, trust is essential if patients are to ask for and accept our help.

In our effort to make our profession better understood, Pier and I bring you to the front lines of modern psychiatry – the inside of the psychiatric hospital where I work, the largest in Canada: its emergency room, Acute Care Unit (ACU), inpatient units, electroconvulsive therapy suite, and outpatient offices. We introduce you to the nurses, social workers, and other frontline staff, psychiatry residents (qualified medical doctors undergoing an additional five years of training in order to obtain specialist standing in psychiatry), and administrative staff with whom I work daily to provide care for the more than thirty thousand patients who are seen in my hospital each year.

We address some of psychiatry's most ignominious past practices but balance these with stories of its heroes: men and women who have worked persistently, creatively, and ethically to push forward psychiatry's scientific research, as well as humane and imaginative treatment innovations that have improved the quality of life for patients. Their stories are part of psychiatry's legacy.

We juxtapose some of psychiatry's most exciting neuroscience with less futuristic innovations that have more immediate practical applications: telepsychiatry, housing programs, and evidence-based psychotherapies.

Most important, you will meet my patients. (In our Authors' Note, we describe the patients in this book: some are real and identified with permission, and others are drawn fictitiously from our many years of practice.) Here, they often appear at times when it was my job to persuade them to accept help but when the barriers to their doing so seemed insurmountable. Why would a middle-aged man hearing voices telling him that he is under surveillance by a militant religious group choose to confide his madness to a stranger, albeit one with a medical degree? Why would a woman struggling to care for a baby from the depths of postpartum depression agree to put a pill in her mouth every day despite her fears of poisoning her breast milk? Why would a physician wrestling with an addiction who knows he could lose his license to practice trust a psychiatrist enough to disclose the truth? What allows a fifteen-year-old Indigenous woman who has been sexually assaulted by a family member to tell a doctor what she cannot even tell her parents? Why would any of them ask for help? The answer? These individuals are suffering, and the right psychiatric care can provide understanding, trust, support, and hope.

I have thought of my meeting with Andrew several times in the intervening thirty years. Psychiatry cannot yet answer the essential question of why our lives took such different directions: why I get to work in a job I love, have a family that supports me, and the physical and mental health to support my activities, while my university squash partner was robbed by psychiatric illness of all those things. As psychiatrists, we have the capacity – and the obligation – to do a better job of explaining our current profession, our understanding of psychiatric disorders, and our treatments; of acknowledging our specialty's past abuses and current mistakes; and of sharing our passion and hope with our patients, their friends and families, public policy makers, potential funders, and the media. It is only by fulfilling that obligation that we will replace fear and suspicion with trust and encourage individuals suffering from psychiatric disorders to seek our help.

This book is our contribution to that process.

Welcome to a week of my life on the front lines of medicine's most misunderstood specialty.

1

Family Medicine

SUNDAY

My mother rubs her eyes. "I can't think why I'm having so much trouble with my vision these days. I keep seeing something moving, almost like a fan turning, but I know there's nothing there. Nancy, what do you think? Should I get my eyes checked?"

My wife, Nancy, and I are chatting after lunch with my parents in the family room of our Toronto home. My parents are visiting from Halifax for the weekend to attend our older son's graduation from law school. Nancy, an ophthalmologist, takes a surprisingly long time to answer.

"I have some ideas, Ruth," she says finally. "Do you want to hear them?"

This is one of those moments when life slows down – when, for example, you know for certain that your car is going to crash into the vehicle in front of you, or you get the message that your child's school is calling unexpectedly. We wait – Nancy, my father, and I: an ophthalmologist, a pediatrician, and a psychiatrist, respectively – for my mother to speak. Usually I focus more on people than on my physical environment, but now I watch the June sunlight coming through the window, lighting up the swirls of dust particles in the air like spun sugar. My diminutive but wildly energetic mother, diagnosed and treated for lung cancer six months ago – successfully, we thought – looks at her hands before flashing a glance at my father, sitting preternaturally still on our sofa.

"I'd like to hear what you think," my mother replies.

My physician wife has realized immediately that my mother's deteriorating vision is most likely caused by lung cancer spreading to her brain. Nancy chooses her words carefully, as she has been trained to do. All doctors have varying degrees of formal training or clinical experience in breaking bad news: Don't convey certainty prematurely when the news is bad and confirmatory tests are pending. Don't take away hope unnecessarily. Nancy talks about possibilities, about brain metastases, about ruling out certain diagnoses, about being thorough. This way, the patient – who on this warm June afternoon happens to be my mother – has time to get used to the possibility that she may eventually hear something that previously seemed unfathomable.

Bad news. It is an aspect of doctors' work that separates us from everyone else except our professional relatives: nurses, ambulance staff, police. Physicians live in a world where the everyday statistical likelihood of bad news is reversed: we see the seven-year-old with fatal leukemia, the mother with two young children killed in a car accident, the grandfather dead of a heart attack after a family dinner where he complained of indigestion. It makes it hard in our personal lives to maintain a balanced perspective. Some of us have to work hard to remind ourselves that not every headache is a brain tumor or a stroke, and that not every child's high fever is meningitis. Others soldier on with cavalier assumptions of their own immortality, a maladaptive coping strategy that lends itself to excessive risk taking. Every physician of my generation remembers a celebrated professor or two who smoked incessantly between patients or surgeries, even in the face of decades of grimly accumulating evidence about cigarettes' extraordinary capacity not just to shorten lives but also to make the days left miserable.

I am more of the second type – assuming that my health and that of my family members will be robust until forced by undeniable evidence to admit otherwise. My experience to this point has largely supported my outlook. Both my parents have lived unusually long and healthy lives into their late eighties, a fact that has allowed my two siblings and me the illusion that we are still young things, barely flirting with middle age, despite being well into our fifties and sixties. We are the children of an optimistic pediatrician father and a tough-minded mother who made a career out of volunteering. As we grew up with the usual childhood maladies, my father exhibited healthy denial, while my mother, uncontaminated by any formal medical education, saw all forms of illness as character flaws.

In the Goldblooms' handbook for life, one written by four generations of physicians, illness is part of the human lot, and anticipatory worrying or feeling oppressed by its appearance in oneself or one's loved ones is not only a waste of time but also a potential roadblock to a good joke.

LATER SUNDAY EVENING, after the convenient distractions of Nancy's composing and faxing a letter to my mother's GP outlining her concerns and recommending next steps, organizing an earlier than scheduled flight home for my parents, and driving them to the airport, I am finally alone with my wife.

"How are you?" she asks.

I know she will not judge. "Fine, I think. Everything's organized. There's nothing more we can do until after the scan."

Nancy doesn't question this ridiculously superficial answer. It's the advantage of having a spouse who has stuck with me for almost forty years and known me since childhood. She knows when to probe and when to allow me my illusions, at least temporarily.

"Yes, we'll take good care of her."

I hug her tightly, thinking of the myriad times in my life when Nancy has nudged me closer toward acknowledging feelings to which I cannot immediately gain access. This probably seems a strange thing for a psychiatrist to write, but as many of my patients, family, and colleagues have told me over the years, I am not the stereotypical psychiatrist.

I have heard the old chestnut that there is nothing like a parent's impending mortality to make you think about your own, but this evening I have no intention of allowing my thoughts to bury either my mother or me prematurely. As I organize my belongings for the next day, I realize I haven't thought for a long time about my decision in 1980 to choose psychiatry as the area of medicine (my version of a family business) that I wanted to pursue. There is – with the striking and influential exception of my father-in-law, Nate Epstein – a dearth of psychiatrists in my family and a plethora of Goldbloom pediatricians across four generations. Given my temperament, which has been characterized since birth by extroversion, a dislike for introspection, a love for performing (particularly comedy routines), and a general chattiness, my decision surprised almost everyone who knew me. These days, that decision comes to my attention only when an eager medical student or psychiatry resident facing his or her own career choice asks me how I made mine. Tonight, it does not take Nancy to point out to me that my reminiscences are an effective distraction from thinking about what news the week will bring.

THERE IS NO DOUBT that psychiatry is a peculiar job. While other doctors ask questions that few others in your life will ever ask – How are your bowel movements? What are your drinking habits? – and enter orifices of your body to which no one else will ever have access, psychiatrists have an even more unusual mandate. We want to know about your moods, your thoughts, worries and preoccupations, your relationships, your experience of school and work, and your grandmother's tendency to put tinfoil inside all her hats to avoid electronic surveillance. We routinely interview police officers, criminals, and homeless people as part of our training, and we spend hours on call in the middle of the night calming individuals who believe that they are the victims of an international conspiracy or that scientists, extraterrestrial or otherwise, have implanted speaker devices in their brains. During the day, we may treat a depressed businessman, a panic-stricken college student, a substance-abusing medical colleague.

Being a psychiatrist also creates a considerable social barrier, at least initially. Announcing one's career as a psychiatrist at social gatherings tends to produce a lull in the conversation while listeners seek to respond appropriately. Some say, "Oh, God, are you analyzing me?" and hastily review what they have previously said; others take the opportunity to divulge highly personal information in the hopes of a quick professional opinion.

Even some of our patients are initially put off by our profession. Very few people wish or believe they or their child will ever need to see a psychiatrist. A family doctor, an obstetrician, and arguably a surgeon to remove a recalcitrant appendix or to fix clogged arteries, but not a psychiatrist. Some patients enter my office and answer my initial questions with the enthusiasm of someone referred to a periodontist for gum surgery. Some are fearful that something said inadvertently will result in being "locked up" or fundamentally transformed by treatment in a bad way. Others dissolve in tears as they sit down for the first time, having waited too long to talk about something private and profoundly troubling.

Medical colleagues also tend to be wary. Medical students considering psychiatry as a specialty usually conceal it from their nonpsychiatric supervisors, surmising correctly that it will be a mark against them. "Why don't you do something really useful?" "Won't you miss real medicine?" "Do you really want to spend your time listening to miserable people?" After one long night on call in the ER during my residency, I met a friend, a resident in another medical specialty, for breakfast in the hospital cafeteria. She marveled, "I can't believe you're in psychiatry. I couldn't do it. I would find it so depressing." She was training in oncology.

It doesn't get better once in practice. Colleagues forced to consult you for assistance with hospitalized patients frequently fail to let their patients know they have done so; as a result, when you appear at the bedside, they and their families are horrified and want to know why Dr. W felt they needed to see you. "Does he think I am crazy, that this is all in my head?" The greatest compliment either a patient or a physician colleague can pay a psychiatrist runs along the lines of "You don't seem like a shrink . . ."

Arguably, the stereotype associated with psychiatrists is borrowed from the far greater stigma suffered by our patients. Patients with mental illness have historically been hived off from the majority of medical patients into asylums and large gloomy psychiatric hospitals built, like prisons, on the periphery of town. It is a relatively recent phenomenon – post–Second World War – for there to be psychiatric wards in general hospitals. Long before film and television, let alone the Internet, Charlotte Brontë's *Jane Eyre*, published in 1847 to instant acclaim, depicted Mr. Rochester's first wife as a violent, fire-setting lunatic, kept locked in the attic. Her caregiver, Grace Poole, resembled her unstable ward in both her demeanor and lack of social graces. Charles Dickens' *Great Expectations*, first published in 1861, was equally well received, with its portrayals of the eccentric and demented Miss Havisham and her troubled adopted daughter, Estella. Neither masterpiece did anything to increase sympathy among readers for the mentally ill or their caregivers.

It hasn't improved over time. In the twentieth century, F. Scott Fitzgerald, in his semi-autobiographical 1934 novel *Tender Is the Night*, described Dick Diver, a psychoanalyst, who marries his schizophrenic patient (modeled on Fitzgerald's troubled wife, Zelda) and almost destroys himself with alcohol. More recently, films such as *One Flew*

Over the Cuckoo's Nest, Frances, and *Girl, Interrupted* have continued the theme of caregivers who resemble their wards in their unappealing psychiatric profiles. Nurse Ratched has entered the psyche of the English-speaking world as the epitome of the sadistic, parasitical torturer of the mentally ill who masquerades as caregiver.

The portrayals have some basis in historical reality. Psychiatry's past has more than its fair share of horror stories: from the overcrowded asylums of the late nineteenth century with their unwashed and uncared-for patients, to the unheeding savage rush toward psychosurgeries in the United States and Britain from the 1930s to the 1950s, and the postwar psychoanalytic community's endorsement of the cruel and unscientific concept of the schizophrenogenic mother. In this sense, psychiatry shares a history with the rest of medicine, which has its own repertoire of horrific treatments enthusiastically endorsed and subsequently abandoned.

There is also some truth to psychiatrists having things in common with their patients. Psychiatrists are more likely to have had experience with mental illness ourselves or in our families than doctors in other specialties. This shouldn't be surprising. Some physicians who experienced insulin-dependent diabetes in childhood, or witnessed it in a close relative, have understandably become endocrinologists, driven by both noble and self-serving goals to improve understanding and treatment of that illness. Others have chosen oncology after a parent or sibling died of cancer.

Educational researchers describe medical students interested in psychiatry as a career as being more reflective and responsive to abstract ideas, liking complexity, and being more tolerant of ambiguity than their colleagues. They also have more nonauthoritarian attitudes, more open-mindedness, a greater interest in social welfare, and a preference for aesthetic values. Psychiatrists are also more likely than their medical colleagues in other specialties to have an undergraduate degree in the arts and humanities.[1]

On a more mundane level, psychiatrists face ignorance about the day-to-day nature of our work. The common image of a psychiatrist's practice is of a middle-aged professorial type – not a "real" doctor – who conducts rambling intellectual conversations with interesting, troubled people in an office resembling a sitting room rather than the workplace of a medical doctor. My working life, and that of the majority of my colleagues, bears no resemblance to the professorial stereotype, appealing as it may be.

Most people don't understand who psychiatrists are and are not in this day and age. We are not predominantly psychotherapists, and were rarely ever so outside North America. This fact causes confusion for the lay public, which has difficulty differentiating among the various types of mental health professionals, most of whom engage in the so-called talk therapies to a greater or lesser extent.

Psychologists are usually graduates of either a master's or PhD level university program whose training includes the acquisition of therapy skills, the study of the mind in health, distress, and disease, and expertise in the measurement of individuals' psychological states and function.

Social workers also train in university programs that focus predominantly on social and cultural determinants of mental health and function, and tend to acquire skills in interpreting families, systems, and relationship dynamics for the purposes of intervening for health.

Other therapists may train outside universities in programs that focus more narrowly on a single type of therapy: art, music, play, and dance, among others.

Psychoanalysts, practitioners of psychoanalysis, historically the best-known talk therapy and the intellectual child of Sigmund Freud and his disciples, have now largely been cast out of mainstream psychiatry. Contemporary psychoanalysis exists in institutes and centers outside hospitals and universities, and is practiced by professionals and academics from a variety of disciplines, including medicine, who have been trained in its origins, theory, and technique and who have undergone psychoanalysis themselves.

Each of these groups of mental health professionals – psychiatrists, social workers, psychologists, analysts, and other types of psychother-apists – has its own history and culture, not to mention professional territory to secure, and relationships among them have shifted at var-ious times and in various countries. There can be frank competition for patients in private practice and a high degree of collaboration and teamwork in hospitals and community agencies.

Psychiatry is the only one of the mental health disciplines that lives within medicine and whose practitioners are all medical doctors. Psychiatrists may, as a result, struggle with a dual identity: on the one hand, they are physicians trained in the traditional model of medical science, and on the other, mental health practitioners who acknowl-edge multiple determinants of psychiatric disease and who work with colleagues from a wide variety of academic and philosophical perspec-tives. Depending on your viewpoint, this has either enriched psychiatry to an extent that it now offers medicine an extraordinarily diverse path forward to bringing mind, body, and society back together, or has led to an inferiority complex where psychiatrists feel the need to prove themselves "real doctors" by focusing on medications or neuroscience to the exclusion of other disciplines. It is probably clear by now that I am in the former camp.

Psychiatry has been a struggle for me, not the natural fit that pe-diatrics or surgery would have been, with their relatively sunny out-looks – at least within the medical profession – and fix-it approaches. The vast majority of children in the West in a post-antibiotic era grow to adulthood, and most surgeons have the satisfaction, at least in the short term, of removing, replacing, or resizing the offending body part that is causing their patient distress. In contrast to these specialties' action-oriented fixes, I found the stereotypical psychiatrist's probe of "Tell me how you feel about that" hackneyed and not particularly help-ful. Patients are usually effective in telling me how they feel, consciously or unconsciously, without my asking. It is also the case that I am a doer, and I like to fix things. I come from a privileged background – both economically and genetically – that was often far from the experiences of my sickest patients, whose illnesses relegated them to society's margins. And I was a bit of a jerk when I chose psychiatry: full of youthful narcissism, arrogant, loving the sound of my own voice, and convinced that I was going to make psychiatric history in some undefined way, coming from a lineage, by blood and by marriage, of people who made their marks on the world of pediatrics and psychiatry.

But from the beginning there was something in psychiatry that brought out the best in me. My natural curiosity and liking for people drew me to the patients' unusual stories, as did the opportunity to spend longer periods in conversation with them than was possible in other faster-moving medical specialties. In psychiatry, the time spent talking with the patient was seen as essential to determining diagnosis and treatment. During the course of those conversations, I learned that the vast majority of patients were not weak or lazy but victims of both genetic and circumstantial bad luck. This misfortune took the form of a strong family history of mental illness, or the loss of jobs, relationships, and even housing. They taught me an understanding of both resilience and defeat that my previously limited experience of life's hardships had not. I also loved the intellectual eclecticism that defines psychiatry's unique mix of neuroscience, social anthropology, psychology, and philosophy. Understanding drug interactions and human interactions were equally important. What's more, thirty years ago psychiatry offered scientific frontiers that appeared wider and deeper to my novelty-seeking nature than any others in medicine. In order to understand my patients' experiences, I was forced to think more broadly.

In retrospect, the timing of my decision to enter psychiatry was a fluke. Even ten years earlier, I probably would not have chosen it. In the 1970s, Freudian psychoanalysis still reigned in North American psychiatry, where it had been imported in the 1930s and 1940s by Central European Jewish refugees fleeing Nazism. Its dominance intriguingly never extended to the rest of the psychiatric world, except in France and parts of Latin America. In postwar Britain, psychiatric treatments continued to be offered predominantly by physicians in hospital settings, or by the growing number of general practitioners. Neither did Australia nor other European countries share the North American experience of a rapidly burgeoning community of medical and lay psychoanalysts. But in North America forty years ago, it was psychoanalysis that became synonymous with psychiatry. I would have found the endless discussions of patients' internal psychic worlds, and the hours spent analyzing both their repressed feelings, assumed to be expressed covertly in dreams, and their every interaction with me, tedious beyond belief.

MY MANY DISCUSSIONS WITH Nate Epstein, my father-in-law, profoundly shaped my view; my opportunities to watch him at work as a psychiatrist steered me into his profession. The composer and lyricist Stephen Sondheim has remarked that when he was a teenager, he came under the influence of a close family friend, Oscar Hammerstein II, and learned the craft of lyric writing from him; he suspects that had Hammerstein been a plumber, he would have followed him into that profession. So it was that Nate became a powerful figure in shaping my career.

Nate, like my mother, grew up in New Waterford, a coal-mining town of nine thousand people in Cape Breton Island. His father, Benny, and my grandmother, Rose, had adjacent stores on Plummer Avenue, the only commercial street in the town, and he and my mother grew up together as friends. Nate's wife, Barbara, also from Cape Breton, also knew my mother and her family well. As a result, at our wedding, most of the relatives across three generations of our families already knew one another.

Nate had learned a tough and plain-speaking style on the streets of New Waterford. It reflected a broader trait of speaking his mind and not beating around the bush. His Cape Breton childhood also gave him an ability to relate easily to a broad range of people, to value family, and to adhere to principles. Nate had trained in medicine in the heyday of psychoanalysis in the 1950s. He relinquished psychoanalytic practice in the late 1960s for an academic career researching family function and family therapy. Its echoes, however, could be found in his willingness to engage in direct conversations with his patients, not to mention friends and family, about the unconscious drives that fueled their thoughts and behavior. Nancy still recalls, as a young teenager at the dinner table, relating a dream she had had the night before about a gun and then listening, mortified, as Nate explained phallic symbols to her.

I had not seen that side of Nate growing up. He had a way of relating to children that allowed them to connect with him quickly; he never pandered or pretended to be their age. From an early age I knew him simply as "Nate."

But what Nate did for a living was largely a mystery to me – as it was at first for his Polish immigrant merchant father. Later, when his father became justifiably proud of Nate's professional success, he gave a superb definition of the trade: "A psychiatrist is someone who knows when you're lying, even when you don't know yourself."

I first experienced Nate's professional skill at age eighteen. As an undergraduate, I found myself uncharacteristically down and irritable. I telephoned my brother Alan, then a medical student at McMaster, where Nate was the founding chair of the Department of Psychiatry. Alan suggested that I come to visit him and talk with Nate. So I called Nate, who said, "Sure, come on up." Within an hour of my arrival, Nate had wormed out of me, much to my surprise, that I was furious with a roommate who had, in my view, treated me badly. Desperately uncomfortable with this novel experience of a negative emotion, I had persuaded myself that it was my fault. The encounter is still a bit of a blur, but what is distinct is my memory of the psychic equivalent of a thorn being taken out of my paw. The relief was quick and palpable. My meeting with Nate that afternoon opened my eyes to the oppressive consequences of unacknowledged feelings and to the ability of a psychiatrist to help someone untangle his or her emotions and beliefs within a relatively short period of time to an extent that brought relief.

It was eight years later that I found myself applying to a psychiatry residency program, but in retrospect my experience that afternoon was the beginning of my path toward a profession that no one who knew me would have anticipated.

One of Nate's other characteristics that made psychiatry seem possible and appealing for me in my early twenties was his irrepressible maleness. Tough, blunt, and unafraid of confrontation, he was infamous throughout his career for using expletives to pepper his expressed emotions and opinions, much to the joy of like-minded trainees but occasionally shocking to his more restrained colleagues. He was impatient with any psychiatric intervention that he did not view to be practical, immediately helpful, and comprehensible to patients. His research on and practice of family therapy was a model of his straightforward, jargon-free approach to family distress and dysfunction.[2] More than fifty years later, the resulting McMaster Model of Family Therapy remains in international use for research and clinical care. I think the underlying message to me from Nate's success in psychiatry was that if this irreverent, impatient, active man could carve a career path within the field, the likelihood of my finding similar rewards was high.

PSYCHIATRY IN MONTREAL, where I trained in the 1980s, as in the rest of North America, was experiencing an inexorable transformation to a modern medical specialty shaped by scientific findings. The majority of physicians entering the field no longer envisioned the practice of the urbane psychoanalyst in a discreet private office, and certainly not that of the white-coated alienist (a historical term used for physicians who looked after mentally ill patients) carrying his ring of heavy keys to the insane asylum on the edge of town. We rejected both the arcane traditions of psychoanalysis and the isolation of the asylum in favor of collaborating with our medical colleagues in shared clinical settings. We had a common goal: mining contemporary neuroscience for treatments to alleviate the mental anguish and socially distressing behaviors of patients with psychiatric illnesses. We hoped for cures but settled in the short term for drugs whose effects were limited to reducing symptoms of illness (sometimes markedly) but that unfortunately produced significant side effects. We recognized the importance of the therapeutic relationship enshrined in psychoanalytic models but were attracted to newer forms of talk therapy that were shorter, problem focused, less expensive, and had scientific research to support their effectiveness.

The contrast between the recent psychoanalytic past and my present as a newly minted doctor entering psychiatry mirrored an intellectual dualism that has characterized psychiatry since its inception. The popular historian of psychiatry Edward Shorter has written of cycles in psychiatry fluctuating between those who ground the specialty in medicine and the laboratory and those who see it as part of a philosophical, even spiritual exploration of the human condition. In *A History of Psychiatry* he writes that since its infancy, "psychiatry has always been torn between two visions of mental illness. One vision stresses the neurosciences, with their interest in brain chemistry, brain anatomy, and medication, seeing the origin of psychic distress in the biology of the cerebral cortex. The other vision stresses the psychosocial side of patients' lives, attributing their symptoms to social problems or past personal stresses to which people may adjust imperfectly."[3]

For a psychiatry resident in Montreal in 1982, psychiatry's transition from an isolated psychoanalytic stronghold to a home within medicine felt as irresistible and irreversible as the Industrial Revolution, though I was soon to discover that this progression was to be far more challenging than it then appeared. In contrast to discoveries such as Prozac and positron emission tomography for visualizing brain function, Freud and his successors' theoretical musings on the human psyche evoked the musty air of a nineteenth-century library.

Fortunately for me, at the time of my residency, psychiatry was clearly moving into a phase favoring the neuroscientific vision, one that suited my liking for practical and measurable medicine. In 1986,

Leon Eisenberg, a well-known and respected leader in twentieth-century American psychiatry – coincidentally a friend of my father's – wrote an article in the *British Journal of Psychiatry* with the title "Mindlessness and Brainlessness in Psychiatry."[4] In it, he argued against the historical distinction that had over the centuries rent psychiatry into warring camps – biological empiricists versus psychosocial theorists – affirming that the two categories necessarily overlap, and that both perspectives are needed to understand and help people with mental illness.

Eisenberg's call to arms – trumpeted from a position clearly within the medical camp – inspired my newly minted fellow psychiatrists and me. In the mid-1980s, when I finished my training in psychiatry and began my clinical and research career, there was no question that I was on the side of those who saw psychiatry as necessarily and beneficially part of medicine. It is only in hindsight that I recognize the naïveté that characterized much of my belief in psychiatry's ostensible progress. It was the famous third edition of *The Diagnostic and Statistical Manual of Psychiatry* (*DSM-III*), published in 1980, that signified North American psychiatry's rejection of psychoanalysis. It took an atheoretical approach to the causes of psychiatric disorders, focusing instead on signs and symptoms that could lead to reliable diagnoses – by which I mean that two psychiatrists, observing the same signs and symptoms, would come up with the same diagnosis. I pored over it as if it were a liturgical text, because it categorized relentlessly and made sense of nonsense. I believed the *DSM-III*'s premise: that reliable diagnosis triggered correct and effective treatment, which in turn led to the relief of symptoms. The linearity of my thinking was youthful and simplistic, blinding me to the complexity that individual differences brought to the process of diagnosis and treatment. Though two people may share the diagnosis of schizophrenia, they will present their experiences through the lenses of their different personalities and backgrounds, and will consider treatments based not on the similarity of their symptoms but on how they relate to the physician treating them.

Then and now, psychiatrists have no laboratory tests, no blood screening or brain imaging to reliably diagnose psychiatric illness. We continue to rely on the symptoms and signs experienced by people, and their similarities and reproducibility. In contrast, we find our ability to treat by explaining these reproducible and generic illness categories in the contexts of individual narratives – narratives written from each patient's genetics and experience, and the impact of these on brain structure and function. Over time, my colleagues and I learned that our attempts to understand a patient's individual experience, belief system, support system, and sense of identity allowed the psychiatric treatment of generic symptoms such as disturbed sleep, depressed mood, and hallucinations to be individually tailored to that patient's needs and preferences, and therefore tended – at least in our clinical eyes – to be more successful. This is the intersect of science and art in psychiatry – indeed, in all of medicine.

When I entered psychiatry, it was also changing in a way that was attractive to me in terms of the type of work and workplace environments that it offered. By the 1980s, North American psychiatry had moved back into the hospitals, both general hospitals and specialized psychiatric hospitals (in the rest of the world the majority of psychiatrists had never left). Fewer psychiatrists were holed up in isolated offices where faded Persian carpets and expensive couches evoked Freud's secluded approach to his troubled patients. The isolation and drawing room atmosphere of such an office held no appeal for me. I could not imagine not being a doctor, and I had loved hospitals since my childhood days of collecting my father at the hospital after school, meeting his colleagues and hanging around his office. As a medical student, I had made rounds with Nate on the acute care general psychiatry inpatient unit he ran. Its scuffed floors and institutional color palette emphasized its utilitarian purpose. This was where the action was – the most severely ill people and the greatest opportunity to make a difference in psychiatry.

When I am asked for career advice by younger people now, I give them three simple yardsticks for gauging possible professions: you like it, it likes you, and you think you will be good at it. All three applied to me when I decided to pursue psychiatry. It continues to suit me: I still enjoy going to work. I still look forward to meeting new patients and learning new things. I still hope that somewhere in my week I will be able to help a patient (preferably more than one!) struggling with the distress and dysfunction caused by his or her psychiatric disorder. But what I didn't – and couldn't – anticipate was how it would change me.

BEFORE SETTLING INTO BED on Sunday night, I scan my BlackBerry calendar to review the workweek ahead. I turn to Nancy, who is reading beside me. "It's a busy week for me. I'll need to make sure I leave time for Mum. I don't want to pretend this isn't happening; I just really need to know what's going on. And if her cancer has metastasized, I mean, she's had an extraordinarily long, rich, healthy life. We all have to die sometime. It'd be ridiculous to think this is unexpected."

"We'll get through it," Nancy says.

2

Listening for a Diagnosis

At eight in the morning, after a vigorous squash game, I pull into the parking lot underneath the ugly 1960s midrise building where I work. It is a concrete fortress that houses one of the three main downtown sites of Toronto's largest psychiatric hospital, known as the Centre for Addiction and Mental Health (CAMH), the result of a complex merger of four institutions in 1998.

Each of the three sites in its own way reflects the city's history of shifting public attitudes toward the hospital. The largest site is in the city's west end, an area that was countryside when the Provincial Lunatic Asylum was built there in 1850. The asylum was part of a larger nineteenth-century trend that crossed national boundaries; many psychiatric hospitals were built outside a city's limits, ostensibly to provide their inhabitants with the respite and quiet associated with such bucolic locations. The United Kingdom's Lunacy Act of 1845 specifically stipulated that an asylum should be placed in a spacious countryside location but comparatively close to an urban setting.[1] Meanwhile, in nineteenth-century New Zealand, small purpose-built asylums were constructed on the outskirts of the main towns and in more remote areas[2]; and in Australia, Adelaide's Parkside Asylum was built in 1870 just beyond the ring of parklands that surrounded the city center, to provide a "modern" alternative to the old overcrowded Adelaide Lunatic Asylum on one of Adelaide's main streets.[3]

The desire to distance oneself from the strange and the unusual is as old as humanity, a trait shared with our animal relatives. It manifests today, despite our supposed sophistication, in the stigma and isolation that many visibly mentally ill individuals suffer. But history defeats our best-laid plans. Today my hospital's western site, once a rural, sprawling campus, is surrounded by one of Toronto's swiftly gentrifying neighborhoods. Large parts of the site are under construction; the plan is to create a state-of-the-art urban psychiatric hospital that brings together the best ideas in architecture, urban planning, landscaping, design, and mental health.

The central site, where I work, is located in a somewhat less fashionable part of the city, just west of its largest university. It is immediately adjacent to the old Jewish immigrant neighborhood, Kensington Market, whose streets over the years have been populated by successive waves of newcomers to Canada. The hospital at this site opened in 1966 as the Clarke Institute of Psychiatry, a younger twentieth-century sibling to the older provincial asylum in the west end. It was conceived of as a place where the university's scientists and academics would mix with psychiatrists and their patients to push forward the frontiers of science. Yet significant advances, such as establishing one of the world's leading brain-imaging centers in psychiatry, focused on positron emission tomography (a way of seeing the function rather than the static architecture of the brain), as well as an internationally renowned molecular genetics laboratory, have yet to trigger a major transformational shift when it comes to providing a biological underpinning to clinical diagnosis – that elusive laboratory test that says "you've got the illness" – or to improving psychiatric treatment outcomes.

MY OFFICE IS IN a corner of the building on the eighth floor, with windows on two sides and a view of the city down toward the lake. It is quiet, tucked away from the main patient areas of the hospital. One corner, with a wingback chair for me and a comfortable chair for patients, is where I do my clinical work with outpatients. There is also a large round table with comfortable chairs where I sit with families or committees.

Simone Rodrigue, my assistant, is not in yet. I am happy to have a quiet hour to catch up on my charts and email before the day begins. The mundane tasks keep thoughts of my mother at bay. Simone and I work well together; we respect each other's rhythms. Last Friday, before she left, she placed all the relevant documents for today's work in a file folder labeled "Monday" and stored it in a discreet cupboard. This morning I have a new assessment, a patient whom I have not met, whose family doctor recently referred her to the hospital's outpatient clinic.

My job, and that of the resident with me for the morning, will be to answer the specific questions that the patient and her family doctor have for us. Most often they are about diagnosis: Why is the patient feeling or behaving in an unusual way? Sometimes the diagnosis has been made already and the questions are about treatment. Why is the most commonly recommended treatment used by the family physician not working? What else can be tried? Sometimes the latter category of questions leads back to the first category: the reason the treatment isn't working is that the diagnosis is incorrect, and the treatment by definition is a bad fit.

I enjoy the process of diagnosis and appreciate its central importance in our care of patients. In psychiatry we rely primarily on listening to and observing the patient, although additional information from caregivers, family, and friends can be essential. This careful process harkens back to an era in medicine when physicians lacked our current sophisticated array of diagnostic imaging and laboratory tests, and were forced to rely on their five senses. Arthur Conan Doyle, a physician as well as the author of the Sherlock Holmes mysteries, used his clinical skills to inform his protagonist's feats of diagnostic observation. A more recent exemplar of the diagnostic virtuosity made possible by acute observation and penetrating history taking is the infamous television medic, Dr. Gregory House. It is true – historically and now – that sometimes a physical cause for the patient's psychiatric symptoms is identified, leading to medical investigations that provide confirmation, but even then the path to diagnosis is determined initially through the physician's history taking and observation. I was taught in medical school, long before I entered psychiatry, that a physical exam or lab tests should serve mainly to confirm what the physician already suspects after taking a careful patient history.

These outpatient assessments for the purpose of diagnosis (and sometimes, if the diagnosis has already been made, for advice regarding treatment) are probably the portion of my work that most fits with the public's largely outdated perceptions of how psychiatrists practice – in an office, probably not part of a hospital, on their own rather than as part of a team, in a one-to-one relationship with the patient, with meetings taking place once to several times weekly, and the psychiatrist asking penetrating and at times oblique questions that unerringly get to the heart of the patient's dilemma. My reality and the reality of most of my psychiatric colleagues today is quite different. Even these outpatient meetings tend to be one-time events, or at most are followed up with widely spaced visits at the request of the patient and the family doctor to review the effectiveness of the suggested treatment or to try something else if the treatment proves ineffective. Even among the patients I have followed for a number of years, there is no "Tuesdays at 4:00 p.m." regularity to the contact. If they are in crisis or relapse, I see them as often as needed, but if they are well, the visits are irregular and more infrequent. I have not practiced open-ended weekly psychotherapy with my patients since my residency.

And while most psychiatrists have some type of outpatient practice, many of us are also based in hospitals, treating patients who come to emergency rooms or who are admitted to inpatient units, working in the same environments in which our training took place. Hospitals are where we see the severely mentally ill: patients who cannot function at all, albeit temporarily in most cases.

In diagnostic assessments, our questions tend to be transparent and focused on the patients' current state of health and their response to treatment. We ask about disturbances in the most basic, animalistic aspects of functioning – energy, appetite, sleep, sexual drive – as well as those that reflect our complex humanity – pleasures and interests, mood, concentration, memory, and motivation.

I flip through the pile of papers that Simone has left for me and find the referral note for this morning's patient. The consultation was requested five weeks ago from a physician in a walk-in clinic, and the cover letter is terse and unhelpful – "Please assess and treat" – reflective of either a busy day or simply an anxiety about managing patients with psychiatric problems and a wish to pass them on as swiftly as possible. Fortunately, most of the time the letters give a provisional diagnosis and an account of what has already been tried. And learning from experience, the hospital now has a referral form that compels the referring physician to address a number of important clinical issues before the patient will be seen here. Most of the boxes on this morning's referral form are sparingly filled with "not applicable" and provide little additional information apart from the patient's age, sex, and contact information.

In some ways, I prefer to see patients "cold," without information that might bias my perspective. But the reality is that I have at least two people to be concerned about – the patient and the referring doctor – and I have to try to meet both their needs. Those needs may not be the same. Sometimes family physicians want clarification and reassurance regarding their diagnoses, and sometimes advice about what to do next in the way of treatment. Other times, they may hope to have a psychiatrist take over the care of a complex patient. Some patients come in somewhat unwillingly, rejecting or dreading a psychiatric diagnosis, while others have had to prod their family physician to initiate a referral. The other reality is the family, who all too often feels blamed or ignored or both. I compromise by telling patients that "I've seen the information your doctor provided and it's very helpful, but there's no substitute for hearing things directly from you."

The outpatient clinic is part of a teaching hospital, so this morning's seventy-five-minute assessment for the purpose of clarifying the patient's diagnosis will be conducted by a senior resident in psychiatry (a qualified physician in his final year of specialty training). I will be in the room observing silently until I can no longer restrain myself. As soon as the resident gets to "That covers what I wanted to ask you about. Now let's see if Dr. Goldbloom has any questions," my self-imposed gag order is lifted. When I am on my own, these initial assessments take less time, generally an hour. But residents need more time as they learn the longhand of interviewing; clinical experience will teach them the shorthand.

Some mornings, based on the training needs of the resident, I do the entire assessment myself and allow the resident to watch. It's frankly easier, in part because it is a less passive experience for me. And it's a chance to provide an observation opportunity that our students rarely get: to see how a psychiatrist works rather than how he or she talks about working. It has always struck me as bizarre that surgical students spend much of their early training watching staff surgeons cut, but most psychiatrists do their clinical work in a more clandestine fashion. The roots of twentieth-century psychiatric practice, as opposed to nineteenth-century asylum care, are in the cloistered dyad of the psychoanalytic relationship, where the peeling back of layers of unconscious thought occurred in a secular confessional, far from prying eyes. While psychoanalysts view this Socratic process leading to self-revelatory disclosures on the part of the patient as a treatment in itself, today's psychiatric assessment uses some of the same techniques –

questions that go beyond the surface response, silence that allows the patient to reflect or muster the words to express inner states – to identify the patient's problem and to gauge his or her willingness (both conscious and unconscious) to engage in treatment. This is the popular image of "seeing a psychiatrist" – a quiet room where the distractions of the outside world are silenced to allow the exploration of the inside world. By contrast, surgeons work in an operating theater, with its implicit and actual audience.

THERE IS A KNOCK on the outside door of the office on the other side of Simone's desk. I open it to see a tall, muscular young man with broad shoulders, dressed in slacks and an open-necked button-down shirt. Josh Leitner is one of several senior residents currently working with me who are completing their fifth and final year of training, before getting to hang their shingle as psychiatrists. We are relatively new to each other, but he has observed several of my interviews, and he participated in my Introduction to Clinical Interviewing seminar some four years earlier.

Josh has an easy charm and self-confidence that I suspect will appeal to or disconcert patients, depending on what they are looking for in a psychiatrist. He is hardworking and eager, determined to achieve and demonstrate mastery of the essential clinical skill of diagnostic assessment. He is ambitious, and I like that. Armed with an impressive academic background in neuroscience, he has already published some basic science research. He bones up assiduously on diagnoses and appears to have committed to memory all the diagnostic criteria (the specified abnormal experiences and behaviors described by and/or observed in the patient) for all the disorders. He is a prolific reader of the major journals, scouring them for articles that relate to the cases we see. It's not hard for me to see that at a superficial level, he is an amalgam of elements reminiscent of my own youth – either real or just aspirational (certainly the latter when it comes to height).

But at the same time, as Josh nears the end of his residency, I get the feeling he is logging time with me as a necessary requirement, unsure if I really have much left to teach him at this point. His sense of his own clinical certainty is unsettling, perhaps because it is familiar to me from thirty years ago, when I took an earlier version of the *DSM* – the American Psychiatric Association's *Diagnostic and Statistical Manual* outlining all the established diagnostic criteria for psychiatric disorders – to be the unvarnished truth rather than the best-possible expert consensus at the time. It makes me realize that there is no substitute for seeing a great number of patients over time to both bolster and also undermine your faith in theory and practice. I worry more about the students who lack doubt at the end of their training than those who feel on the edge of an uncertain career precipice and are hungry for advice and correctives.

Usually, the resident and I meet for a few minutes before the arrival of the patient to review the referral material. Today, however, the advance details are scarce. When I suggest we review the few details we have regarding the patient, Josh says he would like this morning's assessment to be a simulation of his impending licensing exam, meaning he will not have any advance information about the patient and will complete the entire interview in fifty minutes; under other circumstances we have the flexibility to let the interview run longer if clinically indicated.

As is our ritual, we head out to the hallway to introduce ourselves to the patient before bringing her in for the interview. For me, the process of diagnostic observation begins there – how the patient appears and interacts in those first few seconds. Everything is fair game in our medical sleuthing – appearance, clothing, grooming, facial expression, speed of movement, style of interaction – as long as it doesn't lead to premature judgment. There is no blank slate when two people meet, and I know that patients size me up with the same speed, their impressions superimposed on their assumptions (and often Google searches) about me. I hope Josh's antennae are also tingling in the hallway encounter.

In the long corridor, our patient, a woman in her early thirties, is seated, holding her BlackBerry but not looking at it. She is blond, but her clothes – black leggings, a loose gray tunic, and short scuffed black boots – wash her out; she looks pale and tired and has dark circles under her eyes. She is dabbing her eyes with a tissue and starts when I address her.

"Good morning, Ms. Ludovic. I hope I'm pronouncing it correctly."

She nods and manages a smile, but it appears effortful rather than spontaneous.

"Please call me Anya."

"I'm Dr. David Goldbloom, and this is Dr. Josh Leitner, a resident in his last year of training who is working with me today. Please come in."

As we usher her into my office, I recall my own first teacher in psychiatry, Joel Paris, who went on to become chair of psychiatry at McGill University. In my first year of training, Joel would barge into the outpatient assessments I was conducting as an earnest resident, observe for ten minutes, and leave. Afterward, as we debriefed, I found out to my chagrin that he had picked up more in his ten minutes of silent observation than I had in an hour of talking with the patient. I had been too preoccupied with determining what I would ask next to listen carefully and observe.

Anya takes the seat Josh offers her. As he begins a formal but hurried explanation of the interview process, her eyes fill with tears.

"I don't know why I'm crying," she says.

Josh doesn't waver from his recitation of the rules of and exceptions to confidentiality, the letter that will follow to her family physician, and the duration of the encounter. It's like a cop on TV mechanically reciting to a perp his Miranda rights – "You have the right to remain silent . . ." My notepad starts to fill, not with clinical information about the patient but rather with notes about how Josh can refine his interview technique and convey more interest in the patient's experience. It's not about the questions he missed so much as the cues, verbal and nonverbal, that he ignored – the patient's pauses, the averted glances. Whenever he uses an awkward or unclear turn of phrase, I write it down precisely so he can hear how it sounds afterward. My first note concerns one of my particular peeves as I hear Josh warn Anya, "I need to ask you some questions now that I ask everyone, even though they may not apply to you." It irritates me to hear residents dismiss their own questions even before they ask them.

Researchers have provided some sense of what people want to hear at the beginning of a first psychiatric encounter – useful information, since first impressions can be lasting ones. A recent experiment involved three types of introductions – the psychiatrist provided a brief introduction with only his name, professional status, and the statement that the patient had been referred by a family doctor; the psychiatrist provided the same information as well as telling the patient how long the appointment would be and what help would be provided; and the psychiatrist provided all of the above as well as an apology for being late because a personal issue, details of which were also provided (ill relative, lost keys, etc.). Videos of these introductions were shown to a range of patients, who were asked the following three questions: Do you believe each one is a good doctor? Do you think each doctor is trustworthy? Would you like this doctor as your psychiatrist? This was a good litmus test, based on first impressions, of how well the patient was likely to work with the physician. The results were clear: patients want only an explanation of what is going to happen and how long it is going to take.[4]

I usually begin interviews with some small talk to give patients a chance to settle in, and to remind them that in addition to the medical reason for our encounter, we are also simply people meeting for the first time. In today's instance, our patient's name, Anya Ludovic, is Slavic, although in collecting the "identifying data" that is part of the beginning of an assessment interview, Josh has not displayed any particular interest in the ethnocultural background it suggests. This strikes me as a lost opportunity to exercise natural curiosity, to break the ice by talking about something less emotionally overwhelming than why she chose to consult a psychiatrist, and to level the playing field by allowing the patient to teach the doctor something. Whether it's finding out the specifics of a patient's job or financial situation, asking the names of children or pets, it's a couple of moments at the beginning of the encounter that help fulfill part of the stated reason for the assessment: "I'm here to find out who you are."

Anya is thirty-one and single. She works in the human resources department of a midsize corporation in Toronto, a job she has held and succeeded in for almost ten years. She lives alone in a condo and has no children. She's in a relationship with a man eleven years older and quickly states that it's problematic.

Rather than following up on that, Josh asks her why she has come to see us.

"This is a big cycle . . . things seem to repeat themselves," she replies.

In the formal language of medical documentation, this will appear as the "chief complaint." Crucial in what Anya has said is the fact she has already completed on her own one of the psychiatrist's tasks – to look for patterns in human experience, whether of symptoms or of interactions with people.

Josh opts not to explore the pattern she alludes to but rather responds to the tears and palpable sadness, asking her about her mood.

"I think I'm depressed," she says.

This is the "low-hanging fruit" of psychiatric diagnosis, given the seeming ubiquity of depression. One in five women will experience clinical depression over the course of their lives. Any physician, especially a psychiatrist, will have a number of patients who struggle with the all-too-common and recognizable pattern of experiences (both physical and psychological) and behaviors that define depressive illness. And it would be next to impossible for a medical student rotating through a psychiatry service – whether in an outpatient clinic or inpatient ward – to make it through without meeting at least several patients suffering from depression.

"What's different for you between being depressed and being sad?" Josh asks. He is parroting a question he has heard me ask many times. In my experience, people with depression can tell the difference in a heartbeat, often describing their depression as feeling numb, less reactive to things good or bad, and – unlike sadness – not seeming to have resulted from specific triggers or to resolve when external circumstances improve. Family members are often keen observers and valuable sources of collateral information as well, especially when a patient is unaware of or minimizing her symptoms. They pick up on someone's diminished emotional reactivity or withdrawal, whereas sometimes asking the patient to describe the changes in her mood is like asking someone to describe an automatic process like driving.

Anya describes a depression that washed over her in late autumn of last year.

"Fall has always been a rough time for me . . . I don't know why."

I make a note to myself to talk with her about seasonal affective disorder. Autumn is a vulnerable time for many people, possibly due to changes in available light (in contrast to the popular and incorrect perception that Christmas must be "the worst time for depressed people").

"This time it started with not wanting to get out of bed, not wanting to eat, but forcing myself to. Some days I'd oversleep, almost like I was in hibernation mode, up to twelve hours at a time. Other times it took me hours to fall asleep."

Josh interrupts her to ask a series of related questions about the characteristic features of depression. In response, Anya acknowledges a loss of energy and motivation to do things for work and for fun that used to come automatically, trouble concentrating on what she reads, walking into a room and forgetting why she did so, and feeling uncharacteristically overwhelmed by simple decisions. She began to make excuses to avoid friends, letting the phone go to voice mail, and ignoring texts and emails. As she withdrew, her thoughts turned more inward, wheels spinning over mistakes she had made and how she had let herself and others down.

Josh asks carefully and directly about suicide.

"Have you ever felt so bad that you've thought about killing yourself?"

I make a note to tell him I liked the way he asked this. Sometimes residents have trouble getting to the point. The two subjects that make physicians most uncomfortable in talking with patients are sex and death; it's no surprise there are a thousand approximations in questions that are designed to alleviate physician disquiet. I've heard countless students come up with meandering variations on "Have you ever, you know, thought about, well, ending it all? I mean, like, going to sleep and never waking up?" It's as if students are dreading a response of "You know, I hadn't thought of that until you mentioned it, but it would really solve all my problems." In my experience, when you ask plainly, "Have you been thinking about killing yourself?" the usual response is both acknowledgment (it is a widespread symptom in depression) and relief (the patient feels that the doctor understands the problem and doesn't have to be protected from the ugliness of this kind of pain). And it's better than the loaded question, "You're not thinking of killing yourself, are you?" where the desired reply is clearly telegraphed.

Anya says that while occasionally she has felt she would be better off dead, she has never actually thought about killing herself: "The guilt is bad enough already. I already feel like enough of a burden to my family. My mother's sister, my aunt Christina, died of an overdose when I was fifteen. I saw how devastated my parents were. I don't want to put them through that again."

"What about self-harm?" Josh asks. I groan inwardly at a formal descriptive term being asked as a question. For those people who engage in self-harm, it is not usually preceded by the thought "I think I'll harm myself." Self-harm describes behaviors such as burning or cutting oneself superficially, actions not intended to be lethal but rather to distract the person from intolerable moods or feelings. Recent research has demonstrated both growing numbers and a growing awareness of "cutters" among teenage girls in particular.[5] People who cut themselves do not often report pain but more often describe a sense of relief and distraction or of feeling more rooted in reality when they see blood.

"What do you mean?" Anya replies – appropriately, I think. Josh gives some concrete examples. Averting her gaze, she answers that in her late teens and early twenties when she felt overwhelmed or acutely alone, she used to cut herself superficially on her wrists and upper thighs, but she became worried about how she would explain the scars. In recent years, she adds, the same feelings have been more likely to trigger binge eating, although not this time.

Josh picks up the cue about her eating behavior and quickly screens for weight fluctuations, intense body image concerns, and purging through self-induced vomiting or abuse of laxatives. She denies them all, and Josh moves on after satisfying himself she doesn't have a full-fledged eating disorder.

While the residents are generally conscientious about exploring suicidal thinking, they are less comfortable exploring people's sexual interest and function. I've heard many awkward variations, including, "So, how are things . . . down there . . . you know, I mean, in terms of the bedroom . . . you and your partner." They are far less likely to ask about sexuality if the patient is older or not in a relationship (when I ask residents if they've even *heard* of masturbation, they often blush at their oversight). Getting the residents over their reticence about exploring sexuality with patients has to precede any specific teaching about how to ask such questions in a plain, nonjudgmental way. Given the adverse sexual side effects of many antidepressant and antipsychotic drugs, it's an important line of inquiry in understanding why some people are reluctant to take their medication. Josh has not asked at all about her interest in or experiences of sex.

Instead he asks Anya how many similar episodes of low mood she has had.

"I feel like they come pretty much every year and hang around for a couple of months. During the worst ones, I can't get to work."

Josh asks, "Do they seem to happen out of the blue, or have you noticed a pattern?"

Anya pauses. "I am a bit embarrassed you'll think this is trivial. I have noticed they often happen when I'm fighting with my boyfriend, but I also think I'm more cranky when I feel down. So it's hard to say . . ."

What Anya has told us may or may not be true in terms of her depression's causes, but it does tell us how she orders her universe. We all look for explanations of the nonsensical, including depression that comes out of the blue with no obvious cause. And retrospection is unreliable compared to tracking methodically on a go-forward basis. An inexplicable belly twinge may lead us to review the day's eating and consider the wisdom of the two slices of pepperoni pizza five hours ago. Anya has nevertheless linked her depression to problems in her relationship; I hope Josh will explore the possible connection, but instead he zeroes in on her initial episode of depression. On the other hand, it's good to know he pays attention. I had told him last week, "Whenever you're dealing with a patient with depression, you need to know about the first episode and the worst episode."

Anya replies, "The first time I ever experienced it I was twenty-three. I had an abortion the month before, but I actually don't think it was connected. At least I'm sure there was more to it."

She explains that a second abortion at age twenty-seven was not associated with any depressive symptoms. I remind myself to emphasize to Josh post-interview that the context is usually more complex than a simple and recurrent event serving as a trigger. While it is tempting to look for single answers to explain cause, experience has taught me that depression usually emerges from a perfect storm of physiological and psychological stresses but can also come completely out of the blue with its own unknown internal rhythm.

He then asks her, appropriately, whether she has experienced the opposite kind of mood state. He is trying to determine if she has ever been manic. The danger here is that simply feeling good in the wake of depression can be misconstrued as evidence of bipolar disorder, a diagnosis that has grown in popularity and broadened in terms of its diagnostic perimeters. People with classic bipolar disorder (or manic-depressive illness) feel far more than good. They experience a euphoric rush, often likened to being high on illicit drugs, and frequently inter-mingled with a short-fuse irritability that gets them into trouble. And mania can be protean in its manifestations – impulsive and extravagant spending way beyond one's means, wildly grandiose thinking about oneself and one's potential, sleep needs that completely evaporate or reduce to one or two hours per night with the person still going full throttle the next day, and a willingness to strike up a conversation with strangers and to speak a mile a minute.

Anya doesn't endorse this, adding, "I wish I did feel like that."

No, you don't, I think, having witnessed too many personal train wrecks caused by manic episodes. At the same time I understand why someone dwelling in the dark cave of depression would yearn for this kind of bright light.

"Would you describe yourself as a worrier?" Josh asks. This seems to be the standard question I hear from residents as they screen for the presence of generalized anxiety disorder, panic disorder, and obsessive-compulsive disorder. I've met very few unworried patients, and the complete absence of worry can itself be worrying.

Anya describes her worry as a push-pull in relationships. She des-perately wants relationships, worries that men will leave her unexpect-edly, and feels smothered by them when they don't; it leads to volcanic eruptions of conflict and breakups. It's worry all right, but it's not the set of diagnostic worries that Josh was screening for.

Josh checks the clock. He is about twenty-five minutes into this interview and wants to be done in another twenty-five minutes if this observed process is intended to simulate his final exam in psy-chiatry. I'm also tracking the time to make sure Josh allots an ade-quate amount to an attempt at understanding the person beyond the symptoms. Anya seems unaware of our occasional furtive glances at the clocks placed strategically around the room, but maybe she does notice.

Fifty minutes is an arbitrary increment, but it has become iconic as the duration of a psychoanalytic session, allowing the psychoanalyst time to make notes and a phone call before the next patient at the top of the clock. It was even enshrined as a popular book in the 1950s – *The Fifty-Minute Hour*.[6] And it is now part of the billing code in the province of Ontario (actually, forty-six minutes for a consultation) and a standardized time for resident evaluation exams.

It is rare for a physician in any other field to spend fifty minutes with a patient (unless the patient is asleep for a complicated surgery). This time frame is being eroded even within psychiatry (especially in the United States), where insurance-funded visits to a psychiatrist may be for brief checks regarding prescribed medication. The latest version of the *DSM* is accompanied by a pocket guide that teaches how to do a full diagnostic assessment in thirty minutes.[7]

Anya may not have noticed Josh checking the clock, but she certainly notices that he is writing notes as he interviews her. I've tried to dissuade my residents from stenographic note taking during clinical interviews for a number of reasons: it diminishes eye contact; it sets up a two-part cognitive task of talking and writing, which disrupts active listening; and it makes patients curious and uncomfortable about what gets recorded and what gets left out, a code for what is significant. I jot a note of feedback for Josh – *Write less* – aware of the irony.

"I don't drink, and I don't use drugs now. I used to get pretty blitzed on vodka when I was a teenager, and I used ecstasy a few times at raves about ten years ago," Anya replies to Josh's screening questions about substance use. Josh seems more relaxed in the wake of this answer, perhaps thinking the case is less complicated or perhaps feeling less judgmental of the patient. Similarly, her medical history is "clean" apart from a penicillin allergy and the two abortions.

Josh has learned to ask women, regardless of whether they have children, how many times they have been pregnant. He is still surprised by how many women tell of having abortions, sometimes traumatic and sometimes entirely benign. And miscarriages and still-births, which are almost always devastating. Surprisingly, these aspects of women's reproductive and emotional lives are often overlooked. It's important not to presume what the impact has been – but it's also important to ask.

Next on his checklist is "family psychiatric history," a survey of who else among Anya's relatives may have experienced psychiatric illness. She reports that both her mother and maternal grandmother have been treated for depression. He notes this and moves on, missing potentially valuable information about the nature of their illnesses and what, if anything, helped them to get better. As for her father, he died a decade earlier of a severe infection. He was younger than I am now, just another reminder of my impending senescence that undermines my identification with Josh.

This is Anya's first ever visit to a psychiatrist; she has never had a similar assessment and has never been treated with psychiatric medication. She has, however, been in psychotherapy for a year, but she seems surprised when asked about the focus or goals of treatment. She says she can be open with her therapist, who is a good listener, but Anya doesn't seem to have expectations beyond that. I feel my own bias rising; she should expect more than someone who listens well. She should be able to say what it's helping with. But maybe that's just me and my need for tangible outcomes.

Ten minutes remain in the encounter, and Josh steers the interaction toward what will be called in the report "personal history." There is the usual collection of information around the patient's mother's pregnancy with her, the delivery, and her developmental milestones (age at which she first walked, talked, etc.).

This is a time when the interview can soar and become textured or diminish to a hurried visit through nodal events. Josh is accelerating as the remaining time evaporates, asking in a perfunctory way about Anya's parents – their qualities and her relationship to them – about her childhood temperament and friendships, her academic performance and extracurricular interests, and finally her occupational and relationship experiences as an adult.

Performed in this way, the personal history is a ridiculous exercise – trying to summarize the past thirty years of the patient's life in under ten minutes. None of us want to believe that our individual complexity could be distilled so quickly.

I've tried to teach Josh that this part of the interview is not a sequential tour of the greatest hits of someone's life but rather a search for themes, which is what Anya was already noticing: recurring patterns of behavior and experience in relationships and in jobs, and an evolving sense of personal identity across the spheres of human behavior that reflect our individuality – namely, love, work, and play.[8]

Anya reveals that she has had five serious boyfriends, relationships characterized by frequent conflict, breakups, and getting back together. Josh checks carefully to make sure there has been no physical or sexual abuse but doesn't explore whether there is a recurring theme within the conflict from boyfriend to boyfriend. Josh gets full marks for safety but limited credit for depth.

As per our routine, Josh gives me a chance to ask a few questions at the end. He believes his diagnostic checklist is complete, and in a superficial sense it is.

I want to ask Anya more about what is going on in her life right now. "Anya, I want to pick up on some things you've mentioned. How are things with your boyfriend lately?"

She immediately starts to cry and takes several tissues from the box next to her on the table.

"Walter, my boyfriend, has Crohn's [an inflammatory bowel disease]. It's been getting worse and now his doctor's told him he needs multiple operations. Walter's pretty freaked; he wants to get married before the surgeries. I don't want you to think I am a terrible person, but maybe I am. I don't think I want to marry him right now."

She explains that she feels ambivalent in the context of the uncertainty of his medical future and guilty about possibly abandoning someone who is ill. She feels trapped.

I seize her word. "Have you felt trapped before?"

Anya tells me that she backed out of two previous engagements to other boyfriends because she felt claustrophobic. When she was an adolescent, her father became incapacitated after an injury at a construction site; as an only child, much of the burden of caring for him fell to her while her mother was holding down two jobs. He died of a spinal cord infection when she was twenty-one, after years of misery.

"I hated having to go home right after school when my friends were doing sports or going to each other's houses. I knew when I got home that he'd demand that I run errands for him or bring him endless beers. I've never told anyone this, but it was a relief when he died. You see, I told you I was a terrible person."

To my chagrin, Josh is now writing furiously, having relinquished the interviewer's role. I decide my feedback to him about his insensitivity to our patient's visible distress can wait.

"Anya, it's normal to resent having to care for people, even if you love them. And you were a teenager, trapped but doing what you needed to do for him. That doesn't make you a bad person."

A map has started to emerge of Anya's relational universe that a few minutes ago had been terra incognita. The contours of some of the patterns she described as problematic at the outset of the hour are coming into focus. We then ask her to step out so we can put our heads together and come up with a plan for her. She moves to the hallway, where there are magazines and a chair.

"So what do you think is going on?" I ask Josh as the door closes behind Anya.

"Major depressive episode, recurrent, moderate, and without psychotic features; she also has borderline personality traits," he replies, armed with symptom evidence.

Josh's answers are taken directly from *DSM-5*, which was released thirty-three years after the publication of *DSM-III*, which I used as a resident. The *DSM* series (together with its European cousin, the World Health Organization's International Classification of Diseases [ICD]) constitutes psychiatry's ongoing attempts to classify mental disorders. Until biological markers are identified for specific psychiatric illnesses, the *DSM* will continue to be revised.

Both classification systems conceptualize a psychiatric disorder as a disruption in the patient's psychological experience or behavior and functioning that constitutes a source of subjective distress and/or objective impairment. Significantly, the definition of disorder excludes those responses to a loss or stressor that are expectable or culturally approved – it's normal to be sad if a loved one dies or to be stressed by the loss of a job. Similarly, behavior that deviates from social "norms" does not necessarily imply the presence of a mental disorder. The word "disorder," rather than "disease," was used because psychiatrists' patients lacked the objectively measurable pathological signs that historically had been used to define a disease state. But "disorder" comes closer to matching up with "illness," defined by medical anthropologists as the subjective experience of feeling unwell. It has been said that organs – including the brain – get diseases, but people get illnesses. It's common for people to say "I feel sick" or "I feel ill"; nobody says "I feel diseased" or "I feel disordered."

Psychiatry has had many different classification systems over the past two millennia, distinguished by the relative importance they place on phenomenology (the study of things as they appear in our experience; in the case of psychiatry, how we experience mental illness), causal factors, and the natural course of the illness. But none has been as controversial as the *DSM*. The fifth edition was released to fanfare and controversy in May 2013.[9] I attended the launch in San Francisco and witnessed both the protest marches and the long lines to buy copies as if they were tickets to a rock concert.

The *DSM* grew out of late-nineteenth-century attempts in the United States to gather statistics on mental illness drawn from census data. Subsequently, in 1917, the American Medico-Psychological

Association (later the Committee on Statistics of the American Psychiatric Association) and the National Commission on Mental Hygiene gathered more specific information from mental hospitals on diagnoses applied to their inpatients. Given their source, the latter diagnostic categories inevitably focused on the severely mentally ill or neurologically damaged. After the Second World War, an attempt was made to include the types of problems seen in soldiers returning from the war. Thus the first edition of the *DSM*, published in 1952, and heavily influenced by the psychoanalytic background of its authors, added diagnoses that referred to how psychological and social events affected personality formation and development.

Over the six decades it has been in existence, the *DSM* has been an ongoing source of controversy, attacked for its lack of a "true" scientific basis, its reliance on the opinions (and arguably biases) of experts in the field, and its susceptibility to social and cultural norms. One of the most frequently cited – and infamous – examples was the inclusion of homosexuality as a disease category until its removal in 1974 as a result of intense pressure from gay rights groups and members of the psychiatric profession. The position statement documenting the rationale for the change reflected the controversy at the time regarding views of homosexuality but acknowledged that many gay people did not meet the more general requirements for psychiatric disorder of both subjective distress and impairment in role functioning. At the same time, reflective of clinical practice then, the position statement argued that "modern methods of treatment enable a significant proportion of homosexuals who wish to change their sexual orientation to do so. At the same time, homosexuals who are bothered by or in conflict with their sexual feelings but who are either uninterested in changing, or unable to change, their sexual orientation can be helped to accept themselves as they are and to rid themselves of self-hatred."[10] We've come a long way since then.

The accusation of bigotry has continued to plague the *DSM*, with feminist critics decrying a previous category called "self-defeating or masochistic personality disorder" that referred predominantly to women, and more recently the argument that the diagnostic category known as "gender identity disorder" pathologizes and discriminates against transgendered individuals. "Self-defeating personality disorder" was removed in *DSM-IV* and "gender identity disorder" was changed in *DSM-5* to "gender dysphoria," with no mention of disorder.

The *DSM-5* has arguably met with the greatest hostility yet, with psychiatrists in warring camps: the chairman of the *DSM-IV* task force publicly criticized his successors as lackeys for the pharmaceutical industry who seek to extend the reach of mental illness far into the realm of everyday behavior,[11] and the British Psychological Association criticized it in a public statement as exemplary of all that is wrong with psychiatry's narrowly biomedical model of illness.[12] Not surprisingly, the international media has had a field day chronicling the divisions among the ranks of mental health professionals.

Having witnessed the launch of *DSM-5* and reviewed its text, however, I am struck by how incremental its changes are over that of its predecessor. This is not a paradigm shift, and every edition – with the exception of *DSM-5* – has included a longer list of diagnoses than its predecessor, a progression mirrored in the classification of medical diseases in general. We still cannot classify disorders based on their causes or biological markers, so we have to rely on symptom patterns. Beyond that limitation to the science behind *DSM-5*, its release aroused fears that reflect, for me, a more generic fear of mental illness and of psychiatry labeling normal human variation as pathology – with the resulting worry that either the illness or the treatment, or both, will erode an individual's sense of identity.

The limits to diagnosis as a means of understanding patients are not unique to the *DSM*, and certainly not to psychiatry. William Osler, arguably the preeminent physician at the turn of the twentieth century, wrote a caution to medical students: "The good physician treats the disease; the great physician the patient who has the disease."

In my own residency in the early 1980s, my colleagues and I had to present cases to Dr. Herman van Praag, a visiting professor of psychiatry from the Netherlands who was at that time head of psychiatry at Albert Einstein College of Medicine in the Bronx. He was a major researcher in biological psychiatry. After one of the other residents presented an extraordinarily complex case of a man with treatment-resistant depression, outlining the symptoms and every conceivable treatment tried, van Praag asked simply, "What can you tell me about him as a person?" The resident was stumped and mortified. It was a lesson I never forgot, and to this day I try to find out in all interviews what the patients are good at, where their passions lie. Their interests and competencies help to round out a portrait beyond the symptoms that bother them, and I think it's easier for people to feel respected, during what is ultimately a dissection of their moods, thoughts, and behavior, if they feel seen as more than the sum of their symptomatic parts.

I ask Josh what his recommendations would be. He thinks Anya needs to focus in psychotherapy on recurring relationship patterns, and with her permission, he will speak with her therapist. He wonders if she would be a candidate for dialectal behavior group therapy, a relatively new validated technique for people with borderline personality disorder. He also feels she could benefit from an antidepressant.

"Depression" is one of those words in our lexicon that have been diluted of their clinical meanings. We use it to sound more sophisticated when describing normal human feelings of sadness, disappointment, loss, and even despair. People talk about feeling "so depressed" about their favorite sports team's recent losses. But that feeling alone is not a psychiatric disorder and does not require psychiatric treatment.

So when does feeling depressed get formalized as "major depressive disorder, recurrent, moderate, and without psychotic features"? It does so when a set of symptom requirements – impairment in mood, interest, pleasure, appetite, weight, sleep, energy, concentration, and memory; feelings of worthlessness; thoughts of death – endures for at least two weeks and causes significant distress or difficulty in role functioning. It has been recognized and described for thousands of years, although the language keeps getting tweaked.

For patients to whom they give this formal diagnosis, physicians will focus on talking therapies, lifestyle interventions such as increasing physical activity and improving sleep routines, and/or medication, depending upon the severity of the symptoms. Other treatments may also be suggested to target coexisting issues, such as a history of trauma, anxiety, or substance abuse.

Although there is evidence to support the observation that a third of people with untreated depressive episodes will get better on their own within a year,[13] few would suggest that patients suffering from the debilitating symptoms of depression should be left to their own devices, particularly given the risks associated with untreated depression: alcoholism and drug abuse, worsening of chronic medical illnesses, job difficulties, family problems and, of course, suicide. It's also the case that between 50 and 70 percent of patients who experience one episode of major depression will experience further episodes,[14] which in turn are likely to last longer and are less likely to have clear stress triggers, appearing "out of the blue."[15] This potentially unfavorable evolution makes it clear that treatment of an initial episode should focus on prevention, early identification, and management of future episodes.

As for the label "personality disorder," it is a diagnosis sometimes used loosely to describe individuals who are disliked. People find it more palatable to say "He's got a big-time personality disorder" than to say "He's a jerk" or "Whatever the problems are between us, they're his fault." But personality disorders do exist, and the official *DSM* language defines them this way.

An enduring pattern of inner experience and behavior that deviates markedly from the expectations of the individual's culture. This pattern is manifested in two (or more) of the following areas:

1. Cognition (i.e., ways of perceiving and interpreting self, other people, and events)

2. Affectivity (i.e., the range, intensity, lability, and appropriateness of emotional response)
3. Interpersonal functioning
4. Impulse control

The enduring pattern is inflexible and pervasive across a broad range of personal and social situations; leads to clinically significant distress or impairment in social, occupational, or other important areas of functioning; is stable and of long duration, and its onset can be traced back at least to adolescence or early adulthood; is not better explained as a manifestation or a consequence of another mental disorder; is not attributable to the physiological effects of a substance or another medical condition.[16]

What does this mean? First, it's about a long-standing pattern of functioning and feeling, as opposed to an episode of illness. Second, it's about how people consistently view themselves and other people, the "lability," or fluctuation, of their moods, how they habitually interact with others in ways that often lead to difficulties, how impulses overwhelm them and lead to trouble.

Borderline personality disorder is just one of ten principal personality disorders categorized, and it is the one that has caught public attention. It is characterized by mood instability, relationship instability, impulsive and self-destructive behaviors, and disturbances in the person's sense of personal identity. While not definitive, Anya's description of plunges in mood triggered by relationship conflicts, her earlier history of impulsive, risky drug use, her disclosure of past episodes of cutting herself, her chronic feelings of aimlessness, and her sense that her life is not worth living certainly suggest that treatment target these aspects of borderline personality disorder.

In recent years, a therapy for patients sufferering from borderline personality disorder called dialectical behavior therapy has been demonstrated in studies by both its creator, U.S. psychologist Dr.

Marsha Linehan, and other psychotherapy researchers, to be effective and palatable to patients. Dialectical behavior therapy draws on Eastern meditation techniques, recently reinterpreted for Western countries as mindfulness, and uses them to help patients manage their emotions and reactions to others with less distress and volatility. A central goal is to help patients find coping strategies other than self-harm or suicidal impulses to manage their distress. The therapy consists of skills groups, individual therapy, and after-hours telephone support for patients in crisis. It is intensive and expensive in terms of the therapist's time, but it has demonstrated an ability to reduce patient visits to the emergency room and inpatient units that would more than justify its up-front expense.[17] Dr. Linehan's career and integrity in speaking of her own history with the disorder have given a personal face to the therapy, and its potential for success.

Josh's treatment suggestions regarding Anya's depression are appropriate. But I remind him that by diagnosing borderline personality disorder, we are intersecting with Anya at a ninety-degree angle to the trajectory of her life, making assumptions about the course of her illness. Further, such a diagnosis is a highly adhesive one that will dog her clinical record for years, potentially evoking negative reactions from health professionals who have come to understand the diagnosis as one highly resistant to intervention and its sufferers as difficult patients, given their chronic thoughts of suicide and recurrent crises. Finally, depression brings out the worst in people's defenses and interactions; when they are depressed they can be more fearful, irritable, negative, and withdrawn.

I remind him that she mentioned a vulnerability to depression in the autumn, and that her symptoms could also be considered in the context of a seasonal affective disorder that has characteristic symptoms and cycles. Careful delineation of such a diagnosis may suggest effective treatment with high-intensity lights for thirty minutes a day.

It's worth a conversation not only with Anya but also with others who have known her for more than fifty minutes – her family, her family doctor, her therapist. Josh looks vaguely frustrated as I create more work for him, but I want him to expand his thinking at this critical stage of his training. Psychiatry, more than any of the other specialties, is about communication, yet we are often not good at it, hiding behind the skirt of confidentiality or opaque language.

Josh would likely pass his final exam easily based on this interview, case presentation, and plan. He has been thorough, and has screened for possible related diagnoses and for the patient's safety. When, in a matter of weeks, he takes that exam, it will be an evaluation not of whether he is superb, but rather whether he is good enough. But Josh is ambitious and so am I. I want him to be better than good enough.

Anya returns to my office, and Josh gives her his feedback. He tells her she has the symptoms of a "major depression," using the language of the *DSM*. I wonder how this language sits with her. I suppose it beats being told your depression is minor, almost trivial. He explains that she would likely benefit from an antidepressant, and he names several brand names that she might recognize, explaining that all of them work equally well but none works immediately – she may have to wait four to six weeks for a response. He goes on to explain that they all can have side effects, including nausea, headache, sleep disturbance, and sexual dysfunction.

I cringe listening to this catalog of delay and disturbance associated with the proposed treatment, offered in the spirit of full disclosure but in the absence of positive messaging that the medication will very likely help her to feel better. And even positive response to antidepressants can vary among patients. Many people start to experience some improvement within days, while the full effects can take several weeks to emerge – a very different message. If you think how few people actually complete a ten-day course of penicillin for strep throat once they stop coughing, imagine someone expecting to take medication for four to six weeks with no anticipated benefit and the potential for unpleasant side effects.

When presenting information, I always start not by laying out a range of options for the patient to choose from like on a restaurant menu, but rather by saying what I think will help them. As psychiatrists, we offer expertise and experience, not just a catalog of choices. This does not obviate the need to explain the range of options, but I believe we fail in our professional responsibility by not recommending a course of action. And the ultimate yardstick for those recommendations should be "What would you do if this was your brother or sister (presuming you liked them)?" And if you're recommending something different, the question is why?

Josh rushes somewhat over the explanation of borderline personality traits. He clearly doesn't like telling her she has a personality disorder, revealing a common bias against such individuals. This bias ignores the fact that for some people, at least, such an explanatory model helps make sense of nonsense and chaos and provides a path to feeling better. He tells her he would like to speak with her therapist about the direction of her treatment and mentions that a group program at the hospital in dialectical behavior therapy has some openings. He explains that this treatment, drawn from a fusion of Eastern and Western psychotherapies, has proved to help people with her problems.

He manages to avoid a lot of jargon, explaining his diagnosis in plain language but not completely fulfilling what I have tried to teach him about an explanation's critical components: Why do you think she has this problem? How common is this problem? How frequently do people get better? How does treatment make a difference?[18]

This would have been the opportunity to talk about the genetic component of depression given her family history – to link her experience over her father's death with current relationship problems; to tell her that depression is both very common and highly treatable and that she should expect to get better. It is also the chance to tell her that antidepressants work, and that although they all can have side effects, of which she may experience some or none, her physician will monitor carefully for them. This approach better instills the message of hope for recovery and balances the patient's expectations.

Nevertheless, Anya seems relieved by Josh's words and grateful for the time he spent trying to understand her difficulties. She admits she had already Googled some of her symptoms, recognized herself in some descriptions of borderline personality disorder, and wondered if this "fit" her. She agrees to authorize communication with her therapist and to follow up with her family doctor on our medication recommendations.

After Anya leaves, Josh and I debrief about the interview. He expresses chagrin that he had not mined the revelatory information that appeared in her relationship history but also says that the final exam pressure is to confirm and rule out the major psychiatric diagnoses – mood and anxiety disorders, psychotic disorders, and personality disorders – while at least screening for other less common disorders, and at the same time ensuring the patient is safe. He is right, and from a safety and utilitarian perspective, diagnosis is a big priority. But it's less interesting and rich, and it's not an either/or; to be a good psychiatrist, you have to be able to do both. Most of the time, a psychiatric diagnosis can be made handily within fifty minutes. If someone is floridly psychotic, it is obvious in less than a minute. I remember meeting a patient in my office for the first time who was too preoccupied by the voices screaming in his head even to answer my questions.

But sometimes more time and more sources of information are needed. And other times there is no psychiatric diagnosis to be made, though as the range of psychiatric diagnoses expands, it gets tougher to leave an assessment without some kind of official label, even if it doesn't represent an illness or disorder. Indeed, the *DSM-5* refers to conditions ranging from experiencing abuse to having economic problems as "Other Conditions That May Be a Focus of Clinical Attention." In the United States, this category means you don't have to have a mental illness to talk with a mental health professional and have it paid for by an insurer. But in the rest of medicine it is considered reassuring to tell people they don't have a diagnosis, and it should be so in psychiatry as well.

Among the academic papers I provide to my residents is an old one by my father titled "Interviewing: The Most Sophisticated of Diagnostic Technologies."[19] Writing from his perspective as a pediatrician, he describes much of general pediatrics as the treatment of the worried parents of healthy children, noting that the unchanging and primary need of patients and families from their physician is the relief of anxiety. And doctors provide this by devoting time, providing clear explanations, and offering hope. I believe this is feasible within a single assessment, which means it is not only diagnostic but also therapeutic. Anya left the office with a frame for understanding the symptoms that were distressing her as well as a model for relief and the hope that she doesn't have to continue to feel this way.

Despite forty years of intensive research into the brain science of mental illness, psychiatry remains limited to the use of clinical signs and symptoms as the way to establish diagnoses. In that regard, psychiatry maintains its connection to the core diagnostic principle of clinical medicine: pattern recognition. This is our trade secret, our skill that allows physicians of all types to wear the mantle of diagnostic expertise. We rely on the repetitive nature of symptoms – chest pain radiating down the left arm as indicative of a likely heart attack – to guide us through the morass of someone's distress, to make sense of it, and to help us provide a coherent explanatory model (even if time proves it to be incorrect) that offers some kind of meaning, relief, and hope. It would be a terrifying experience for any physician if he reacted to every patient's story with "Oh-oh, I've never seen this before." By the end of a day at the office, he'd be a wreck. But if he never experiences that doubt, then complacency and sloth have overtaken curiosity and concern.

The flip side is that experience can lead to premature judgment or even tedium. I spent the first seven years of my career doing research in the field of eating disorders (anorexia nervosa and bulimia nervosa), looking at possible biological abnormalities in hormone systems, metabolic systems, and even blood platelets, as well as evaluating psychological and biological treatments. To develop my clinical familiarity and to recruit research subjects, I saw in clinical consultation more than five hundred women with such disorders. While I felt competent in doing the assessments, I worried that I was starting to make assumptions or take shortcuts – or worse, feel that I had heard it all before. So I made a concerted effort to vary my clinical practice by also running a general psychiatric inpatient unit for people with psychoses, mood disorders, and other problems that lead to emergency hospitalization. I knew I needed the variety and the novelty, and the next phase of my career involved creating a General Psychiatry Division for the university, perfectly suited temperamentally to someone who likes not to know who's coming next.

In the domain of clinical medicine outside of psychiatry, a careful patient history remains a powerful diagnostic tool and a source of comfort to patients. This devotion of time, questioning, and concern to someone in distress was captured eloquently by Arthur Miller in his play *Death of a Salesman*, when Willy Loman's wife says, "Willy Loman never made a lot of money. His name was never in the paper. He's not the finest character that ever lived. But he's a human being, and a terrible thing is happening to him. So attention must be paid. He's not to be allowed to fall in his grave like an old dog. Attention, attention must finally be paid to such a person." Psychiatry is about understanding, diagnosing, and treating – but, like all good medical care, it is also about paying attention.

One of the lessons learned over thirty years of clinical work – and Josh will have to work to accumulate such learning – is the mismatch between what we psychiatrists think is important and what patients view as critical. Some patients have told me years after we met that "when you said that, it made an enormous difference," but what they remember is usually something I do not recall and the impact of which I hadn't considered. And it generally isn't an atom-splitting revelation either (not that I've ever uttered one, anyway). It's that convergence between a patient's experience in the moment and a psychiatrist's clinical and personal response that fuses intuition, skill, and experience;

we've all had such encounters that endure for us, but it is rare for both individuals involved to have one simultaneously.

Josh is listening to this feedback, but I can tell by the glazed look on his face that he is likely dismissing my ramblings as those of a frustrated thespian or just a yammering sentimentalist. I encourage him to read a book by Eric Kandel, psychiatrist, neuroscientist, and Nobel laureate, titled *The Age of Insight: The Quest to Understand the Unconscious in Art, Mind, and Brain, from Vienna 1900 to the Present*[20] – if only to see that breadth and depth are not incompatible, and that the fun in psychiatry is the opportunity to integrate biology, psychology, and the sociocultural into the context of a person's life. He jots down the title, gathers his papers, and leaves me with the tail end of the morning.

3

Coping but Not Cured

For most physicians on a busy clinical day, lunch is a stolen moment in the office between patients. It's a time to look over the mail or read a journal article, often with bits of chicken salad dropping out of the sandwich onto the pages. The quickest path to food for me is a visit to the ground-floor coffee shop by the hospital's main entrance. It stands in stark contrast to the expansive food courts in general hospitals that feature chain restaurants and gourmet coffee outlets. Ours is a drab counter with a terse menu of options. There's always soup of some sort, and it's hard to go wrong with a toasted bagel.

As I wait for my order, I glance around at the people seated at the handful of Formica-topped tables. At other hospitals, this scene would include people in hospital gowns hooked up to intravenous drips on rolling poles, looking ashen and uncomfortable. Photo ID cards on lanyards, white coats, and nurses' multicolored uniforms would clearly distinguish the staff from everybody else. It's different at our hospital, although the stigmata of illness are sometimes still there. But there are no uniforms for staff – nurses and doctors wear "civilian" clothing, and increasingly the dress code has devolved to every day being "casual Friday." When people ask me how to tell the staff from the patients, I always say, "It's simple – the patients get better."

I notice a bulky man in his late twenties sitting at a table near the window. The hospital tag on his wrist makes it clear he's an inpatient. With him is an older man who bears a clear family resemblance. The patient, who has a shaved head, numerous piercings, and tattoos, wears a torn plaid shirt, its buttons awry, pulled over a T-shirt, baggy, dirty track pants, and unlaced running shoes. His companion, whom I assume to be his father, is immaculately groomed, with the type of wavy gray hair usually seen on men in advertisements for high-end European watches. Collecting my soup and bagel and heading toward the elevators, I see the father reach over and take one of his son's hands gently into his, placing both on the table and cupping his other hand over them.

We have a rudimentary coffee shop, but we have no gift shop, no way station where visitors can pick up a token that expresses to patients support, hope, and community. We have more than five hundred inpatient beds at our hospital, always running at greater than 95 percent capacity. That's a big facility these days. Yet the smallest community general hospital, with fewer than a hundred inpatient beds, has cheery volunteers running a gift shop near the entrance. We don't have the same stream of visitors to support the business model of a gift shop – a sad reality that has been echoed in research on how few get-well cards and flowers populate psychiatric wards compared to medical or surgical inpatient units.[1] It's a reflection of shame and stigma, how the suffering of mental illness itself can be compounded by isolation and lack of support.

When I return upstairs, Simone is talking on the phone. I wave at her, pick up my mail from her desk, and walk toward the inner door to my office. It's a relic of an earlier era in psychiatry that my office has one door leading in from Simone's office, through which patients enter, and another leading directly to the hallway, where patients can exit. The idea was that patients shouldn't see each other – in contrast to the crowded waiting rooms in clinics where people cough all over each other and hear their names called out loudly by the receptionist. The separate-doors arrangement also signaled that seeking psychiatric help was more secretive and shameful than getting any other kind of health care. What do you say when you run into a friend entering or leaving a psychiatric hospital? "Hi, what are you doing here? Is everything okay?" Those would be easy and obvious questions at an encounter in the atrium of a children's hospital or the waiting room of a family doctor's office. But it remains a loaded set of questions in a mental health setting. Under the noble umbrella of confidentiality, embarrassment and even a sense of personal failure are protected from exposure.

Simone puts the caller on hold and greets me with her familiar "What up, G?"

"Anything in the mail? Anyone looking for me?"

"Nothing thrilling in Goldbloom land," she replies, reassuring me that I can eat my lunch in peace.

Monday afternoons are devoted to appointments with patients whom I have been seeing for anywhere from weeks to years. But none of them has a fixed, recurring appointment. My work schedule doesn't allow for that, and often neither does theirs. If they are in crisis, I see them often; if they are doing well, many months may pass between encounters. It's what allows me to see six to ten new patients in assessment every week, providing consultation or short-term treatment.

My practice also reflects my view that a specialty like psychiatry needs to be more accessible to more people. If my practice were limited to seeing the same people every week (or, if they were in psychoanalysis, three to five times a week) for an hour at a time on an open-ended basis, it would consist of a small group of people I would know very well. It is still the stereotype of the psychiatrist, and some psychiatrists – now a minority – still do work that way, but the majority of us now work in institutional or community settings, and we see many of our patients only for a consultation, for a short course of treatment, or for irregular longer follow-ups. This is a twenty-first-century model of psychiatry, but it also reflects who I am – drawn to newness and variety.

Sitting at my desk and glancing at today's schedule, I note that the patients booked for this afternoon are all reasonably stable except for the last one of the day, Daryl Orzech, who was recently discharged from the hospital. The five before him, despite the struggles that led them to seek psychiatric help in the first place, are currently not in crisis; they are either doing pretty well or stuck at a long-standing level of disability. Sometimes just achieving stability is a triumph. None of them is "cured." All patients with major psychiatric disorders, such as depression, bipolar disorder, and schizophrenia, must anticipate and plan for the possible return of their most disturbing symptoms. Part of our work is to be vigilant for early symptoms and to encourage individuals and their families to recognize clues that a relapse may be happening, as well as to reinforce those treatments, supports, and activities that help people stay well. Other patients must deal with residual minor symptoms most days. And all of them need help to manage the wreckage that a disruptive episode of illness has wreaked on their lives. On the other hand, most of my patients are coping, and some are moving forward in their work and relationships.

I STEP OUT INTO the hallway where Ben Young, my first patient of the afternoon, is seated, leafing quickly through the pages of a magazine but not appearing to read it. He's wearing the same rumpled clothes as the last time I saw him – a frayed lumber jacket and pants his lean frame can't fill. I think of him as young, even though he is now thirty-eight, perhaps because when I first met him he was twenty-six, or perhaps because I am resisting my own aging. But the other reality is that Ben's illness has frozen his progress from young adulthood to early middle age, derailing him from the tracks of traditional expectation and success.

Ben, the scion of a successful and ambitious family, has had a harrowing journey. After completing university and looking forward to a career as an economist, he tumbled into paranoid schizophrenia in his mid-twenties. Although men and women are equally vulnerable in terms of the one in a hundred people who will develop this illness, it hits men at an earlier age, often during their late adolescence and early twenties. Ben's illness first included an explosion of paranoid delusions, a belief he was under surveillance by government agents and under continuous threat of torture and death. He heard voices inside his head laughing and yelling at him, and telling him not to go outside. After several hospitalizations, the most terrifying aspects of these symptoms were successfully extinguished with antipsychotic medications, but the Ben his family knew prior to his illness – the young man who loved parties and family gatherings, and who was an avid canoeist – did not resurface.

As I show him in, I remind myself that today I need to talk with him again about a transfer of his care from me to a specialized multidisciplinary outpatient team at our hospital. The team includes psychiatrists, nurses, occupational therapists, social workers, recreation therapists, and peer-support workers – the latter being people who have experienced major mental illness themselves and now help others. We've touched on this subject before, and Ben always says, "I'll think about it." He is reluctant to make any changes in his life, which at times is hard to reconcile not only with my therapeutic zeal but also with my belief that this team approach is the best option for helping him. Loss of motivation can be one of the debilitating aspects of schizophrenia. But beyond his seeming resistance, I realize I am also one of the few people he ever talks to.

As he enters the office, his body odor is potent. I am already thinking about how to air out the room for the next patient. The reinforced windows in this 1960s psychiatric hospital don't open – for obvious reasons – although in our new buildings, in an effort to create a more homelike atmosphere and catch a breeze, the windows have been designed to open a couple of inches. Ben looks vaguely bewildered, and his face registers little emotion.

"What's up?" I ask.

"Not much," he replies blankly, a minimalist answer that conveys volumes about his experience. Despite living in a major North American city, his world is very small. He lives on the margins of human interaction, spending his days in libraries and malls, sheltered from the elements and from intimate human contact. He lives alone in a small apartment in a seedy part of town, supported by public assistance that goes mostly to rent; he usually visits food banks in the final week of the month before his next check. He rarely speaks to his parents now. We call them from my office sometimes, since otherwise they would never hear from him.

"Are you still hearing those voices talking about you?"

"No, they're gone."

"What about when you walk down the street – do you feel like people you don't know are staring at you or talking about you? Do you ever overhear things about you when you walk past a group of strangers?"

"No. But some days I just don't go outside."

"Why?"

"I don't know."

As we talk about his daily routine, I am looking for evidence of change or the emergence of his old symptoms. He works at a community center one half day per week but doesn't want to increase his time there or get to know the other people, although he concedes "they're all right." Progress is slow. It's a struggle to engage him. My job is to help keep his psychosis at bay with medications – in Ben's case, one of the newer generations of antipsychotic medications, risperidone, which he takes nightly – to keep him connected to people, and to provide that space in my office he seems to want. And I need to monitor him for the side effects of his treatment; antipsychotic drugs can sometimes produce symptoms of Parkinsonism, with stiffness or tremor in the arms and legs or an inability to sit still. After long-term use, there is also the risk for a movement disorder called tardive dyskinesia, which can include facial tics and grimacing. On most of Ben's visits, I do a neurological exam that takes only a couple of minutes to screen for these side effects. When risperidone and other newer antipsychotic medications were introduced in the 1980s and 1990s, there was hope that they would induce far fewer side effects than their predecessors. That initial optimism was not borne out; the side effects that have emerged with the newer drugs are simply different, some of them equally off-putting for patients. A more helpful shift has resulted from research showing that much lower doses of the old medicines than were used previously could be as effective for patients with psychosis and are associated with significantly fewer side effects.

As I type my progress note, I realize – again – that I haven't talked with him enough about the transfer of care from me to the community clinic. Even though I know that his needs would be best served by a different model of care, I am either reluctant or stunningly forgetful. My reluctance likely stems from multiple sources: sensing his connection to me and not wanting to sever it, and avoiding my own sense of failure that he is not getting better.

Between appointments I have a ten-minute gap that allows me to type a note in the electronic clinical record. I tell residents that there is never an excuse to not document a clinical encounter when it is fresh in one's mind; even a couple of hours later, important details will be lost. I also frighten them with horror stories of procrastinating colleagues who were threatened with the loss of hospital privileges because they left mountains of unfinished documentation languishing in the medical records department.

I briefly summarize the key points of each encounter in my note, written in the SOAP format common to hospital charts for any medical problem, whether pneumonia, cancer, or depression. *S* stands for "subjective," the patient's perceptions. *O* represents "objective," what I have observed. *A* is "assessment," which includes not only the formal psychiatric diagnosis but also what the patient is currently dealing with, such as job problems, relationship issues, money. *P* indicates "plan," whether it is medication, psychotherapy, or other intervention.

Ben's note reads:

S: No concerns or complaints. He continues to attend Progress Place one half day per week, doing filing, and says it is "good." He does not want to increase his involvement. Remainder of time is spent in malls and libraries, looking in magazines and at store windows. No contact with friends or family. He denies any delusions or hallucinations. Claims to eat twice per day and says he takes his meds regularly. Denies problems with sleep or appetite.

O: Malodorous, disheveled, but punctual and cooperative in answering questions. No obvious weight change. Affect severely constricted. Marked thought poverty evident. No evidence of delusions or hallucinations. Not suicidal or aggressive. Aware of diagnosis and rationale for treatment. No evidence of Parkinsonism or tardive dyskinesia.

A: Schizophrenia, residual type – prominent impairment of affect and motivation.

P: Continue risperidone 4 mg at bedtime.
Continue efforts re transfer to case management team.
Return 4 weeks.

It's an admittedly terse summary of a complex illness and journey, but the purpose of such documentation is not to weave an elaborative narrative but to communicate critical information about the person to another clinician, and to remind the author of the note at the next appointment what happened the last time. It's not possible to do justice to the distorted course of Ben's life in a necessarily short clinical note, and part of me wouldn't want to try, perhaps because I would have to confront the limits to the benefits of both the treatment he is receiving and our therapeutic relationship, neither of which has led Ben to re-engage with the world around him and with the person he was before his illness.

MY NEXT PATIENT, JOANNA DaSilva, is a graduate student in Renaissance literature who has a diagnosis of bipolar disorder type II. I think she meets the fashion definition for hipster, at least according to the tutelage I have received on matters sartorial from my younger son: she sports a straw fedora, black-framed heavy glasses, a plaid skirt, and black leggings. She removes her white earbuds as she walks in and powers down her mobile phone. She was once embarrassed (appropriately, I thought) when someone called her during our appointment. That is in contrast to other younger patients who not only leave their phones on but also take the call, if only to say, "Hey, listen, I'm at the doctor's office. Can I call you later? What time is good for you? I'm going to be tied up for the next hour . . ." as thin trails of smoke emanate from my ears.

Joanna has never been hospitalized, but she struggles with mood instability. It seems most recently to be enmeshed in problems she has encountered finishing a doctoral dissertation that she has been working on for the past four years. When she gets depressed, Joanna is unable to make progress in her writing, and this in turn fuels her sense of failure and incompetence. When her mood is elevated, she thinks she will finish her thesis in a month and hurtles ahead to imagining the graduation ceremony, only to face disappointing reality when her mood becomes level and she appraises her own work more accurately. It's another example of illness getting in the way of life, blocking her completion of a milestone that is important to her and for her.

I first met Joanna when she was twenty-one and her family doctor asked me to see her in consultation. After the consultation, I referred her to the student health service of the university for ongoing help in the form of both psychotherapy and medication. Six years after my initial assessment, and having seen three other psychiatrists in the interim, she came back to me. She asked if I would now treat her. Her request coincided with some availability in my schedule – as well as that hard-to-define essence of a therapeutic relationship when you feel the moment is ripe to be of help to someone. I have followed her since then, usually at intervals of several weeks to several months when things are going smoothly for her.

Now thirty-two, she has looked for multiple sources of relief, from yoga to psychotherapy to medication trials. She has experienced side effects of drug treatment, from nausea to loss of sexual drive, and has mustered the courage to try again when treatments fail her. Fortunately, the mood stabilizer lamotrigine, one of the anticonvulsant drugs commonly used to control seizures but also used by psychiatrists to regulate mood swings, has produced a level of calm that allows her to feel herself. What's more, she has no side effects from it.

She grins and laughs while describing the simple pleasure of feeling well. "This may sound stupid, but it just feels like me, physically and mentally. I can tell the second I get up, and it's a feeling I haven't had in a long time. It's hard to explain; it's easier to tell you what feeling sick is like!"

I remind her she is "allowed" to see me when she is feeling okay, both to share her good news and to let me see what being well is like for her. It helps me to know her baseline. At the same time, I have to be vigilant that her good mood isn't "too good," as can be the case in hypomania, a milder form of mania. I probe carefully about changes in her sleep patterns, energy, and speed of thinking.

"Don't worry, Dr. Goldbloom. I'm not manic. I know why you're asking, but really, I'm okay."

Within psychiatry, "mood" has a specific meaning – a subjective emotional state that is sustained over a fixed period of time.[2] Psychiatrists investigate a patient's moods through a combination of the patient's subjective report and the physician's assessment of the patient's affect or series of affects – moment-to-moment external presentations of his or her emotional experience. While mood and affect are distinguished within psychiatry as subjective and objective aspects, respectively, of the patient's experience, they are also distinguished by longevity. I think of a patient's mood as her climate: her mood pattern, month to month, year to year. Affect is the weather: the day-to-day, minute-to-minute oscillations in a person's expression of her internal state.

While mood and affect can be related, this is not always the case. For example, psychiatrists refer to "inappropriate affect," which might describe someone who smiles repetitively while chronicling the death of a loved one. "Blunted affect" describes someone whose facial expressions and speech remain unvaryingly neutral while he or she describes experiences that run the gamut of emotional peaks and lows. A patient with "euthymic affect" has an external presentation within the midrange of emotional states, neither euphoric nor melancholic, neither subdued nor agitated. It is easy to see why critics point to the subjectivity inherent in this supposedly objective assessment; the psychiatrist's notion of an appropriate representation of emotion may play a role in descriptions of a patient's affect.

"Euthymic" is also the technical term for "okay," so as Joanna leaves to tackle the next chapter of her thesis, that's what I write in my note under "Assessment."

These days, Joanna's diagnosis of bipolar disorder runs the risk of dilution as a clinical label. Outside medicine, the term "manic" is sometimes used casually – and caustically – to describe high-energy people, much in the same way that "depressed" is used to describe normal feeling states of sadness, disappointment, and loss. Years ago, a colleague observed me busily and happily working and teaching, and said, "Did you forget to take your lithium?" She managed, in one fell swoop, to pathologize my temperament and trivialize people who are ill. The memory still irritates me.

Within psychiatry, the criteria for making a diagnosis of bipolar disorder have loosened. As a result, more people with milder forms

of the illness are likely to be diagnosed with it by a health professional, or to diagnose it in themselves after reading about it.[3] Classical
bipolar disorder, historically called manic-depressive illness and even
manic-depressive insanity, affects 1 percent of the population, men
and women equally. This more severe form, also called bipolar disorder
type I, features sustained and severe episodes of mania and depression.
These people can lose touch with reality and become psychotic. They
may need hospitalization, and some – as many as 15 percent over the
course of the illness – may end their lives by suicide.

In recent decades, however, another group has been identified who
experience both recurrent depression and periods of less intense and
more subtle mood elevation, or what is called hypomania. This group is
labeled bipolar disorder, type II, Joanna's diagnosis. Mood-stabilizing
drugs like the one Joanna takes can be more helpful than antidepressants. But as the margins of diagnosis widen, the risk increases of en-
croachment onto normal variants of human experience. This includes
people with the far more common illness of depression, whose merciful
respite from symptoms runs the risk of a bipolar diagnosis if they feel
just a little too happy for a couple of days. I'm reminded of my father's
definition of a healthy person as "someone who hasn't been adequately
investigated."

Bipolar disorder has become almost fashionable, with celebrities going public with their diagnoses, and films such as *Silver Lin-
ings Playbook* offering a soft-pedaled version of the disorder. But there
have also been searing accounts of the experience of the illness that do
not sugar-coat the consequences. One such is Kay Redfield Jamison's
memoir about her illness, *An Unquiet Mind: A Memoir of Moods and
Madness*, all the more memorable because she is an internationally renowned researcher in bipolar disorder.[4]

MY DEFINITION OF GERIATRIC patients keeps shifting as I get older. As
I stare into the headlights of my sixtieth birthday, it's only my patients

in their eighties whom I think of as elderly. Betty Thomson, my next patient, is in her late seventies, with recurring episodes of depression since the birth of her second child fifty-odd years ago. Her sons, both now comfortably middle-aged, usually come to their mother's appointments and are here today. They provide valuable information about how she is functioning. So does her hair color. One of the clinical tips I learned in editing my textbook *Psychiatric Clinical Skills* came from two geriatrician colleagues. In their chapter on assessment of older adults,[5] they describe the "white-roots sign" of depression in older women. According to them, it is possible to calculate how long an elderly depressed woman has been neglecting herself by mentally measuring the length of her white roots. Every half inch of white growth indicates one month of depressed disregard for a previous standard of appearance. They noted that this is increasingly relevant for men as well, confirming my "dark" suspicion that my head of gray hair in my fifties is more common among men than it sometimes appears. Betty is well coiffed today.

I usher her into my office. Her sons wait outside, knowing I will bring them in once I have had a chance to explore how Betty feels.

"Fine, thank you, and how are you?" she responds to my initial inquiry, reflecting the social graces she has maintained from an upper-crust childhood. I think of my late paternal grandmother, Annie Goldbloom, a woman of propriety and formality who held on to these overlearned behaviors for some time after dementia robbed her of the details of a rich life. It was easy for her civility to obscure her deficits until later in the disease's progression. I realize sharply that my mind has drifted to my grandmother because I am concerned that Betty may be slowly dementing.

Whether through well-heeled social graces or lack of awareness or forgetting, Betty tends to minimize her symptoms. It reminds me of a favorite *New Yorker* cartoon where a nurse ushers a patient into a physician's office, saying, "Mrs. Perkins, the doctor will see you now. Please try not to upset him." When Betty is depressed, she seems surprised by her symptoms, describing them as if they are unfamiliar and baffling to her despite their predictability to her children and to me. It is this bafflement that leads me to worry that in addition to her mood problems, she may be experiencing symptoms of dementia – two disorders that can be challenging to distinguish in the elderly. Fortunately, colleagues in geriatric psychiatry and neurology are involved in her care, helping to navigate the muddy diagnostic waters.

Today, mercifully, she is well and her self-appraisal as "fine" is later echoed by her sons, who are palpably grateful she is better. Depression in people her age is often too readily dismissed by some younger clinicians, along the line of "I'd be depressed, too, if I was that old . . . if all my friends were dying off . . . if I didn't have work anymore . . ." This easy dismissal denies the suffering and the treatability of depression in the elderly; I have seen many such patients recover and enjoy life again.

As part of the visit, I ask Betty to draw the face of a clock, complete with numbers, and to place the hands of the clock at ten minutes past eleven o'clock. This is a well-recognized quick screening test for cognitive impairment, and Betty completes it slowly but accurately, commenting as she draws that forty years ago her father left engraved Patek Philippe watches for both his grandsons. Chronologically, she is in the zone of risk for dementia, but so far, the memory disturbances that have been part and parcel of her depressions have resolved as her mood has lifted. I still don't understand why she never recognizes her depression when it returns, and I wonder if it is a merciful forgetting of past suffering or a more subtle cognitive problem that eludes our standard screening tests. As she and her sons leave, I remind myself that time will answer my uncertainty.

Betty, like both Anya and Joanna, is among the significant number of women of all ages who experience depression. I see more depressed women than depressed men. When I tell people this, the response is often "Of course. Women seek help for depression, and they're more likely to talk about how they feel than guys are." As a guy, I know this to be true. But it's an insufficient explanation. Surveys conducted in communities rather than in clinic offices, where people are not asking for help, have repeatedly demonstrated that depression is at least twice as common in women. The relative contributions of biology, psychology, and social role remain a topic of research and debate but have not yet yielded a definitive answer that explains the gender differences.

I AM RIGHT ON time for Stephane Nguyen's appointment.

I don't like to be kept waiting, and I don't like to keep others waiting. It is rude. In other areas of medicine, it's pretty routine for people to show up for a scheduled appointment and not be seen until an hour or more has passed. There's a reason they call it a waiting room. But in psychiatry, where time is such an obvious commodity, it's easier to stay on schedule. And as someone who likes setting up challenges for himself (efficiently getting a maximum number of errands done in a finite amount of time, getting a string of green lights while driving, purging files to keep them current, and other minor life victories), the clock is an excellent governor and reward mechanism – "Whatever else you might think of Goldbloom, at least he's punctual."

"*Bonjour, mon vieux!*" I greet him in French, because it was the language in which he was schooled growing up in Montreal, the hardworking son of Vietnamese refugees who fled communism to come to Canada. Unlike his parents, who spoke Parisian French, he speaks a Quebec patois, although he is equally comfortable in English and Vietnamese. He is slight, slim, and short-sighted.

Stephane is a scientist, a researcher in nanotechnology, who has had significant academic success despite an intermittent illness that causes him to become suddenly, severely, and disablingly paranoid. During these periods, which can last for weeks, he suspects people of making critical, devaluing comments about his Asian heritage wherever he goes. He hears remarks from strangers about him when he walks past them and picks up references to him in the most benign contexts. He can't function at work when he is ill.

But when he is well, he is a prolific and celebrated scholar, with grants from funding agencies in Canada and the United States. He has worked in three top-level research laboratories in North America, but his location seems to make no difference: his illness has followed him between cities and across borders.

This rare type of illness, where a single paranoid or other type of delusion is the only sign of illness and where the person's long-term ability to function well in terms of work and relationships is often preserved, is called a delusional disorder. It's an example of how someone can be psychotic – experiencing symptoms of unreality such as delusions – without having schizophrenia. In fact, amphetamine abuse, brain tumors, prescribed and illicit steroids, and many other conditions can result in someone's becoming psychotic. That's part of the diagnostic challenge when someone experiences a symptom like a paranoid delusion – understanding its larger context, looking for other related symptoms, and coming up with a diagnosis and a treatment. Whereas Stephane's delusion is persecutory, a person who is certain that a distant celebrity is in love with him would be said to have an erotomanic delusion. Although Ben and Stephane have both had paranoid delusions, their overall journeys have been stunningly different. Ben's schizophrenia has included many more symptoms and impediments. The paranoid delusion is the only symptom of Stephane's condition.

"How is work?" I ask him. Work is everything to Stephane, and it's a great barometer of his mental health. He answers earnestly, like a scientist describing his latest data analysis. The world of nanotechnology is one about which I knew nothing before meeting Stephane, who has a geeky enthusiasm for what he does. He wants to improve my understanding, which when we met was limited to a vague sense that he worked at the atomic or molecular level. In fact, at our first meeting, when he told me he was a nanotechnologist, I joked, "You seem pretty big for a nanotechnologist." He thought that was funny – fortunately, since I had instantly depleted my nanotechnology joke repertoire.

Stephane's illness responds well to the antipsychotic medication risperidone. It is the same medication Ben takes, but Stephane takes a much smaller dose, and he tolerates it well. I ask him about various side effects: muscle stiffness or tremor, restlessness, weight gain, his ability to get and keep an erection, and whether he is having any problems with ejaculation. He denies them all. Nevertheless, I will send him for blood tests after our visit to check for hormone and lipid changes that can be induced by his treatment.

Stephane knows he has an illness. This understanding improves his adherence to treatment, which is often a challenge in psychiatry and throughout all of medicine. Long-term adherence for all chronic physical and mental diseases in developed countries averages about 50 percent, with lower rates in developing countries.[6]

Why don't people stick with treatment, even when it works? I think there are several reasons. One, paradoxically, is that if the treatment works and the symptoms are alleviated, the personal incentive to continue the treatment diminishes. Many people with strep throat, given a ten-day course of penicillin, stop taking the antibiotic after a couple of days when the cough subsides – the problem is that though the symptom is gone, the underlying infection may linger. Two, and this particularly affects those with psychotic illnesses, is a patient's inability to recognize that he or she is ill. This is not the same as choosing not to take treatment despite knowing the illness and the consequences of the decision, which some people with terminal cancer do. Three is side effects, and psychiatric drugs, like all drugs, come with many different and difficult ones, such as significant weight gain, agitation or sedation, and the movement disorders I described earlier. All physicians need to watch carefully for side effects and help patients manage them. Four, and this is a pragmatic reason for nonadherence, is medication's cost and access; newer drugs can be ferociously expensive, despite often being no more effective than their cheaper antecedents. But we tend to think that newer is better, a belief promoted by pharmaceutical companies that spend millions on marketing campaigns to persuade both physicians and patients that this is the case. For people without an insurance plan that covers prescriptions, it may come down to a choice between paying in full for rent and food or getting a month's supply of medication.

Some patients feel uncomfortable disclosing that they have not been taking their meds, worrying they will be embarrassed or judged by their doctor. An effective door opener to discussing adherence is "It's hard for many people to take their medication like clockwork every day; most people miss days. What about you?" Stephane, however, is supremely organized and has programmed a special alert on his smartphone.

He books his next appointment with Simone, using voice-activated technology to enter the information into his smartphone calendar. Since he seems well and is tolerating his medication, I will see him again in three months unless something comes up.

"*A bientôt!*" he says cheerily as he heads down the hall toward our clinical laboratory for his blood work. He walks past Arthur Silver, my next patient, who keeps his eyes glued on his newspaper.

"Give me a minute," I tell Arthur, who always arrives early. I know it will be five minutes (which I've budgeted for) before I finish typing my clinical note and checking my email for any news of my mother.

There is none, and I tell myself there is no benefit to my worrying, and yet it gnaws.

ARTHUR COMES INTO MY office with a purposeful stride and nods silently as he sits down. He always has an agenda for seeing me, and after a few seconds he launches in.

"The stupidest things keep reminding me of her."

"It's normal, even if it catches you off guard. Why would you want that to end?"

He is a landscaper coping with his wife's death in a car accident eighteen months ago, after thirty years of marriage. He had come to me for help with his depression eight years earlier, long before his wife died, and treatment has evolved from relief of his symptoms of depressive illness to adjusting to the impact of a devastating loss. Bereavement itself is neither a psychiatric illness nor a cause for psychiatric treatment, although many of its sufferers undoubtedly benefit from the support of family and friends and some may need professional therapy. I wouldn't be seeing Arthur had he not struggled with a recurring depression when his wife was still alive. Back then, he needed regular treatment. Now he comes infrequently – precipitated either by the need to renew his medication or by his worry about relapse.

Arthur's current grief is not depression but a painful journey nonetheless, even as he ventures into the mysterious terrain of new relationships. Friends have fixed him up with women, but after three decades of marriage he finds courtship ritual to be unfamiliar terrain. And there's the issue of his mental illness as it affects dating. Like many single patients, he wonders on which date the issue of his illness will surface and whether this will determine that it's the last date. He will find his way, but he likes to check in with me on occasion to make sure he isn't completely off course. He doesn't want to be overly secretive, he doesn't want to scare someone off, but also he ultimately doesn't want to be with someone who can't accept his mental illness as one dimension of who he is. I ask him to tell me how he would tell a date about his diagnosis. It's a useful role-playing exercise, because for all the years he has lived with this illness, he has rarely articulated it. I ask him to imagine the response and consequences as he tries out different versions to find one with which he is comfortable.

Differentiating the grief of bereavement from depression can be challenging at times, and the latest version of the *DSM* has been roundly criticized – excessively, in my view – for potentially pathologizing normal sadness after loss by a change in the diagnostic criteria. In the previous edition, *DSM-IV*, a diagnosis of depression could be made *only* if the symptoms were not better accounted for by bereavement, *only* if the symptoms lasted for more than two months after the loss, or *only* if there was "marked functional impairment, morbid preoccupation with worthlessness, suicidal ideation, psychotic symptoms, or psychomotor retardation."[7] Arthur has none of these, but his grief has extended well beyond two months, and his heart is broken.

The *DSM-5* dropped the earlier two-month duration for grief that exempted its symptoms from diagnosis as depression. This caused an uproar over concerns that many simply bereaved people might be diagnosed as suffering from a mental illness and be prescribed unneeded psychiatric medications. But *DSM-5* devotes more text than its predecessor did to differentiating grief from depression, not by its two-month duration (which always seemed arbitrary anyway) but rather by its qualities – the experience of pangs of grief associated with thoughts of the deceased and the ability of the bereaved to experience positive emotions and humor in a way depressed people cannot. It states, significantly, that the differentiation "requires the exercise of clinical judgment based on the individual's history and the cultural norms for the expression of distress in the context of loss."[8] It's a terrible reflection on the practice of medicine in the twenty-first century that someone has to state formally that a diagnosis requires "the exercise of clinical judgment." The day it is no longer required I might as well take down my shingle, as caring for patients will be a dull, mechanized process rather than one of building a trusting relationship within which diagnoses can be ascertained, treatment tailored to the person's needs and preferences, and support given. The latter is what I signed up for thirty years ago.

My clinical judgment is that Arthur is not depressed according to either *DSM-IV*'s or *DSM-5*'s criteria, based on both the times prior to his wife's death when he was depressed and on how he is currently functioning overall. He is still getting caught off guard by his grief, but the antidepressant that he has been on for several years, after multiple episodes of depression, is not intended to – or able to – block his profound sense of loss. What Arthur needs from me is not a different medication or a different dose but the sounding board and understanding that our therapeutic relationship provides. While depression was his original ticket of admission to my office, he faces something different now and needs intermittent help with the inevitable challenges of re-building his life without his wife and inviting new people into it. Given his long-standing capacity for self-criticism and self-loathing, some of the help comes from guiding him to see that he is not the "fuckup" that he dreads being.

THE AFTERNOON IS GOING quickly. For each of these five patients, the duration of the encounter is roughly fixed, and they know that my question "Do you need a new prescription?" is a prelude to the finale. All of them are on some kind of psychiatric medication, which likely reflects both my orientation and the severity of illness in the patients I see working in a tertiary-care psychiatric hospital. But if the treatment was just about dispensing pills, I could courier these to patients after they faxed me a symptom questionnaire. In person I offer them at least three things: a defined period during which we work together to un-derstand where they are in the course of their lives and their illnesses; a review of their symptoms and the impact – both benefits and toxicities – of their treatments; and a plan for the next steps to help them address identified symptoms, crises, and life problems. It's not a friendly chat about whatever is on their mind, but it's also not a mechanical check-list of the presence or absence of specific symptoms or side effects. It's an engagement that includes screening for problems, understanding context, promoting skills and strengths, and reinforcing hope. If done well, it may look and feel like a "natural" conversation, but its purpose is diagnostic and therapeutic, not social.

THE DOOR LEADING TO Simone's office is slightly ajar as I type my note about Arthur. It's not open enough for me to see the speaker, but it allows the clear transmission of a familiar voice:

"Goldbloom, are you ready for me? Ya wanna coffee?"

I don't need to check my schedule. Daryl Orzech has arrived for his appointment. I wave him into an office he knows all too well. Daryl has been my patient for more than a decade. I've known other patients longer but few as well. I have been his doctor through stormy hospitalizations, years of outpatient encounters, and many meetings with his close-knit family. Today he is the patient I am most worried about because of the rocky road he has endured over the past two months, including two hospitalizations – once, briefly, for depression, and then more recently for a manic episode that plummeted rapidly into the familiar mud of depression. These two hospitalizations came hard on the heels of the death of his friend Pat from a malignancy just over two months ago. But Daryl's bipolar disorder has had its own internal rhythm over the years, and sometimes the search for precipitants of episodes comes up empty-handed. This last appointment of my day is not one to rush.

A trim man in his midfifties, just a few years younger than me, with a receding hairline and a pockmarked face covered by a short beard, today Daryl is wearing a Hawaiian shirt and khakis. Some days he wears a fedora that gives him the air of a *flaneur* on the streets of Toronto, but today he is bareheaded.

"Hey, Goldbloom. Have you missed me?" he says as sits down in the armchair my patients use. His voice is always raspy, sounding as if he spent the last few hours shouting but more likely reflecting his heavy smoking.

I like Daryl. I like him a lot. He is, like me, a bit of a *tummler*, a Yiddish word describing a noisemaker or clown. We enjoy each other's company, recognizing our shared liking for the stand-up role, while still constrained by the formalities of the doctor-patient relationship. I have to find something I like in patients I see; otherwise, I would dread their appointments. With rare exceptions, I do, but it's definitely easier with some patients than with others. It's very easy with Daryl – except when he's severely manic. Otherwise, he is a sweet, surprisingly shy but warm man, with an irrepressible sense of humor.

But Daryl doesn't see me for laughs. He sees me because of his struggle with severe bipolar disorder, an illness that has played horrendous havoc with his life since his diagnosis forty years ago at age seventeen. It has resulted in countless hospitalizations and overwhelming roadblocks to the kind of life he wanted but has not achieved. I see a large part of my job as a psychiatrist as helping my patients get their lives back on track after an episode of illness has derailed them. More than almost any other area in medicine, psychiatric disorders wreak collateral damage: on relationships, employment, finances, even housing. In the midst of crises, law-abiding citizens with mental illness may find themselves encountering the police as first responders. While we do not have cures yet for the majority of psychiatric disorders, we do have the ability – and the obligation – to help patients put back together these essential building blocks of a good life. And success in these domains may diminish the severity and frequency of future illness episodes. A lot of my time and that of my colleagues therefore is spent on referrals to vocational counselors, social workers for housing and financial support, and community groups for increased social contact.

Today my main goal is to assess whether Daryl's two recent back-to-back hospitalizations – both initiated by me – and the electroconvulsive therapy (ECT) given during those stays have stabilized his mood sufficiently, and whether the decision for his most recent discharge four weeks ago, which he pushed for, was appropriate or premature. A secondary goal is helping him to find work, something he desperately wants.

I start with the second goal. "How did it go with Melissa last Friday?" I ask. "Did she have any suggestions for you?"

He tells me about his assessment with Melissa Yuen, an occupational therapist I had asked him to see about increasing his productive activities and securing part-time work. I have already reviewed Melissa's note in the electronic chart, a detailed account of Daryl's skills, interests, activities, and obstacles – including his doubts about himself. They have scheduled a follow-up meeting for next week, and Melissa has connected him to a specialist in employment opportunities for people with mental illness.

Daryl replies that he likes Melissa's enthusiasm but wonders if he can live up to it. Daryl being Daryl, he also can't help commenting, with an arch of his eyebrow, "Doesn't hurt she's good-looking!" I silently agree, since Melissa is undoubtedly attractive, but also because I hope this will provide some additional incentive for Daryl to continue seeing her beyond the help he clearly needs. In any case, he needs Melissa's enthusiasm; it is a professional as well as a personal trait and one of the reasons I like occupational therapists so much. In contrast to many other mental health professionals, OTs are less preoccupied with people's limitations and more focused on their potential.

Working in a major hospital that has more than three thousand employees, I am lucky in that I can easily call on colleagues within and beyond the hospital for advice, a second opinion, and additional treatment for my patients. At various times, I have sent my patients to social workers, nurses, occupational therapists, psychologists, addiction counselors, and other psychiatrists. Working with these skilled people provides me with relief from clinical isolation and offers my patients an array of services to help them.

In an effort to find out if Daryl has been using his supports since discharge, I ask him about his cousin Stan, who often provides Daryl with work opportunities and occasionally pays for Daryl's travels. Daryl is grateful but worries about being a burden to him. Stan occasionally comes to appointments with Daryl and is both ebullient and loving toward him. A big man, often tanned and with wavy silver hair, Stan's optimism and energy are a source of strength for Daryl. Today Daryl tells me that he did two days' worth of clerical work at Stan's office last week, for which he was paid, and that Stan took him out for a steak dinner as well.

It's good news, but it doesn't show in Daryl's face. Normally, the impact of a good rib eye in his belly and some cash in his pocket would cheer him up. But today his depression overshadows any good news, and he views these acts of giving as a sign he's not going to get better and become independent.

I move on to my primary goal with Daryl, assessing his brittle mood state. With him, my exploration of mood symptoms and screening for risky situations takes little time; we know each other well and a shorthand communication has evolved. The appointment with Melissa evoked some painful realizations for Daryl. She asked him to fill out questionnaires about his interests and skills; he is frustrated that he is not in step technologically with the rest of the world, that he never learned to use a computer – "I feel like Rip Van Winkle." In some ways, he is right. The toll of more than thirty years of treatment-resistant bipolar disorder and dozens of hospitalizations has been heavy, interrupting his development and progress as an adult. We've been down this path before; he's reluctant to take computer courses because he gets frustrated. He also despairs of the fact that in his fifties, he doesn't have a job or a stable and intimate relationship with a woman.

"I gotta get going, I gotta accomplish something," he insists. It has become a familiar refrain, and I feel both the need to act – hence the new OT referral – and my own frustration that he rejects out of hand some suggestions for engaging in volunteer work.

I understand his point, his sense of being suspended in time like Beckett's perennial anticipators, Vladimir and Estragon, in *Waiting for Godot.* I've heard it from him before. We both had high hopes when Daryl enrolled in the Assistant Cook Extended Training Program at a community college, a program designed for people recovering from mental illness or substance use disorders. I had lobbied hard for him to enroll and visited the program when he was there. He seemed pleased to be working in a phalanx of multiple adjacent kitchens, dressed in a white uniform. After nine months, he graduated despite a couple of episodes of illness, during which he was hospitalized. His instructor was understanding and a great cheerleader. I was touched when Daryl invited me to his graduation, and I cheered with his family in the auditorium when he accepted his diploma. In that moment, I felt a part of his extended family. Frustratingly, however, he was not able to turn his training into sustained employment. The realities of the marketplace were not as accommodating as his training program. Maintaining consistent employment is challenging for many people with severe mental illness. The reasons are complex: outmoded work skills, inadequate accommodation by employers, and episodic flare-ups that cause employment interruptions.

Now, as he sits a few feet away, Daryl's sadness radiates across the room despite his efforts to contain it, to protect me. But he is talking in coherent sentences, and he continues to engage me in conversation, something he is not able to do when his depression is at its worst. After discussing his current mood symptoms with him, I therefore conclude from this "tell" that the discharge decision was reasonable. The rest of our time together is devoted to a fairly pragmatic discussion of his functioning and quality of life, including the odd jobs he thinks he can do for neighbors and family members, and his need to get a real mattress instead of a sofa bed in his apartment.

DARYL HAS CLASSIC BIPOLAR disorder in terms of symptoms, severity, and duration, unlike Joanna's less dramatic experience of bipolar II. Bipolar disorder is one of psychiatry's so-called three major mental disorders – the other two are depression and schizophrenia – and they constitute the most potentially destructive experiences for patients. I imagine them as forces of nature, like tornadoes or tsunamis, lifting people in their wake and twirling them upward until they either are set down safely or crash-land and break into tiny pieces.

The symptoms of classic bipolar disorder had been described in the literature for millennia prior to the *DSM*. One of the earliest to write about this was the Greek physician and follower of Hippocrates, Arataeus of Cappadocia (CE 150–200), who is more widely known as the first physician to describe diabetes. He wrote about his patients in his book *De Causis et Signis Morborum* (On the Causes and Indications of Acute and Chronic Diseases): "And they also become peevish, dispirited, sleepless, and start up from a disturbed sleep. Unreasonable fear also seizes them . . .They are prone to change their mind readily; to become base, mean-spirited, illiberal, and in a little time, perhaps, simple, extravagant, munificent, not from any virtue of the soul, but from the changeableness of the disease."[9]

Arataeus added that "some patients after being melancholic have fits of mania, so that mania is like a variety of melancholy." Similarly, he noted that in other cases a person previously euphoric and exceptionally lively "has a tendency to melancholy; he becomes, at the end of the attack, languid, sad, taciturn, he complains that he is worried about his future, he feels ashamed." And the cycle continues, with the patients bouncing from their melancholy to "show off in public with crowned heads as if they were returning victorious from the games; sometimes they laugh and dance all day and all night."

The patient when sick might become grandiose; for example, "without being cultivated he says he is a philosopher . . . and the incompetent [say they are] good artisans." Arataeus pointed out that mania was often euphoric, with the sufferer having "deliriums, [where] he studies astronomy, philosophy . . . he feels great and inspired." Only at its worst, where the victim of mania is overcome by furor, is there a risk that the mania escalates to a point where the ill individual "sometimes kills and slaughters the servants."

It amazes me now, almost two thousand years later, to recognize verbatim the phases of mania that the majority of patients who come to psychiatric attention experience – the initial burst of energy, restlessness, feelings of expansiveness, mastery, and self-aggrandizement, followed by sleeplessness, increased irritability and, often, the spiral down into psychosis and breakdown. Almost thirty years ago, I was asked on live television, during a morning show segment on illness, to define a nervous breakdown. I said, "There's no such thing – and they happen all the time." My strained effort to be clever may have obscured my attempt to convey that, technically speaking, there is no specific disorder called a nervous breakdown. But when people become severely psychiatrically ill – with any one of a variety of disorders – it sure feels like a nervous breakdown. The building blocks of the nervous system – neurons – are not working properly, and the consequence is that the ways we think, perceive, feel, and act may be knocked off their foundations.

Bipolar disorder is a state where a person's moods swing between sustained highs and lows, well beyond normal variations, to an extent that places the person at risk of severe and even life-threatening consequences, disrupting work, school, relationships, and even the most basic of our survival functions – eating and sleeping. Daryl suffers from bipolar disorder type I, where the highs can cross over into loss of contact with reality in the form of delusions and hallucinations, and dangerous behavior, rather than type II, Joanna's diagnosis, where the highs are less pronounced but may still cause the patient to court dangerous risks by inciting uncharacteristic behavior – sex with multiple partners, spending beyond one's means, leaving safe employment to start what the patient is convinced will be an exciting, lucrative new project. Joanna's diagnosis doesn't include bizarrely irrational thoughts and actions that are clearly outside the norm. Depression can look the same with regard to severity in both types of bipolar disorder, although in my experience if the manias are less pronounced, so are the depressions.

It is hard for people who have not seen someone in a manic state to understand how a mood can disrupt a person's life to the extent that it has Daryl's. But mania at its zenith has almost nothing in common with most people's experience of an "up" mood. It is characterized by an intense and sustained mood change that can be euphoric, irritable, or both, but is well beyond the normal range of experience for most of us. Most of us don't buy a couple of cars or a house in an afternoon on a whim or take a twenty-four-hour walk along a highway because we have energy to burn. Under its influence, people may become convinced they are about to be recognized as the world's greatest singer or that they need to contact the nation's leading scientists to share their sudden understanding of the cosmos. But as happens intermittently to Daryl, it may be associated as well with volatility and anger. For him, the irritability and impatience lead to confrontations with people and an uncanny knack for pushing their buttons. I have had some patients who, when manic, made criminal threats or physically assaulted strangers – and then were agonizingly remorseful when their moods stabilized.

Mania is accompanied by a surge of energy that can lead people to stay awake for days or get by with just a couple of hours of sleep a night. They may engage in reckless behavior in social and sexual situations. This is not just an elevated sex drive but also a loss of restraint that can compromise an individual's social life, health, and safety. Thoughts race, making it hard for the mouth to keep up. People may talk more loudly and quickly than usual and be harder to interrupt. What comes out of the mouth can reflect paranoia and grandiosity. The paranoia can range from an irritable suspiciousness to full-blown delusions indistinguishable from those seen in schizophrenia, including a firm belief that one is being monitored and persecuted by the government or other religious, racial, or political groups. The grandiosity is not the garden-variety self-importance of jerks but rather a sense that one is the most talented, accomplished, attractive, and admired person with limitless potential. In fact, paranoia and grandiosity can fuse. I had a patient who believed that he had composed all the pop tunes claimed by the Beatles, and that these had been stolen from him.

In its milder forms, manic people can be the life of the party – but the mania doesn't end when the party does. Mania can persist for weeks or even months, playing havoc with people's lives and those of their families and friends. Virtually all people who experience mania will eventually plunge into significant clinical depression – hence the term "bipolar." There must be people out there who experience only manic episodes and who would technically still qualify for a diagnosis of bipolar disorder, but I've never met one.

I'VE SEEN IT ALL with Daryl.

Daryl first got ill at age seventeen with symptoms of depression. Initially he was treated as an outpatient with antidepressants, showed a rapid improvement, and seemed to have fully recovered. Within several months, however, he was evaluated by a colleague of mine, who wrote in Daryl's hospital chart:

> [Daryl] noted a great increase in his self-esteem and resumption of a goal to be a millionaire by age 30. He had difficulty falling asleep and then would be awake until 6 a.m. full of energy . . . Initially he went on a spending spree, buying $1100 worth of clothing. In the four weeks since then, he feels he has settled down and made a success of his life. He has taken a job selling jeans and claims to have made $88,000. In addition, he owns an expensive car and has made a brief trip to Florida where he claims he was robbed. His parents, however, feel these claims with regard to money are not correct and that Daryl has not made more than $1300 since taking his new job. The only other change that Daryl suggests is that he may be somewhat more extroverted in recent weeks. Several weeks ago, he successfully performed onstage as a comedian and claims he now has an audition set up for this week to be a performer.

Arataeus would have confirmed Daryl's diagnosis of bipolar disorder based on the earlier depression and his subsequent manic state.

Over the next twenty years, Daryl bounced in and out of the hospital for periods of weeks to months, with outpatient follow-up by a succession of psychiatrists. Most of his hospitalizations were for mania because that was the state that caused him the most trouble and led him to be threatening or confrontational, stripping away his normal shyness (sometimes he even stripped away his own clothing). Some of these hospital stays required him to remain in our ACU, a secure ward where people are closely observed. It has a high ratio of staff to patients and was chosen for Daryl when his volatility and intrusiveness made him react to things going on around him that weren't necessarily related to him – such as a noise, a color, or someone making eye contact for a fraction of a second too long – or when he was too agitated and disruptive to manage on a more open inpatient unit. Daryl's irritability was compounded by nicotine withdrawal when the hospital first limited smoking in the building and then banished it entirely. Because he was involuntarily detained in the hospital, he couldn't even go outside for a cigarette, which only fueled the agitation that had led to him being an involuntary patient in the first place – a real catch-22.

At first, in an attempt to prevent future episodes of his bipolar disorder, Daryl's doctors tried the traditional treatment: mood-stabilizing drugs, the prototype being lithium. Lithium, a naturally occurring salt from the table of the elements well known to high school students, has been in used in medicine for various ailments for more than 150 years. It was introduced into the treatment of mania in 1948 by Dr. John Cade, a psychiatrist in Australia who made a great clinical discovery based on what turned out to be a flawed theory. He believed there was a component in the urine of manic individuals that reflected a metabolic disorder, and he conducted a series of experiments in which he injected patients' urine into the bellies of guinea pigs. The animals died much more quickly than those injected with urine from healthy controls. He wondered if the uric acid in the urine might explain the rapid deaths of the guinea pigs and tried to modify its toxicity by adding lithium. The guinea pigs grew calmer. That, remarkably, was the end of the animal phase of the experiment! Cade next took lithium himself and, finding it to be safe, treated ten manic patients with it. That process was a far cry from the years of research that precede the development of new drugs now, but he got lucky: the effect was dramatic.[10]

Awareness of lithium's benefit caught on broadly, but belatedly, in the late 1960s. Since then it has been a godsend to many people with this illness, but like all treatments, it doesn't work for everyone and it has side effects, especially involving the thyroid gland and the kidneys. There wasn't much money to be made from lithium by drug companies, because you can't patent a salt. When more lucrative drug alternatives to lithium were found, they were heavily marketed, which resulted in a decline in prescriptions of lithium despite enduring evidence of its relative benefits in mood stabilization and reduction of suicides in people with mood disorders.[11]

Lithium worked for a while for Daryl, and then it didn't. He overdosed on it once, requiring kidney dialysis to recover. Other mood-stabilizing medications were tried. Neurologists had noted in the 1970s that the use of anticonvulsant medications in their patients with epilepsy resulted in unanticipated and unintended improvements in their moods. Their clinical observation led to formal clinical research trials, with the result that antiseizure drugs such as carbamazepine, valproic acid, and lamotrigine broadened the range of options for mood stabilization. This doesn't mean that epilepsy and mood disorders are the same thing. Rather, it means that drugs in medicine get classified by the first condition for which they work. Most of us think of aspirin as something we take for a headache or other pain, because that's what we knew it worked for long before it was discovered that it also helps prevent strokes.

Daryl traversed the range of mood-stabilizing drugs before proceeding to antipsychotic drugs because his manic episodes included severe agitation and irritability as well as paranoid and grandiose delusions – for example, that he was involved with and pursued by the Mafia or was on the cusp of limitless fame. As his escalating mania crossed the boundary between reality and psychosis, he needed antipsychotic medication. But he also needed it to contain the limitless energy and short fuse that led to volatile encounters with other patients and staff. The drugs tried ranged from the very first antipsychotic ever discovered, chlorpromazine, to more recent ones such as olanzapine and risperidone, as well as one reserved for treatment-resistant psychosis because of its potentially lethal side effects, clozapine.

Daryl's depression showed similarly limited response to antidepressant medications, ranging from early versions like imipramine and tranylcypromine, discovered in the 1950s, to the wave of more popular antidepressants triggered by the release of fluoxetine (Prozac) in the 1980s. They sometimes helped him briefly but never held him.

Buried deep in his old chart is a single line in a twenty-seven-year-old note, where it was written: "ECT x 9 for depression . . . – good result." Daryl had electroconvulsive therapy again a few years later for depression, with benefit. Earlier, someone had noted in his chart under the section titled "Family Psychiatric History" that his maternal great-aunt had suffered from bipolar disorder and was treated with ECT.

Daryl's treatments were not limited to the biological sphere. He underwent psychological testing of his IQ, thoughts, and emotions. The famous inkblots – the Rorschach test, first developed in 1921 – were not used at that time and are now largely historical relics. Instead, the Thematic Aperception Test, developed in the 1930s, was used to explore his unconscious thoughts. He was shown standardized drawings of people interacting and asked to create stories to explain the images as a way of revealing prominent underlying personal themes. In response to a picture of a child, Daryl said, "Sad. He doesn't think he's good. He's afraid of how he's going to come across [in front of others]. That's me. If you can't do something well, you don't do it. You cover it up with humor . . . make light of the situation, even at the expense of making a fool of yourself." I recognized both of us in this description.

The psychologist recommended long-term psychodynamic psychotherapy for Daryl, the type of individual counseling that examines unconscious conflicts that are felt to govern mood, thought, and behavior, and searches for their origins in early life experiences and relationships. This therapy is part of the iconic image of counseling, which in this case happened to match the professional skills of the psychologist. (Our efforts to understand people are, of course, shaped by our biases, our training, and the professional lens through which we view individuals. To push a tools metaphor, if all you have is a hammer, everything looks like a nail.) Psychodynamic psychotherapy is the technique I learned as a resident in psychiatry in the early 1980s. At the time I saw its value as a vehicle more for understanding than for change. The evidence for its benefit in the treatment of severe bipolar disorder is lacking, but its theoretical underpinnings colored how I tried to understand Daryl's relationships to other people, including me. For example, I spoke with Daryl about his tendency to idealize his male friends and relatives, and indeed me, while denigrating his own attributes. We discussed this not as an inevitable part of his illness but rather as it related to a challenging relationship with his father.

When I first met Daryl fourteen years ago, he was forty-one and had already had twenty-eight psychiatric hospitalizations in twenty years. He was once again an involuntary patient in our ACU, where I was then the attending psychiatrist. After being brought to our hospital emergency room by police, Daryl had been placed on a Form 1 by one of the physicians there. A Form 1 is a legal document that gives any Ontario physician the power to detain in the hospital for seventy-two hours patients viewed as posing a risk to themselves or others because of a presumed mental disorder, in order to receive a full psychiatric assessment. Known colloquially in Canada as "being formed," this process is known in the United Kingdom as "being sectioned," in the United States as being "civilly committed," and in the Netherlands as "being placed at disposal of the government." Whatever its name, the majority of member countries in the United Nations have some sort of legal framework that allows physicians to detain psychiatric patients when their symptoms pose an immediate risk to themselves and/or others. Interestingly, despite similar criteria for involuntary admission, rates of detention of mentally ill individuals differ widely across countries, differences that have been attributed to mental health professionals' ethics and attitudes, to sociodemographic variables, to the public's perception of risk, and to a country's specific legal framework.[12]

Before meeting Daryl for the first time, I reviewed his chart with the resident and medical student working in the ACU. The documentation was daunting and lengthy; the actual interview was daunting and brief. Daryl was pacing in the unit, where he waited for the opportunity to talk with me. But his irritability and impatience took over when he realized I was not going to accede immediately to his request to leave the hospital for a smoke, a walk, and a meal. Swearing and yelling, parroting my questions back to me, he stormed away.

My clinical note in the chart describing that encounter reads, "I saw the patient and noted that he is well known to [this hospital] from more than 28 admissions over 20 years for bipolar disorder and was last discharged two days earlier against medical advice. He was most recently treated with gabapentin [an anticonvulsant] because of the ineffectiveness of or intolerance of various mood stabilizers and antipsychotics. He was brought to the ER today by the police who reported him 'walking in traffic.'" Seeing Daryl's agitation, loss of inhibition, and impulsivity, I felt he was at risk, if discharged, of getting hit by a car or an enraged pedestrian.

I had enough information from others as well as my own observations to determine that his mental illness would put him at risk of harm to himself outside the therapeutic setting of the hospital. I completed the paperwork to continue his status as an involuntary patient and placed him on a Form 3. Unlike a Form 1, which is valid for only seventy-two hours, a Form 3 allows for a detention in hospital for up to two weeks. It also needs to be completed by a different physician from the one who filled in the Form 1, adding an automatic second clinical opinion.

Unlike a Form 1, which cannot be contested, under Ontario law the Form 3 is subject to speedy legal review at the request of the patient. Later that day, Daryl exercised his legal right to question my findings. Within a couple of days of his request, a hearing was held in the hospital. The panel presiding at the hearing consisted of a lawyer, an external psychiatrist, and a community member.

After hearing my testimony on the risks that his untreated illness posed to himself and others, Daryl leaned in toward me. With a confiding tone, he said in a stage whisper, "I would have stayed, Doc, if I'd known you were so worried about me." Maybe that was the beginning of our therapeutic relationship, when he heard me express my concern for him. It was certainly the beginning of the comedy that has colored our relationship, despite its moments of anger and worry.

It probably influenced the panel's decision making when, at the end of the hearing, unable to contain himself, Daryl asked a female member if she had any daughters at home as beautiful as her. It also likely didn't help his case that one of his aunts who attended the event had, coincidentally, grown up with the legal aid lawyer who was advocating on Daryl's behalf. As the lawyer tried to make a stirring case for why Daryl should be released from the hospital, why in effect his right to liberty was a nobler thing than his health, Daryl's aunt could no longer contain herself. "Murray, how can you say such things?"

In any case, my clinical view prevailed, and the Form 3 was upheld in a legal decision delivered the next day.

On this inauspicious note, our doctor-patient relationship began. Daryl got well enough in the ensuing weeks to no longer be certifiable under the Mental Health Act. The use of antipsychotic medication had calmed his manic fury to the extent that the balance between liberty rights and health rights now tipped toward the former, but he was still not well when he insisted on leaving hospital.

No blood test or reliable clinical method has been developed that determines when someone's illness has reached a severity where fundamental civil freedoms – movement and choice – should be temporarily suspended to restore his health and mental autonomy and to protect him and others. It is, in the end, a clinical judgment call, with a system of legal checks and balances. But if the "on" switch is not easily defined, neither is the "off" switch. When is someone well enough to have his or her legal rights fully restored? Here, the crucial words are not "well" but "well enough." Many devastated families and disappointed clinicians have witnessed the release of patients who have made sufficient improvement that involuntary hospitalization and treatment can no longer be justified, but for whom recovery is still a vague and distant goal.

Although Daryl ignored my best efforts to persuade him to stay in the hospital, he did agree to see me as an outpatient. At my suggestion and with his family's encouragement, Daryl also declared a series of advance directives regarding his care. These are statements made when a patient is well and capable of making informed decisions regarding what treatments he would want if he were to lose the capacity to provide or withhold informed consent. The words "capable" and "competent" are used interchangeably to describe an individual's ability to make an informed decision to accept or refuse treatment. In the United States and Canada, these directives are frequently called "Ulysses contracts," referring to the king of Ithaca and hero of the Trojan War who tied himself to his ship's mast and told his sailors – whose ears were plugged – not to release him however much he pleaded or struggled as they sailed by the Sirens' isle. The Sirens were infamous for their irresistible singing, which lured unwitting sailors to deaths on the island's rocky shores, an evocative metaphor for mania's ability to seduce reasonable persons into madness.

Our relationship over the years has not been without its challenges. His frequent hospitalizations have led to unanticipated encounters on hospital grounds, occasionally coinciding with times when I have been escorting potential donors to the hospital on walking tours. More than once, I have seen a distant figure hurtling toward me across the parking lot. As it draws closer, I recognize Daryl, his hoarse voice yelling, "Goldbloom, I need to talk with you. RIGHT NOW!" I try to explain calmly that I am busy at that moment, to which he replies, "Oh, you're so important now, Mr. Big Shot. Well, guess what, Goldbloom, YOU'RE FUCKING FIRED."

Daryl inevitably "rehires" me once the mania passes. He is always later humiliated by aspects of his mania that he recalls. He is concerned that people will think that the manic Daryl – who can be engaging and funny before he becomes explosive – is the real him and that they will be alarmed or disappointed. He doesn't need to worry, as I often try to point out to him: when his mood is stable, he has an innate warmth and charm that endears him to people.

For Daryl, the frequency of our contact is more important than the length or even the content. He comes to see me as often as weekly, more rarely monthly. It took me a while to understand his need for the regularity of these short appointments, but he explained to me that "checking in" was necessary insurance for him against what he most dreaded – getting sick again. "Even if it's five minutes, I don't care," he would tell me whenever I tried to widen the interval between appointments. The schedule gives shape to some of his formless days. His hunger for connection includes not only me but also Simone, and his encounters in the hallway or elevator with various staff, from housekeeping to clinicians, whom he has come to know over the past thirty-four years.

TODAY IS MY THIRD visit with him since he was discharged. There is no trace of the mania. There is, however, the equally familiar and palpable burden of his depression – not paralytic but oppressive all the same. Although I hesitate to cause him pain, I know what I need to ask Daryl.

"How are you dealing with Pat's death?" I am referring to his close friend whose death from cancer preceded Daryl's recent hospitalizations.

In response to my question, his eyes fill with tears. "I feel useless. He was such a good guy."

Unemployment has always been a source of frustration for Daryl, but during Pat's final weeks in palliative care, it provided Daryl with time to spend with his friend, sitting at his bedside, talking with and comforting him. He felt useful and knew he was doing something that others could not. Five days after Pat's death, bereft not only of his friend but also of a purpose, he felt back to square one and brought himself to the ER, saying, "I'm falling apart . . . I've had enough." Although he denied any plans for suicide, it was clear he needed the support of an inpatient admission. He spent almost a month in the hospital, receiving intensive support from staff who know him well, and he resumed ECT. He seemed to respond well to ECT during the first of the two admissions, but once he was discharged, its impact faded almost immediately, and he was swiftly readmitted. During the second three-week stay, he was agitated, threatening to hit another patient, and manic. Nevertheless, he agreed to resume ECT, and after three treatments his mood improved remarkably. This time the plan is for him to continue his treatments as an outpatient. I make a note to myself that his next ECT is booked for this Wednesday, two days from now.

As he turns to leave my office, Daryl places a hand on my shoulder. "It's hard," he says quietly.

I know Pat's loss has been an enormous blow. A lonely man, despite his outward effusiveness, Daryl values the small circle of long-term friends who have stuck by him during the ups and downs of his illness. Pat was one of the closest of these, and his loss is only the most recent of many losses that the severity of Daryl's illness has meant for him: occupation, marriage, children, and economic security. I watch him go out the door; he seems smaller than usual, although he had told me earlier that he had eaten well and gained weight in the hospital.

As soon as the door closes after Daryl, I type my electronic note describing the appointment. I have to disconnect from the intensity of the encounter in order to document it. I have learned to shut the valve, much as an oncologist or a surgeon has to do in the wake of delivering bad diagnostic news or losing a patient on the operating table. Without the valve, I wouldn't be able to do my job. But if the valve were welded shut, I wouldn't be able to interact with patients emotionally. And if I couldn't do that, I wouldn't be able to fulfill my patients' or my own need for connectedness.

In the note, I describe Daryl's mood as depressed but emphasize that he is able to complete sentences (unlike during periods when he is overwhelmed by depression). He is dealing with loss. I note the absence of suicidality, irritability, grandiosity, or psychosis. I list his diagnosis – bipolar disorder, current depressive episode. And under "P," I document that he will continue his current course of ECT later this week. P stands for "Plan" but not for prognosis – what his future holds. His prognosis is guarded given the frequency of his relapses into mania and depression, the resistance of his illness to treatments that succeed for many people with bipolar disorder, and the challenging reality of his life, where regular employment and a sustained intimate relationship have eluded him.

TO MY MIND, THE recent history of psychiatric neuroscience resembles an online magnifying function: with each decade, another layer of the previously invisible structure and function of our brains is made visible. Each decade, the scientific magnifying glass' painstakingly slow progress takes us a step closer to understanding the clinical implications of genetic and neurophysiological anomalies that put us at risk for or may reflect the damage of mental illnesses. For researchers, these advances are paradigm-shifting. For patients like Daryl and their families, who are waiting for this research to translate into substantial clinical progress, the pace is nowhere nearly fast enough. Meanwhile, in the absence of any ability on my part to predict reliably what lies ahead for Daryl, my job is to not give up on him.

The public understandably clamors for cure, but the reality is that cure is rare in all of medicine. People are not cured of chronic disease or even given absolute guarantees of prevention of a future episode. But it is gratifying as a physician to witness and to help people emerge from the darkness of an illness episode, to find their way back to where they left off or to forge an entirely new path, to reduce the risk of getting sick again or to minimize the intrusion of persistent symptoms on their feelings, thoughts, and actions.

Simone has already gone, leaving a few phone message slips and prescription renewals for me. Nothing looks urgent. Nothing about Mum.

4

Shocked

O n Tuesdays, my morning squash ritual is trumped by an early start to the day at the hospital – specifically, my weekly shift at its suite for electroconvulsive therapy (commonly called ECT or, more colloquially and sometimes dismissively, "shock treatment"). On any given morning, five days per week, my colleagues and I treat fifteen to twenty-five patients. Although the service, Canada's busiest, is housed in one of our older buildings slated for demolition in a few years, the connected network of rooms is adequate to our needs and has been gussied up with bright paint and patients' artwork.

Of the various things I do in the course of my workweek, my role in administering ECT seems to be the one that evokes the greatest amount of eyebrow raising and glance shifting. A majority of people outside and even within medicine seem to have filed ECT away in their personal folder of archaic, abandoned, and likely evil treatments. They think of cinematic references, from *Frankenstein* to *Frances* to *One Flew Over the Cuckoo's Nest*. Those who have real-life knowledge of ECT have frequently obtained it from relatives or family friends whose treatment occurred decades earlier. It's like judging today's version of cardiac bypass surgery on procedures conducted fifty years ago. Of course, there are also people whose concerns are based on accurate reports from contemporary patients who have had significant memory loss as the result of this treatment. I never want to minimize ECT's potential side effects, but I do believe they need to be taken in context with its exceptional effectiveness and ability to save lives. As part of my job, I spend a lot of time explaining ECT to skeptical strangers, friends, and colleagues – time I view as worthwhile.

This morning, I walk through a waiting room of ten people, all outpatients and their friends or family, who arrived at 7:30 to await their appointments. Because of the fast pace of the treatment and the vagaries of downtown traffic, people are asked to arrive early and wait their turn; inevitably, some of them are punctual and eager to get the treatment over with, while others invariably arrive late. The flat-screen TV, donated by a grateful patient who was often bored waiting for his treatment, is tuned to a local news station. A cheery broadcaster is reporting a puff piece about a mobile food vendor; the news banner at the bottom of the screen provides a chilling summary of a car bombing in the Middle East; and a weather forecast populates the left border. In passing, I wonder how much the ubiquitous presence of such simultaneous and unmatched stimuli in our public spaces fuels the rising claims for attention deficit disorder.

The patients and their families are chatting or leafing through magazines. The only ones who appear nervous on my quick scan of the room are those who don't look at all familiar to me, those for whom this is the first in a series of treatments.

I enter the treatment room where ECT is delivered. Its cinder-block walls are covered with cupboards and counters storing monitoring and treatment equipment, medications, and other supplies. An empty stretcher with clean sheets and a pillow, the wheels braked, sits in the center of the room. The anesthetist for today, Rick Cooper, has preceded me and is already at work, mixing up batches of medication and preparing syringes. We have administered ECT together for twenty-eight years. He is a trim long-distance runner, dressed in green scrubs in preparation for his return to the general hospital where he works in the afternoon; he is the only one among us who looks like a doctor. I suspect his TV doctor appearance is comforting to patients as he inserts needles in their veins and gives them oxygen.

Rick is fastidious about his work and always respectful to patients, polite to a fault. I sometimes remind him of a patient with whom we worked together years earlier – a professional comedian in the grips of a severe manic episode for which he was receiving ECT.

Rick formally introduced himself: "Mr. Freedman, I'm Dr. Cooper. I'll be giving you your anesthetic this morning."

The patient, reclined on a stretcher, bolted upright and responded at high speed, "Dr. Cooper, I'm Mr. Freedman. I'll be receiving your anesthetic this morning."

Slightly ruffled, Rick took Mr. Freedman's left hand, tapping it gently to make a vein pop up. As he prepared to insert the needle, he gently warned the patient, "Okay, a little prick now."

Mr. Freedman once again sat up with lightning speed and said, "What did you call me?"

It was hilarious, but if Mr. Freedman's mania had been confined to his comic gifts, he would not have required any treatment. Rick himself is a receiver rather than teller of jokes; he is always ready to hear my latest, which he jots down carefully so he can tell his wife later.

Rick is not the only other person in the treatment room this morning. Joanna Burns, an ECT nurse, checks that all the monitoring machinery that records patients' pulse, blood pressure, oxygen saturation, and heart rhythm are in place and turned on. She and I are the same age (she looks younger) and she has been part of the ECT service for decades. Although I have never met her mother, husband, or children, I feel as if I know them from the small conversational exchanges that have taken place prior to the arrival of patients each morning over the past decade. Her mother's illness, her daughter's travels, her son's studies are all familiar to me. It contributes to a sense of family among us on the ECT team as well as a smooth choreography as we execute our roles. I wonder for a moment if she will ask me about my parents' visit. My hope that she won't is fulfilled when she introduces me to two student nurses who are here this morning to observe ECT, reducing the available time for chat.

From the treatment room, I peer into the adjacent recovery room, a larger room with windows that look out onto the playground of our on-site day-care center. Two nurses are preparing to receive a stream of post-treatment patients who will be arriving every ten minutes throughout the morning; a phalanx of empty stretchers with fresh sheets awaits them. A clean and empty stretcher from the recovery room replaces the one occupied by a patient after each treatment in the two-way traffic between the rooms.

Today I am training one of our residents in ECT administration. She and I talk easily, but the student nurses are shy, standing off to a corner and whispering.

"Have you seen ECT before?" I ask them.

They shake their heads. One of them says bravely, "I don't even know what ECT stands for or why it's called shock therapy."

While part of me appreciates her honesty, together with the shift in health-care education that encourages her to admit to what she doesn't know, my inner curmudgeon remembers nostalgically the days when nursing or medical students would not have dared to turn up in the ECT suite without reading up on the treatment beforehand, if only to survive the inevitable interrogation from their supervisor.

"ECT stands for electroconvulsive therapy. Electro because the treatment depends on an electrical stimulus to trigger a seizure, and convulsive because convulsion was the word that historically described a seizure, because it produced the convulsions, or body tremors and movements, you see with a seizure."

Emboldened, the other student reminds me, "So it's called shock treatment because of the electrical shock?"

"Not originally, although people think of it that way now. When it was invented, it was one of several different types of treatment that were thought to treat mental illness by inducing a physiological crisis in the patient. 'Shock therapy' is an aggressive term. It's interesting to me that although we also use electrical shocks to reboot the heart back to a normal rhythm, most people don't call that shock therapy but use its medical term, 'cardioversion.' Cardiologists aren't viewed as attacking their patients when they try to save them."

The students look confused. They are not here today for a lecture from me on the stigma that clings to ECT and psychiatric treatment but for more practical teaching.

"Have you ever seen someone have a general anesthetic before?" I've learned to ask this since one student several years ago fainted at the sight of someone being rendered unconscious by a drug; there was a loud *thunk* as she slid down the wall to the floor. Fortunately, these two reply that they have both been in the operating room as observers.

I next ask if they have ever seen someone have a seizure. Both of them have; one has a relative with epilepsy and the other witnessed a stranger having a seizure at a shopping mall. They describe people lying on the floor, unconscious, with arms, trunk, and legs jerking violently and repetitively, saliva drooling from their mouths. I suggest they keep those visual memories in mind as they observe ECT.

The psychiatry resident, Angela Ricardo, here for a mandatory morning of training, replies that she has seen ECT before and administered it twice during the junior years of her training, but she readily admits she doesn't feel competent to do it on her own. She is now in her fifth and final year of training. It's frustrating to me that upon graduation residents aren't adept at providing what is arguably the single most effective treatment in our field for people with acute and severe mental illness. Twice, ten years apart, I conducted national surveys of training in ECT across Canada and found the results to be highly variable and often substandard.[1] The stigma about ECT exists not only outside the profession.

I look at the mountain of patient charts piled on a shelf; we will treat twenty people this morning, starting with the ten outpatients, then moving on to patients currently in the hospital, whose illnesses have made it impossible for them to manage at home. Most of them have moderate to severe depression that has not responded to medications and psychotherapy – or they haven't been able to tolerate the other treatments. A few have schizophrenia and have not benefited from antipsychotic drugs and other interventions. While the research for ECT in schizophrenia is less extensive than for mood disorders, research studies indicate that it may still help patients where all existing drug treatment options are insufficient.[2]

Over the past thirty years, various "decade of the brain" announcements have heralded neuroscience advances. Several generations of new antidepressants and antipsychotics have been launched. Clinical practice guidelines for the treatment of severe mood disorders – depression and mania – have recommended any number of combination drug therapies be given prior to ECT, although sometimes ECT is recommended "when the rapid relief of symptoms is required." This restriction has always struck me as odd; why would the slow relief of symptoms be preferred to the rapid? But I know the answer. Many people see ECT as modern psychiatry's most invasive intervention and therefore an "end of the road" treatment, the last resort when everything else has failed. As a result, I see ample evidence of people who have endured long journeys through other treatments, supported by varying levels of evidence, before arriving in the ECT suite.

ECT wasn't always relegated to the ranks of last-resort treatments. In fact, it emerged from an unprecedented period of scientific optimism in psychiatry. It's a historical era I find fascinating and I encourage residents to read up on it, since it was one of psychiatry's most fertile scientific times. Its optimism derived from a discovery made in 1917. The Viennese psychiatrist Julius Wagner-Jauregg became convinced – after decades of painstaking research involving patients with psychiatric symptoms who experienced improvement following an infectious illness – that psychotic symptoms could be cured by inducing high fevers.[3] This led him to use malarial fever to treat neurosyphilis, a variation of syphilis that attacked the spinal cord and brain, causing incurable paralysis and psychosis, and eventually premature death. It was responsible in its advanced form for about one in ten admissions to psychiatric hospitals. Understandably, there was enormous interest in Wagner-Jauregg's treatment.

Wagner-Jauregg had based his supposition that fever could alleviate mental illness on earlier physicians' descriptions of patients whose mental illnesses had apparently improved following attacks of malaria. Influenced by these case studies, as well as contemporaneous research on vaccination, Wagner-Jauregg had previously tried injecting patients with infectious agents, including an extract of *Mycobacterium tuberculosis* (the bacterium that causes tuberculosis in humans), in the hope of inducing therapeutic fevers. Although some patients responded favorably, the majority relapsed.

Disappointed, Wagner-Jauregg injected blood taken from a malaria patient into two patients with neurosyphilis. He then injected blood from the infected men into seven more neurosyphilitic patients. After the patients experienced repeated malarial fevers, Wagner-Jauregg treated their malaria with quinine. As Wagner-Jauregg reported in a 1917 article, six of the nine patients he had infected showed marked improvement; however, all but two went on to relapse. After a yearlong hiatus following the deaths of several of his patients from malaria, Wagner-Jauregg resumed his research, and in late 1921 had published an article in which he claimed that he had treated more than two hundred patients with advanced neurosyphilis, of whom a quarter had recovered to an extent that they could return to their occupations. A further paper by one of his research assistants published a year later claimed that over 60 percent of 400 patients followed over a two-year period had experienced some degree of remission.[4]

Wagner-Jauregg's studies were nonrandomized and uncontrolled, hardly meeting today's criteria for acceptable scientific evidence. None-theless, psychiatrists saw his work as a game-changing discovery for what had previously been seen as a hopeless disease. A 1923 editorial in the *American Journal of Psychiatry* commented, "It may be that every large hospital for mental disorders may have to maintain one or more malarial patients as sources of infectious material."[5] Malarial therapy ignited hope among psychiatrists that other biological, or so-called physical, agents would prove effective in treating patients crippled by mental illnesses, liberating their doctors from a frustratingly limited repertoire of rest and seclusion from the outside world, together with behavioral regimens focused on marshaling the patients through their activities of daily living. Wagner-Jauregg was awarded the Nobel Prize for Physiology or Medicine in 1927, but his scientific contributions were subsequently overshadowed by the postwar discovery that he had been a strong supporter of Nazism.[6]

However, in the twenty-six years following his Nobel Prize, phy-sicians and scientists, inspired by Wagner-Jauregg's work, continued to explore various physical agents as possible treatments for psychi-atric illness, including the so-called shock therapies that were ECT's precursors. "Shock" has multiple meanings within both medicine and common speech that can appear contradictory. ECT is a highly visible example of the linguistic confusion to which this may lead. "Shock" in medicine most often refers to the impact of cardiovascular collapse on the body – the clammy, sweaty cooling of a body that is not receiving adequate blood supply; it has no relationship to the concept of electric shock. The early so-called psychiatric shock therapies were attempts to use physical agents that would mimic the symptoms of shock of car-diac origin in their patients, based on the theory that this would affect the brain and central nervous system in a therapeutic way.

One of the first psychiatrists adventurous enough to try a version of "shock" therapy was a determined, ambitious, and disciplined woman, Constance Pascal, who had overcome her lowly status as a woman and a Romanian immigrant to become the first female psychiatrist in France.[7] Described by her contemporaries as beautiful and enormously charming, she was a member of the elite group of psychiatrists placed in charge of the country's large asylums. In 1926, Pascal wrote *Traitement des maladies mentales par les chocs* (Treating Mental Illness with Shock) with a male colleague. In it, she describes mental illness as deriving from mental anaphylaxis (an allergic reaction), which required an equivalent physical shock to the brain and the autonomic nervous system in order to regain equilibrium. She suggested abscesses, blood derivatives, vaccines, or Wagner-Jauregg's fever therapy as possible sources of shock.[8] (Intriguingly, her theories anticipate the work of contemporary researchers into schizophrenia whose research suggests that some forms of schizophrenia may be related to patients' mothers' immune response to a viral illness during pregnancy.) Significantly, Pascal was looking to induce a type of shock in her patients that at least superficially resembled a picture of cardiogenic shock. She had no intention of causing seizures, or convulsions, as they were more commonly termed, with which she would have been familiar from epileptic and neurosyphilitic patients. In fact, she was at pains to avoid inducing seizures in her therapies.

By the end of the 1920s, a number of clinician researchers were employing insulin, a hormone used in the treatment of diabetes that had been discovered in Toronto in 1922, to induce brief hypoglycemic comas in psychiatric patients, a different type of shock. Insulin dramatically reduced patients' blood sugar levels and left them in a coma that lasted from one to three hours.[9] Patients experienced the same confusion, weakness, sweating, low blood pressure, increased heart rate, and fast breathing that a modern-day diabetic can experience if he or she takes too much insulin, a clinical presentation that may be mistaken for cardiogenic shock.[10] After the coma, the patient would be revived by a glucose infusion. Patients were described as calmer and less agitated following the insulin treatment. Seizures, which were seen as dangerous, were avoided.

The risks of insulin coma therapy were significant. Up to 10 percent of patients failed to emerge from the coma. And in terms of effectiveness, as with malarial therapy, it is difficult to know whether those patients who appeared calmer post-coma did so simply as a result of the natural course of their psychiatric disease or as a direct consequence of the treatment.

Manfred Sakel, an Austrian physician born in 1900 and a leading advocate of insulin "shock" therapy, was the first to induce a seizure – albeit inadvertently – in the course of its application. Sakel began experimenting with insulin comas in patients with schizophrenia, among them the famous Russian ballet dancer Vaslav Nijinsky, who had two hundred insulin coma treatments for a psychotic illness.[11] In the course of Sakel's experiments, one patient who had experienced florid paranoid delusions and auditory hallucinations had an unintended seizure following an injection of 50 units of insulin. Following the seizure, for approximately an hour and a half the patient could not remember the period immediately preceding it. As his memory returned, however, so too did his sanity. He was discharged from the clinic and was able to resume his job; Sakel reported the results in the Viennese medical literature.[12]

A contemporary of Sakel's, László Meduna, a Hungarian who trained as a neurologist and neuropathologist at the Interacademic Institute for Brain Research in Budapest, was the first modern physician to use seizures deliberately to induce a bodily "shock." In the course of his work as a neuropathologist, Meduna performed autopsies on the brains of patients with epilepsy and with schizophrenia. He believed his autopsies demonstrated a "biological antagonism" between the two diseases.[13] He then further considered the possibility that seizures resulting in a shock-like clinical crisis might have a therapeutic impact on psychotic patients.

In his efforts to find a substance that would induce seizures in animals, Meduna experimented with strychnine, caffeine, absinthe, and other substances, all to no avail. Finally, he stumbled across a scientific paper on the use of camphor to produce artificial convulsions. Camphor is known today primarily as an ingredient in both Vicks VapoRub and mothballs, and is manufactured from turpentine oil. Historically it was made from the bark and wood of the camphor tree and was a widely used folk remedy for numerous ailments.

Meduna injected camphor into guinea pigs, with good results. Encouraged by this success, he gave the first camphor injection to a patient with schizophrenia in January 1934. The patient had been in a frozen state of catatonia, not moving or eating by himself, and incontinent, for four years. Meduna described the first modern use of convulsive therapy and his own anxiety:

> After 45 minutes of anxious and fearful waiting the patient suddenly had a classical epileptic attack that lasted 60 seconds. During the period of observation I was able to maintain my composure and to make the necessary examinations with apparent calm and detached manner. I examined his reflexes, the pupils of his eyes, and was able to dictate my observations to the doctors and nurses around me; but when the attack was over and the patient recovered his consciousness, my legs suddenly gave out. My body began to tremble, a profuse sweat drenched me, and, as I later heard, my face was ashen gray.[14]

The patient reportedly went on to have a full recovery. Meduna's next five camphor-treated patients also improved. He reported that in his first year of using convulsive therapy, ten out of twenty-six patients with schizophrenia recovered, and three others improved significantly. These results were unprecedented in the days before the development of modern antipsychotic drugs for schizophrenia.

Later, a safer and more effective medication-based convulsant, pentylenetetrazol, replaced insulin-coma therapy and camphor-induced seizures. But the medication had significant side effects that made it unpopular with patients.

It was not until 1938 at the Clinic for Mental and Nervous Diseases in Rome, headed by Dr. Ugo Cerletti, that electric currents were used to induce a seizure. After years of experimenting with electricity to induce seizures in dogs and pigs, Cerletti's juniors urged him to let them try the treatment on patients. The professor, known for his prudence as much as for his brilliance, finally let them know in the spring of 1938 that he was ready to proceed. The team awaited only an appropriate patient.

That patient, Enrico X, was a thirty-nine-year-old who had been found wandering in the streets and was unable to give any information about himself. He was clearly suffering from advanced psychosis. Ferdinando Accornero, a junior doctor on Cerletti's team, later described Enrico X as delusional, speaking in a made-up language and demonstrating a thought process that was both disorganized and illogical. He also characterized him as unemotional and passive. Enrico X had not come willingly; he was brought by the police. Nor could he consent to treatment. In an era where the ethical importance of patient consent in medicine was not yet anticipated, Accornero pronounced the patient as "ideal for the trial."

Accornero described the tension in the room as the first two currents were applied to the patient. There was evidence of some muscle spasms but no generalized seizure. Finally, Cerletti commanded that the current be set at the maximum voltage. Felici, another junior physician on the team, pushed the button to activate the current. Enrico X had a tonic spasm of his muscles, as he had during the prior two applications, but this time he did not immediately relax. Rhythmic spasms, manifestations of a full seizure, followed. The patient stopped breathing, and his face was pale and then blue-tinged with lack of oxygen. Cerletti and the rest of the team silently watched the shaking, discolored patient, counting the seconds while Accornero monitored Enrico's heart with his stethoscope. His heart rate kept increasing but the shakes became more sporadic and his muscles relaxed.

At the 48th second, the patient emitted a stertorous breath and became less cyanotic, and his pulse normalized. We sighed with relief. It was not hot, but our foreheads were wet with perspiration. Now the patient breathed regularly, was sleeping and was calm; there was no evidence of abnormality in the cardiovascular or respiratory systems. We glanced at each other; in our eyes, there was a new shining light. With a calm and decisive voice, the Maestro [Cerletti] said, "I can therefore assume that an electric current can induce a seizure in a man without risks." This short sentence summarized 2 years of work.[15]

Accornero reported that Enrico X emerged from his psychosis and indifference after nine treatments, and improved to an extent that he was discharged home to his wife, who had been searching for him. He was reported to be well at follow-up two years after his initial treatment, but it appears that Cerletti later covered up the fact that the patient was admitted to a hospital in Milan in 1940 with virtually the same symptoms. The patient's wife contacted the Roman physicians to get in touch with his Milanese treatment team, but Cerletti apparently ignored the note from her, despite the fact that a junior colleague had marked it "Urgent and Important."[16]

Electroconvulsive therapy spread rapidly throughout Europe, in part due to a wartime shortage of insulin but also because it was considered relatively safer than previous versions of "shock" therapy achieved by insulin, camphor, or pentylenetetrazol. I should emphasize "relatively" here, given that in its infancy, patients experiencing ECT were not anesthetized or given muscle relaxants. As a result, the seizures could literally be bone and teeth cracking.

As I had discussed earlier with the nursing students, ECT is known today as shock therapy because of its electrical charge, not in reference to the medical term connoting a physiological crisis used to characterize the historical versions of shock therapy that preceded it.

My own history with ECT began as a junior resident in psychiatry in 1982. My first exposure proved memorable, as it is for many medical students and residents. I saw a married woman in her thirties restored from a catatonic depression – she had stopped eating, drinking, sleeping, and talking – to a warm, pleasant, interactive adult after six ECTs, or about three minutes' worth of electrically induced seizure activity and the poorly understood brain chemical changes that follow.

Like many others in my profession during the 1980s and 1990s, I eagerly awaited the release of each new antidepressant and new form of psychotherapy. I have seen many benefits of both. But thirty years after I first observed ECT, I remain convinced that it is one of psychiatry's most effective treatments. Each Tuesday when my shift ends at 11:00 a.m., it occurs to me that these three hours have been the most good per minute that I will do all week.

THIS MORNING, ONCE THE staff have completed their preparatory rituals, Joanna goes to the waiting room and escorts in our first patient, fifty-six-year-old Mustafa Sayed, originally from Egypt, who has been battling recurring episodes of depression. Today is his sixth treatment over the past two weeks, and he is wearily familiar with the routine. He places his coat under the stretcher and climbs aboard without instruction, lying comfortably in his street clothes. Joanna drapes a sheet over him to keep him warm.

"How are you doing?" I ask, resting a hand on his shoulder.

"Better. My family says so."

They would know. Mustafa had become progressively more withdrawn for several months prior to starting treatment, no longer engaging with his family, especially the grandson he adored. He stopped eating and lost twenty-five pounds. He slept poorly and seemed in a fog. He would not have said he felt depressed; he would have said he felt nothing. He began to worry his family would become impoverished, despite their evident financial security. Soon he felt security in nothing. These symptoms had occurred for the first time three years earlier. At that time his doctors prescribed five or six antidepressants, with little success, before suggesting a course of ECT. After ECT, he was able to go back to work and once again enjoy his family and his talent for carpentry. He had been well from then until, seemingly out of the blue, depression hit him again – square on, savagely and quickly. The difference was that this time he and his family recognized what was going on and were keen to move quickly to the treatment that had helped him three years earlier.

I open the top buttons of his shirt to attach two heart monitor leads to his chest, then raise his left pant leg to stick a third on his shin. As I clip to his finger a monitor that measures the oxygen saturation of his blood, we continue to chat. He is engaged and animated, ignoring the now-familiar procedures and focusing on the conversation.

"How are you tolerating the treatment?"

"It's okay. There are headaches, but the Tylenol works."

"What about your memory?"

"My wife told me our nephew visited last week. I didn't remember that until she reminded me. It's embarrassing."

I explain to Mustafa that the difficulty he is experiencing is retrieving memories rather than memories being erased – although both can happen. We talk about strategies to improve retrieval, like keeping a list of whom he sees and what he does on the days prior to treatment.

As we talk, Rick gently takes Mustafa's left hand and with a single smooth move inserts an intravenous needle. He then releases the tourniquet around Mustafa's arm, and tells him that he will grow sleepy and feel a slight burning sensation in his arm as the medication is injected.

After the anesthetic is administered, it takes about ten seconds for Mustafa to fall deeply asleep. Before he does, the last voice he hears is Joanna's, as she holds an oxygen mask over his mouth with one hand, her other on his shoulder, and says, "You're going off to sleep now. We'll take good care of you." Many patients have told me how reassuring her words and voice are, especially given the fear they have of loss of control under a general anesthetic.

Once Mustafa is asleep, a muscle relaxant is administered. This drug makes his arms and legs like limp noodles, so that when a seizure is triggered, the physical signs of it are minimal. The therapeutic benefit of ECT comes from its effect on the brain, not the body. But one of the muscles that relaxes is the diaphragm, which moves our lungs when we breathe. And that's why the general anesthetic is given first. It is a terrifying sensation to be awake but unable to take a big breath. The oxygen mask is used to raise the patient's oxygen level before and throughout the treatment.

Mustafa is asleep and his muscles are completely relaxed – he is a far cry from the talking and gesticulating man he was seventy seconds earlier. Joanna applies the stimulating electrodes to his head, and Rick inserts a disposable foam "bite block" between Mustafa's teeth to prevent him from biting his tongue or breaking a tooth when his jaws contract with the seizure. I do a final double check to ensure that the particular electrical stimulation parameters that work for him are set on the ECT machine.

Mustafa's treatment involves a technique called right unilateral ultra-brief ECT. This means that the stimulating electrodes are placed only on the right side of the head – one on the temple and one near the top of the head – and the duration of the bursts of electrical stimuli – or pulses – is much shorter than the standard procedure of past decades. The reason for this placement of the electrodes and for the shorter stimulation is to minimize the negative effects on memory. In his case, each pulse lasts one-third of one-thousandth of a second, and there are fifty pulses per second during the five seconds he receives treatment.

Then, after I exchange looks with Rick and Joanna to confirm our readiness, I press the button that delivers the predetermined electrical stimulus. Three warning beeps are accompanied by a message on the screen of the ECT machine saying WARNING: STIMULUS ABOUT TO OCCUR. They are followed by a long beep as the machine delivers the stimulus, creating a local current across the front of the brain between the electrodes on Mustafa's temples. The stimulus lasts for five seconds, disrupting the normal electrical activity of the brain and triggering, among other changes, a seizure.

The result is immediate; my hand is on Mustafa's arm and I feel the tonic phase of the seizure, where the muscles simply stiffen for a couple of seconds, followed by the second phase of the seizure, rhythmic movements of muscles contracting and relaxing repeatedly, called clonic movements. This second phase is what people see when someone with epilepsy has a seizure, arms and legs jerking wildly. Of course with ECT there is a profound difference: patients have received a muscle relaxant purposely to minimize or even eliminate any muscle movement at all. The resulting seizure, which typically lasts twenty to forty seconds, is most often manifested by fluttering movements of the toes and slight movements of muscles north of the feet. Sometimes there is no movement at all, and the seizure is evident only on the electroencephalogram that monitors brain activity.

In ECT the seizure almost always ends spontaneously, and about one minute after that, the patient resumes breathing on his own as the muscle relaxant wears off and he starts to wake up. If it does not end by itself within 120 seconds, we end it within a few seconds by the injection of midazolam, a muscle relaxant and sedative commonly used for medical procedures such as a colonoscopy. Throughout the treatment, until he starts moving his lungs again, steady puffs of oxygen keep Mustafa's oxygen level in the normal range.

Although Mustafa's physical seizure lasts only thirty-four seconds, the electrical seizure activity in his brain, which we are also recording, lasts forty-eight seconds. While the physical seizure, or convulsion, is something one can "see," it is the invisible effects on neurotransmitter function and interactions between brain regions that are thought to account for the benefits of ECT. Studies of ECT in animals, where the impact on the brain can be more easily ascertained, show striking similarities to the effects on the brain of antidepressant drugs.

As Mustafa opens his eyes, Rick tells him, "I'm going to help you with your breathing," and gives him some puffs from an oxygen bag. A minute later, when Rick is confident that Mustafa is breathing comfortably on his own, Rick and I wheel him through the narrow doorway into the recovery room, where the nurses there will take over his care.

By the time Rick and I return to the treatment room, only six minutes have passed since Mustafa walked in.

"That's it?" says one of the nursing students, surprised not only at the short duration of the treatment but also the minimal physical signs of seizure.

"How did that compare to your earlier experiences with people having seizures?" I ask.

"It was totally different," one of them says, and the other nods.

Their answer doesn't surprise me. The actual experience bears no relation to the seizures, usually epileptic, that people have seen outside the ECT suite. Nor does it resemble the "shock treatments" depicted in films and television shows, where the patients flail around in obvious discomfort and are often left in a zombielike state.

When I visit patients in the recovery room post-ECT, they are similarly surprised by their treatment's speed and lack of obvious impact. They often ask if they've even had the treatment, a reflection of both the anesthesia and the amnesia that ECT induces.

Angela Ricardo, today's resident, has been carefully shadowing my movements to get the sequence down; it is only when I watch her prepare for and administer ECT later that morning that I can appreciate the sequence of steps that now seem so automatic to me. It makes me think of playing the piano; if I were to focus consciously on what each of my fingers is doing, they would never be able to play together.

While we wait for Joanna to bring in the next patient, I ask Angela to tell me the absolute medical contraindications to giving ECT – in other words, which patients should not have ECT under any circumstances whatsoever.

She thinks for a minute and then says apologetically, "I don't know. I can't think of any."

"Sorry, it was a trick question. You're right: there aren't any – except if you don't have informed consent from the patient or a substitute decision maker. Having said that, there are a number of medical conditions that would make ECT a treatment of last resort. For example, patients with brain tumors and other space-occupying lesions in the brain or those who have had a recent heart attack or unstable heart rhythm disturbance would not be candidates." A seizure, even when induced for therapeutic reasons, causes a transient increase in pressure inside the skull, which could cause problems if the patient already has an increase in such pressure for other reasons like a tumor. And the increase in adrenaline immediately following a seizure could aggravate an abnormal heart rhythm.

I CHECK THE SCHEDULE and see that the next patient is Frederick Chen. I first met him last week when he came in for a consultation to decide whether ECT was appropriate for his situation. Every patient who is referred for ECT is first assessed by one of the five psychiatrists at the hospital who constitute the ECT Service. It is an important check and balance for the appropriateness for the patient of perhaps our most invasive intervention. We reassess the diagnosis, consider the treatment alternatives, evaluate the risks, explain the procedure, and determine whether the patient is capable of providing meaningful informed consent to treatment. It's not a rubber stamp; some patients are sent back to their referring physician with suggestions of other ways to help.

At forty-one, Frederick should be looking forward to decades of professional productivity as well as the joy of watching his teenage daughters become young adults. He has built his own information technology consulting company, and business is good. But he isn't. Normally capable of making quick and important decisions, he now feels stuck in molasses. It started insidiously, with his being uncharacteristically late for meetings and taking sick days for a general sense of unease. He stopped looking after himself. He revised his will and upped his life insurance. And then, with the same methodical approach he brought to his business, he designed a plan to kill himself in a way that he thought would minimize the impact on his wife and daughters. In the moment, it all made sense to him.

His alarmed psychiatrist, who for the past four years had helped Frederick weather less severe episodes of depression that had responded well to psychotherapy, followed the dictum of "If that's not working, add something else." He put Frederick on two antidepressants, an antipsychotic, and lithium for a total of four months. (This aggressive treatment reminded me of an experience from my time as an intern when I was told to give people who had raging bacterial sepsis a course of triple therapy intravenous antibiotics – "the three-gun salute to the unknown infection.") But despite these medications, Frederick's worry intensified, taking the form of endless rumination about the pointlessness of his life. So antianxiety medications were added, and his doctor recommended that he consider ECT.

When I saw Frederick last week, he was understandably nervous and showed me his dosette – a plastic tray with twenty-one lidded compartments, each housing an array of multicolored and variously shaped pills, at least a dozen for each day. As I spoke with him, the diagnosis of depression was not difficult to make. Both his father and grandfather had struggled with it, and his grandfather shot himself at his farm, a reality Frederick had learned about only as an adult. Neither the father nor the grandfather was ever treated; Frederick said that instead his father had "crawled inside a bottle of rye and stayed there."

I asked him, "What do you know about ECT?"

"What I read online, and it scares the shit out of me."

"What are you most afraid of?"

"I'll forget everything. I'll never be the same, a vegetable."

"How is your memory now?"

"Totally fucked. I walk into a room, and I have no idea why. My wife is pissed with me. She has to tell me the same stuff over and over. It just doesn't sink in. I've told my manager to run the business."

"What would you be like if I had met you four months ago?"

Frederick readily painted a portrait for me of an engaged business-man, an involved father and husband with a fondness for trivia contests at a pub he frequented with other members of his pickup hockey league. But he dismissed it with equal speed, saying, "This is the real me now. That was an act, and I think I fooled a lot of people. I fooled myself."

"Do you think it's possible you could get better?"

"I don't know. I'm here, so I guess that says something."

When depression becomes severe and hope is gradually extinguished, the ability to appreciate that any treatment could be helpful progressively erodes. But to provide informed consent for a treatment, the person needs to understand and appreciate that the treatment could improve his mental health. The phrase "understand and appreciate" refers to an intellectual understanding as well as the ability to apply it meaningfully to oneself. For instance, someone could understand that ECT helps a significant majority of people who receive it but at the same time believe it will not work for him because he is too far gone or deserves to remain ill. Depression can magnify guilt out of all proportion to reality, leading people to believe that their suffering is justified, punishment for imagined transgressions. Frederick was able to understand and appreciate the information regarding ECT; he was therefore capable of consenting to or refusing the treatment.

Frederick's wife, Colleen, had come to the appointment with her husband, but I had asked her to wait outside while I spoke with him first. I now asked her to join us. Then I began a step-by-step explanation of what Frederick could expect, from the time he walked into the treatment room until he was wheeled out of the recovery room. Colleen was surprised by the short time frame; she had thought the treatment would take hours.

In response to her question "How does it work?" I explained what we do know – that it works, usually well and quickly – and what we don't know – how it works. They were more interested in the former than the latter, as they were already familiar with a panoply of treatments that hadn't worked.

We then moved on to the benefits and risks. I always start my explanations of any treatment by outlining the benefits. With ECT, the potential benefit is the rapid relief of depression and its associated symptoms. The first risk I describe is that the treatment won't work. No treatment in medicine works for everyone. To me, it's important to start with that risk because it's central to why patients see me in the first place. Then I describe the common side effects – headache, nausea, fatigue – and how we prevent or remedy them. I go on to explain memory disturbance from ECT, that it can be both retrograde (typically difficulty recalling events of recent days and weeks prior to ECT) and anterograde (trouble retaining newly acquired information). Although these disturbances are usually temporary, resolving in several months after completion of ECT, there is the real risk of permanent memory loss. This is not forgetting who you are; it is rather a series of patchy holes in the memory bank. I address Frederick's concern about ending up as a vegetable by assuring him that it has not been our experience over decades with ECT, and that depression, rather than its treatment, robs people of their ability to feel, think, and react. Finally, I describe the risk of general anesthesia itself: whether it is used for a tooth extraction or open-heart surgery, there is always the possibility of not waking up. But that happens rarely, in only one in ten thousand cases where people get a general anesthetic for any reason; in my thirty years of giving ECT, I have never seen it happen. Nevertheless, telling people about this rare but lethal risk is part of informing them before obtaining consent.

Frederick and Colleen looked at each other, then at me. Frederick asked whether the treatment would be painful. I reminded him that he would be asleep for the procedure, but I told him that later he might experience headaches and some muscle stiffness; however, I added that pain is not commonly a significant issue. Colleen wondered whether we would be sure that Frederick was really asleep. I explained that our anesthetists are very careful to ensure the anesthetic has been effective before we proceed with treatment. In response to Colleen's concern about what she would say to her friends if Frederick went ahead with the treatment, I asked her what she had told them to this point about his illness. She looked down and said, "I tell them he has severe migraines. I don't think they believe me, but they're not saying anything. I think they know what's going on." I replied that it's usually harder to maintain a lie than to tell the truth, and that severe depression is a tough truth to share.

I suggested they talk it over and let us know. The ECT service has a video as well as handouts, so people can think about their decision. I also told them that if Frederick were my brother, ECT would be the treatment I'd recommend for him – and that if I were severely depressed, it's what I would want for myself. They nodded silently, and I wondered whether, after the barrage of necessary "consumer information" I had provided for them, this final endorsement was the most important thing they'd heard. Over the years, many patients have told me that the "what I would want for a member of my family" recommendation was pivotal.

To this day, scientists' understanding of how ECT works remains vague. Part of the reason is that we don't know the precise cause of depression. After all, you can't say how a treatment works unless you know the faulty mechanisms it corrects. We could say the same about other treatments, from psychotherapy to medications. The same is true about many cancers, the causes of which remain a mystery. We can, through animal and human studies, observe what treatments do to the brain, but that may not explain why they work. The practice of medicine is littered with examples of treatments that have been discovered to be effective long before we knew why.

Recently, the popular media rhapsodized over a so-called groundbreaking discovery regarding the neurological mechanisms that may be responsible for ECT's effectiveness. The scientists, who were admirably modest in their report, had used brain scans to look inside the heads of patients before and after they received ECT. Their research looked at the connections between collections of cells constituting networks or circuits in specific regions of the brain. These areas had previously been shown to be "superconnected" in patients with depression. Patients who showed reduced connectivity between circuits on scans after receiving ECT showed significant improvement in their depression.[17] I am not sure that I agree with the media's sensationalist description of the study's findings, which to my mind are promising but fairly crude. I suspect that we are still working at a level of analysis that will prove primitive in the light of future research.

Having said that, brain imaging that supports the theory that depression is a problem of excessive connection between certain networks of brain cells, and that the same connections can be pruned by ECT, provides a far more sophisticated theoretical model than we previously had. Prior to the era of new techniques for observing the structure and function of the brain, such as magnetic resonance imaging and positron emission tomography, depression was described as a disturbance of the brain's chemical soup, with ECT providing some sort of extraculinary catalyst to return the recipe to its rightful proportions.

Brain imaging has also contributed to the debate about whether ECT causes permanent "brain damage," its opponents' most ubiquitous criticism. MRI scans have shown no evidence of ECT effects on brain anatomy. In 2001, German researchers demonstrated that the brain scan of a patient who had undergone more than sixty ECT treatments in the preceding five years was no different from scans performed on healthy individuals.[18]

While this research remains rudimentary, it is helpful to be able to share it with patients like Frederick who are considering ECT. A core aspect of my job is to interpret the science behind a treatment for my patients and to attempt to clarify where ideology, fear, or sometimes profit-fueled corruption has distorted medicine's scientific base. This requires me to plod through existing studies to the best of my abilities and to ask for help from colleagues more expert in a specific field when my skills are not up to the challenge. I look especially for studies that include patients' subjective experiences of the treatment. Fortunately, we have a number of such studies for ECT.

I gather from my admittedly not-very-sophisticated understanding of contemporary law on this that I am responsible for conveying to my patients everything known about a treatment that a reasonable person would want to be told. I – and I like to think of myself as reasonable – would want to know not only what physicians and scientists think but also what people who have undergone the treatment have to say about it. Reasonable people want to know whether and how a medication or treatment can kill them; they want to know which side effects may occur and how uncomfortable these will make them; and they want to know what is likely to happen to them if they don't pursue the treatment option under discussion. Most patients don't want to read pages and pages of medical legalese, and neither do I. There is a huge literature on how patients understand risk depending on the way descriptions are worded and quantified, but for my purposes I need to be sure that I have conveyed to my patients the extent of my knowledge – innate, learned, and borrowed – so that if something goes wrong (and I devoutly hope it doesn't) neither my patient nor I will feel we have been taken by surprise.

Beyond my obligation to distill and translate scientific information, I also feel a duty to recommend what I think will be most helpful for the person sitting in front of me. Simply relaying data and conclusions without presenting a strong therapeutic recommendation reflects, to me, an abandonment of the larger role of the physician: to advocate for the health of each patient, leveraging expertise and experience to provide hope and comfort.

TODAY, A WEEK AFTER our initial consultation, Frederick is here for his first treatment. He has seen an anesthetist for a consultation, and she has determined that there are no outstanding medical issues beyond his depression. His blood tests and electrocardiogram are all normal – it's just his mind that is broken. Since this is his first treatment, our explanations of the procedure are perhaps more elaborate than they are for veterans.

Frederick is now on the stretcher and hooked up to the various instruments. Looking at the cardiac monitor, I notice that his pulse is fast, hardly surprising given his obvious anxiety. I try to distract him with conversation as Rick expertly locates and cannulates a vein. Joanna takes over the dialogue with Frederick as the medications take effect.

I turn to the ECT machine and adjust the settings that control the number of electrical pulses and the duration and amplitude of each pulse. The settings required to cause a seizure and to provide relief from symptoms vary substantially from person to person and are determined individually. Electrical activity occurs naturally in the brain and can be recorded with an electroencephalogram, which is also used for sleep studies and identification of seizure activity. But that natural electrical activity doesn't usually cause seizures. In order to trigger a seizure, the intensity of the electrical stimulus from the machine has to be higher than the brain's own threshold of resistance to spontaneously occurring seizures. One person's seizure threshold can be quite high; another's much lower. Therefore, for a first treatment, we determine each patient's threshold by starting with a low-intensity stimulus until we reach the threshold, at which point a seizure occurs.

This is done in the brief period during which Frederick is anesthetized, and it takes less than sixty seconds. Following a protocol based on age and gender, I start with extremely low electrical stimulus settings. Nothing happens. On the second, slightly higher stimulation, Frederick has a modest but perceptible seizure. It lasts twenty-eight seconds and stops. The next treatment will incorporate a stimulus setting tailored to his threshold. ECT is far from one size fits all.

After the seizure subsides, Frederick resumes breathing and nods hazily in response to Rick's questions. I make a quick trip to the waiting room to tell Colleen that his treatment is over and everything went fine. It's not something I do routinely throughout the course of a person's treatment, but there is no getting around the fact that the first treatment can be terrifying for patients and their families and they appreciate reassurance.

"He's all done. He had his treatment and everything went as expected. He'll be in the recovery room in another minute or two."

"Already?" she responds, her tone reflecting relief and concern. I tell her the names of the nurses in recovery and indicate that she can go in there in a couple of minutes to chat with Frederick. I know my reassurance pales in comparison with her seeing and talking with him.

THE NEXT PATIENT, Richard Braudo, needs no encouragement or assistance to come into the treatment room. He has had many courses of ECT over the past twenty years and has gone public with his experience in the media. I'm the psychiatrist giving him ECT today because it is my shift, but I was also the first one to give him ECT.

Richard has kept a detailed chronicle of his illness and treatments, and has reviewed his clinical records. He has summed up his clinical history succinctly:

> 54 major depressions since 1972; 47 different psychotherapeutic medication regimes (only last regime effective); 30 courses of inpatient (all brought major depression into remission) and 2 courses of outpatient maintenance ECT (neither prevented relapse) since 1991 (119 bl, 179 rul; 298 ECT treatments) [Note: bl = bilateral ECT; rul = right unilateral ECT]

A handsome, extraordinarily articulate man with the lithe grace of a competitive athlete, a deceptively tentative smile, and a lilting accent that is part South African and part American Midwest, Richard has been profiled with regard to his illness and experiences with ECT in two national newspapers. When well, he is a tireless advocate for individuals living with mental illness and, more recently, a legal representative for some.

Richard has told me that as a child he was a sunny baby nicknamed Little Buddha by his parents and caregivers, and the last person anyone would have expected to suffer from depression. As a teenager, Richard saw his two older brothers struggle with crippling, suicidal depressions. He made himself and his parents, who also suffered from mood disorders, a promise that he would never fall prey to the disease.

Shortly after beginning college, however, Richard, like his brothers, entered the exhausting, life-threatening cycle of repetitive depressions. But despite hospitalization and poor responses to both medication and psychotherapy, he somehow managed to complete an undergraduate degree and embark on a doctoral degree in economics. Then, in his late twenties, a prescription for antidepressants unmasked his underlying bipolar disorder, switching him from the depths of depression into an episode of hypomania, a mild form of mania. The medication also seemed to increase the frequency of Richard's episodes of depression, which led to his trying to ride the waves of his mood disorder with psychotherapy alone for a number of years. Finally, after difficulty establishing a consistent career path despite his obvious intellectual and personal abilities, he was forced by his illness to move back into his parents' home.

In his early thirties, Richard moved to Toronto, where he had a close relative who had acted as a surrogate father in the face of Richard's father's mental illness, and enrolled in law school. His first year in Toronto was spent in a state of hypomania, after which he crashed and ended up in the hospital, the first of what would be many hospitalizations over the next eighteen years.

By age thirty-five, Richard was desperate. His oldest brother, Martin, a brilliant man who had graduated from a competitive American MBA program to a successful career as foreign currency reserves manager at a Fortune 500 company, died by suicide at age thirty-two. Richard has told me he felt anger that his brother left him to battle their shared illness alone, but no sadness. "He had had enough, he said. He always said to me that I was the one who would figure this illness out. He made a choice. I made a different choice."

I met Richard during his fourth hospitalization. His doctors were starting to despair of their ability to stabilize his moods and were fully aware of the impact repeated hospitalizations would have on his ability to complete his law degree. They also knew that Richard's family history was not on his side; in addition to his brother, three other close relatives had died by suicide. ECT was not widely used in Toronto's general hospitals at that time; I was one of the few physicians trained to administer it at Toronto General Hospital, where I had started my career. Richard's doctor asked me to meet with him to discuss it as a possible treatment option.

Meeting me in hospital for the first time as "the doctor who is here to talk to you about ECT," he did not subject me to the detailed interrogation about statistical outcomes and side effects that he would have had he been well. He was disheveled, with none of the immaculate grooming I later came to know was characteristic for him, made little eye contact, and showed minimal interest in me. Richard says now that he knew immediately he trusted me and didn't feel the need to ask a lot of questions. I was to discover that he makes firm decisions about people and tends to stick with them. Richard has kept his close friends for a lifetime and has shown no desire yet to fire me as his psychiatrist after more than twenty years.

I have little memory of what was said at that first meeting; Richard's recall is far better, despite the many ECT treatments he has had since. He tells me that we talked for an hour while he told me his story, a superhuman effort for someone as mired in depression as he was at the time. Then I apparently said, "I think you should have ECT." I don't remember, but I suspect his pain was so palpable and overwhelming that it seemed like an emergency. Having witnessed many of his subsequent depressive episodes, I know now that he has the capacity to go from health and mild anxiety to immobilizing depression in a matter of days. When that happens, he walks hesitantly into my office, his voice a whisper, his eyes filled with tears, telling me this time it's different, that there is no hope. When he is like this, we both know he needs ECT immediately. More than once, Richard has clung to me physically, as if the torrents of his despair might otherwise sweep him out to sea. His distress is difficult to endure – for him and everyone around him. Hospitalized in this state, he simply lies awake on his bed, not engaging with others, unable to read, barely able to eat.

By the same token, he usually responds equally quickly and dramatically after six to eight ECT treatments over two to three weeks. He becomes cheerful, interactive, and convinced depression will not return as he prepares to resume life where he left off. ECT has never failed him, and successive medical students and residents who have witnessed Richard's treatment have been struck by the "before" and "after" changes within a few weeks.

In the twenty years since our first meeting, ECT became Richard's lifeline, the only treatment we found that could draw him out of the hell of his recurrent mood swings without precipitating mania. We experimented with right unilateral versus bilateral electrode placement – reflecting a debate within the psychiatric literature on ECT as to the relationship between effectiveness and the dose of electrical current and placement of the electrodes. Richard found that bilateral worked faster but made him groggier, so he elected for right unilateral.

Unfortunately, as the years progressed, we started to see the same clinical phenomenon that Richard had experienced with medication – his episodes became more and more frequent with less and less space between. ECT has different effects on patients. Some people have one course of ECT and are never ill again, while others need regular and more frequent boosters. We don't know why. Nonetheless, ECT remains a mainstay of his treatment, together with medication, allowing him to pursue a legal career, to return to the punishing tennis schedule that he enjoys, and to maintain relationships with his numerous close friends.

Richard sees the administration of ECT as part of his self-care routine. He's said that for him it is "just like taking a shower." Other patients have described the treatment as better than a visit to the dentist.[19] In Richard's favor, he has always tolerated the general anesthetic exceptionally well, and he has been known to head off to play tennis within a couple of hours of undergoing a treatment. He is not cured, but he is definitely coping.

When Richard first told me a decade ago that he intended to publicize his positive experience with ECT in a newspaper article in an effort to inform the public and to combat stigmatizing stereotypes, I had mixed feelings. Over the years I have seen the tangible benefit of his and others' decisions to speak up, despite personal costs. When people who have had ECT come forward to talk about their positive experiences,[20] it provides tremendous hope for others contemplating the treatment – often it is of more value than wads of scientific data on its efficacy. But it takes courage to do so, because despite the help it provides, the treatment – as well as the people who have it and the people who give it – is still shunned.

Richard is not the only one who has spoken out. The case that ECT can be used ethically and effectively has been helped enormously by the decisions of prominent individuals to write or speak about their struggles with life-threatening mood disorders – among them Kitty Dukakis, the wife of former presidential candidate Michael Dukakis; the surgeon and writer Sherwin Nuland; Leon Rosenberg, the former dean of medicine at Yale University and U.S. head of pharmaceutical research for Bristol-Myers Squibb; and the writer William Styron. All have recounted that ECT was the only treatment able to pull them back from the underworlds of depression and suicidality.

I watched in awe as Nuland, a tall, white-haired, charismatic, and confident surgeon, who has written on various humanistic aspects of medicine, described on *TED Talks* his descent to the depths of self-hatred, obsessionality, and suicidality. After years of unsuccessful treatments, his psychiatrists believed he could not be helped and should be given brain surgery simply to put him out of his misery. Equally extraordinary was his reflection on how ECT, used as a last resort prior to neurosurgery, pulled him swiftly from those depths and set him on a new path as husband, father, surgeon, and writer.[21] Nuland would not have had ECT had it not been for a twenty-seven-year-old psychiatry resident on his treatment team who argued with the senior staff of the hospital that his patient deserved a course of ECT prior to consideration of a lobotomy. I can imagine Josh making the same purposeful argument and standing up to older clinicians.

Richard always says in his public talks about his illness that having a relationship with his psychiatrist and his treatment team – a personal relationship that encompasses mutual knowledge and trust that transcends the technicalities of the doctor-patient or nurse-patient relationship – has been fundamentally important and therapeutic. He describes the ECT team as a central part of the experience's safety for him. Over the years, he has come to know the nurses, the group of psychiatrists who perform ECT, and the anesthetists well, exchanging quips and updates as they prepare him for the treatment. Importantly, they provide him with trusted feedback about the effectiveness of the treatment, letting him know when they see a response. Joanna, whom he has known for more than twenty years, can predict with astonishing accuracy, based on their early morning chats pre-ECT, how many more treatments Richard is likely to need.

When Richard speaks to fellow patients considering ECT, he tells them that he has only one complaint: "It doesn't prevent relapse. That's the worst thing. You feel better, back to normal, and you think that the depression won't come back. But then it does."

He has also told me in our appointments that it is important I remind him – both when he is well and when he is in the midst of a depression and convinced once again that this is the one that he will never recover from – that we have treatments that work for him, maybe not forever, maybe not without side effects, but that work. While he doesn't like the fact that he has lost some memory for periods during his depressions, he is not sure whether this is the result of illness or ECT, and he's sanguine about either possibility. He once told me that even if ECT had caused the memory loss, he still saw it as a better deal than a lot of the psychiatric medications that he tried. Many of those had obesity and cardiovascular damage as side effects. As he said, "You know, with the meds it's as though you're exchanging one kind of chronic illness for another."

On this day, as Richard relaxes on the stretcher, he tells me about his most recent tennis match as well as his opinion of some of the leading players on the professional tour. ECT seems an annoying distraction. It is only the overpowering anesthetic that interrupts the flow of the detailed tennis anecdote he is relating to me. He drifts off to sleep, ready for the treatment that has rescued him repeatedly from the grips of depression.

"He's so much better," Joanna observes as I prepare to press the button. "How many more treatments are you planning on giving him?" Her not-so-veiled clinical observation is a reminder to me that when Richard reaches a plateau of improvement, it's time to stop, that there is no added insurance value of several further treatments. Half an hour later, as I chat with Richard in the recovery room, we agree that this course of treatment has met its objectives and is over. But Richard's treatment to come – a new combination of medications – will result in a sustained wellness few could have predicted.[22]

OUR LAST OF TWENTY patients this morning treated, I say a breezy "See you next week" to Joanna and Rick as a quiet voice in my brain reminds me I may need to reschedule plans for next week depending on the news about my mother. I make my way through the waiting room, noting that Richard and Mustafa have already left. I wonder if Richard will win his tennis game, and I remind myself I need to consult with a colleague about whether we should consider a maintenance regime of ECT for Mustafa. Given the frequency with which his depressions recur, it may be that he should come in weekly or monthly for an indefinite period for "top-up" ECT.

My stomach grumbles with some urgency that it is time to refuel, but I see Colleen sitting beside Frederick, holding his hand. He could probably have gone home an hour ago, but the nurses likely kept him in the recovery room longer than the others. They have an unerring instinct for knowing which first-timers — and their family members — will benefit from extra solicitousness. As I hear Colleen quiz Frederick on the date and time, I agree with their assessment.

"Are you sure you don't know what day it is?" Colleen asks Frederick anxiously.

Frederick, who is wearing a hunted, slightly dazed expression, shakes his head.

"Frederick," I say, "how are you feeling? You've come through really well." I shake his hand and smile at Colleen.

She smiles back tremulously. "Dr. Goldbloom, he doesn't remember what day of the month it is. Will that pass?"

I make sure I am looking at both of them. "Any initial memory loss usually clears, except sometimes for the time immediately before the treatment. And today he had two stimulations in order for me to figure out his seizure threshold, so that could also make things more fuzzy. It will be only one stimulation next time. It's too early to say if Frederick will have other memory loss. Best to have a relaxing day and a good night's sleep before probing."

Frederick looks relieved not to face more questions he finds difficult to answer, and Colleen leans back in her chair, still holding his hand.

I remind Frederick that I will see him later in the week at my office to find out how he is responding, but I tell him to call me before then if there are any concerns.

"By the time of our appointment, you may already begin to see a difference in how you feel," I tell him, "although of course we will probably need eight to twelve treatments before we see a full effect. Today was a good start."

Heading for the door, I turn back for a moment and see that they are sitting with their heads close together in comfortable silence. I hope Frederick is a rapid responder. Both he and Colleen need some good luck.

As I leave the building, I picture my father later this week, sitting next to my mother in a similar posture as she waits to see her doctor. Not that my mother is ever silent. She will inevitably be running social plans by my father or discussing one or another of their children or grandchildren. My father will nod, smile, and feign interest, while his brain runs over for the thousandth time possible causes for her vision problem that won't mean a death sentence.

Hospitals, doctors' waiting rooms, and X-ray suites are lonely, disorienting places. You are lucky if you have people there with you, luckier still if your stay turns out to be transient. Richard has come to terms with his need for frequent visits for ECT; Mustafa may have to reach a similar place. It is too early to say whether Frederick will be able to make a definitive departure after a single course of ECT. Too early to say what my mother's future holds? Probably not a useful question to ponder at this juncture.

It's not like me to brood; I am clearly in need of sustenance. My route back to my office takes me directly past the Harbord Bakery, where I stop for cabbage borscht and an egg salad sandwich.

5

Bridging Distances

"Boss, just a heads-up before you sit down," Simone calls to me from her office. "You've got to do two televideos downstairs at the studio this afternoon. Kenora and Sudbury. The files are on your desk. Anything you need before I go? Did you remember I'm leaving early today?"

I hadn't, actually, but then I recall that she is on a mission of mercy for one of the animals she rescues. I have lost track of how many birds and cats Simone has saved from untimely deaths. I thank her and let her know I am fine for the telepsychiatry consultations. Two assessments is a relatively slow Tuesday afternoon, but bad thunderstorms in northern Ontario have made it difficult for patients to get to one of the local clinics that constitute the many nodes in the Ontario Telemedicine Network. This network serves a province whose landmass, at nearly four hundred thousand square miles, could accommodate both England and France, with ample room left over for another country.

"Telemedicine" – of which telepsychiatry is a part – is a term used interchangeably with "telehealth" and "televideo." It fascinates me, appealing to my liking for both gadgetry and armchair travel. I also admire its effectiveness in providing care to mentally ill people who would otherwise have to travel huge distances to receive it – or, sadly, be deterred by the cost and stress of the journey and not bother.

Telemedicine, which has been used since the 1970s, has four defining aspects. It (1) provides clinical support, (2) overcomes geographical barriers by connecting users who are not in the same physical location, (3) involves various types of information and communication technologies, and (4) improves health outcomes.[1]

The first recorded case of medicine practiced at a distance occurred in 1906 when a doctor in Nice sent electrocardiographic data over telephone wires to a doctor in Paris. The Parisian physician was able to confirm that the patient in Nice had suffered a heart attack. Today, surgeries can be streamed from local operating rooms to expert consultants far across the world who can watch the surgery and advise the team in the operating room.[2] So can radiological images, pictures of pathological specimens, and images of blood cells.[3] Surgeons have used multimedia messaging to receive videotaped reports on their patients' recovery at home after shoulder replacement therapy and to give treatment reminders.[4] The horizons seem boundless.

In the online mental health arena, psychotherapists now offer therapy via email, instant messaging, websites for sharing materials, and teleconferencing from personal computers.[5] I am not of the generation that will make much use of these treatment modalities, although I do email patients regarding nonclinical issues such as scheduling appointments or referrals. I hear the residents who have facility in social media celebrating these sites' potential to offer new treatments for patients housebound by anxiety or for whom traveling to a physician or therapist's office poses major challenges, either for financial reasons or as a result of physical or psychological disability. I don't see a problem with any of this if the patient accepts the potential risks to confidentiality, and the therapist understands he or she is responsible for maintaining the same level of professional behavior online as in person. But they are not for me. I am too wedded to meeting patients in real time and in the flesh. My telepsychiatry consults are a form of service that I see as necessary and helpful given the lack of psychiatrists in northern Canada, but I miss the immediacy and intimacy of the in-person encounter. This is not to say I don't appreciate the utility of online mental health resources, simply that in the same way I cannot imagine turning on an e-reader ever fully replacing the pleasure of opening the pages of a book, a videoconferenced or online encounter with a patient will always be a second best for me. But having spent countless hours and dollars flying in and out of northern Ontario communities earlier in my career to provide clinical care, I get why this makes sense. And it is now part of my weekly routine.

Conducting a psychiatric interview via teleconference is an acquired skill. Trying to read a patient is demanding at the best of times, requiring simultaneous assessment of many aspects of the person – spoken and unspoken communication, facial expression, body language, dress and grooming, social skills, cognitive ability, and general level of organization in terms of both his or her thoughts and behavior. To do that via teleconference is a little like communicating with someone behind a translucent shower curtain – blurred at the edges, with the nuances and subtlety lost. At least now there is virtually no lag in the transmission of sound; the visual image isn't the high definition to which we've become accustomed with network television, but it's good enough to pick up nonverbal nuance. In the earlier days, I felt as though I were communicating with the patient underwater. I have learned to adapt over the years. I slow down, ask shorter, more focused questions, and leave longer silences so we don't overlap verbally.

Of course, this model of communication has become less strange in the fifteen years that I have been doing telepsychiatry. There are few people under fifty who have not yet used Skype or FaceTime or been involved in meetings or education conducted via teleconference. Communicating with other people at a distance mediated by technology has become ubiquitous. Perhaps in the not-too-distant future, meeting face-to-face in a room with a psychiatrist will seem foreign.

It remains to be seen how the mobile electronic wizardry of the early twenty-first century will reshape patients' ability to gain access to psychiatric services outside the current realm of telepsychiatry, but I have no doubt that entrepreneurial types are currently exploring such options. At my own hospital, plans are afoot to extend our telepsychiatry service to provide emergency psychiatry consultation so that rural and remote emergency rooms and after-hours clinics can access specialty assessment and care. Psychoanalysis is already being provided by Skype from America to China, so why not acute psychiatric evaluation and treatment?[6]

MY RELATIONSHIP WITH long-distance psychiatry dates back to the 1990s when I volunteered for the real thing, joining the psychiatric outreach program of the Department of Psychiatry at the University of Toronto. I became a regular fly-in visitor to mining communities such as Timmins and Kenora, spending a week at a time seeing patients at the hospital and in clinics. I also consulted with local health professionals, both on patients whom they found challenging and on community mental health issues that might benefit from a big-picture approach and an outsider's perspective. I encouraged trainees in psychiatry to sign up for the trips, telling them that it would expose them to the "real world" of mental illness outside the confines of big-city teaching hospitals. For the adventurous residents who did come along, the trips provided me with unparalleled time to get to know them and for us to talk about their careers as well as life beyond psychiatry.

In addition, our university's department of psychiatry has for many decades delivered psychiatric services to the people of Baffin Island, now formally part of the Territory of Nunavut in Canada's Arctic, in the form of small rotating cadres of psychiatrists visiting the island's remote communities for a couple of weeks at a time. As much as possible, the same psychiatrists attend to the same communities. They go two to four times a year, over the years building relationships that I visualize as similar to the rope bridges that adorn adventure playgrounds – unsteady but surprisingly durable.

Though I made regular trips to northern Ontario, I got to Nunavut only twice, filling in for regulars. Both times the destination was Baffin Island itself, the largest island in Canada and the fifth-largest island in the world. Baffin is home to a population of Inuit who are among the Indigenous peoples of Canada. I loved my visits to Baffin; each one broadened my experience of being Canadian in unpredictable ways. Ever hopeful of being asked to return, for years I renewed my annual Nunavut medical license; it was like being in the minor leagues of hockey, waiting to be a draft pick for the National Hockey League.

These trips began with a short flight to Ottawa to catch one of only two airlines that flew to Baffin Island. I realized on my first trip how dim my sense of geography was. When the travel agent told me on the phone that the morning flight leaving at eight o'clock arrived in the north at eleven thirty, I gasped in awe of a fifteen-hour flight. There was a silence at the other end of the line. "Do you own a globe?" she quietly asked. It turns out that south to north is much faster than east to west. I would arrive in Iqaluit, the capital of Nunavut, three and a half hours after leaving Ottawa.

When I first arrived there in May 2001, Iqaluit (previously called Frobisher Bay after Sir Martin Frobisher, the Elizabethan explorer who in 1576 "discovered" what he thought was the long anticipated Northwest Passage to China) was a bedraggled collection of modular buildings surrounded by dirty snow in the winter, and by the rock of the tundra and grasses in the brief summer months. The city itself has just over six thousand inhabitants, but as home to the government of Nunavut, and serving the entire territory's population of over thirty-two thousand citizens, it also features an impressive legislative building, as well as some hotels and restaurants.

On that first trip, the resident and I spent a couple of days consulting at the general hospital in Iqaluit and at the jail, the Baffin Correctional Centre, before heading out to more remote communities. The communities all had dual names – their Inuit names and the colonial leftovers. Presumably the colonial residue will wither eventually, but those names have become famous internationally for their communities' art, textiles, and sculptures – Cape Dorset (Kinngait), Resolute (Qausuittuq), Pangnirtung (Pannirtuuq), Lake Harbour (Kimmirut), and Broughton Island (Qikiqtarjuaq).

I clearly remember my first patient at the BCC. Jim Kusugak was a twenty-five-year-old Inuk man in jail for hitting his girlfriend. He did so not long after the suicide of his youngest brother – the third of his brothers to kill himself, in addition to six cousins who had done so. The jail nurse was concerned that Jim was suffering from severe depression, which might require antidepressant treatment, and asked that I assess his condition before he was released.

Jim was initially reluctant to talk with me, a white doctor wildly unfamiliar with his territory, his people, and his traditions; he may also have been worried about the impact of my assessment on his release from prison. But he warmed over the course of the hour. Maybe the age and cultural differences actually helped – or maybe he sensed I wasn't making an immediate judgment and was listening intently to his story.

Whatever the case, he eventually told me about his family – a two-year-old son with his girlfriend – and his job as a part-time heavy equipment operator, together with an account of recent events. It soon became clear to me that he was not suffering from depression in terms of the usual signs and symptoms we use to make a diagnosis. Instead, he had gone through a period of rage and grief in the wake of extraordinary loss. His symptoms were explosive and intermittent, and had culminated in his being jailed. In that isolated environment, away from his family and from access to alcohol, he had time to think. Ultimately, recognizing that he was his parents' last surviving son, he reached a level of calm and a sense of his responsibility. He wanted to return to his parents in the community of Pangnirtung, learn to hunt like his father, and raise his son. He spoke glowingly of the help he had received from the nurse at the jail and how he liked his male nurse in Pangnir-tung. "He is like a father to me," Jim said.

When our hour was over and I offered my hand, he embraced me, and the spontaneity of the gesture surprised me. It was an auspicious introduction to a new culture.

My next jailhouse consultation was Joanasee Etuangat, a twenty-six-year-old Inuk man from Cape Dorset, in jail for mischief and utter-ing death threats. He was pleasant and cooperative with me. Whereas Jim was able to connect with other people easily, Joanasee had dif-ficulty making friends in his local community, had not progressed through school, and had not otherwise found his way. He had strug-gled to complete fifth grade and was functionally illiterate. Although he professed to watch TV a great deal, the only show whose name he could remember was *Top Cops*. He had a history of hallucinations and aggression since age nineteen and a family history of hallucinations and suicide. By age eighteen, he was drinking twenty-four beers a day and experiencing memory blackouts and alcohol withdrawal seizures.

Although he minimized his aggression, the nurse and guards told me he had been a handful, and his rage appeared completely unpro-voked before and after he was jailed. He had been given injections of antipsychotic drugs and responded well to them. "I feel better with the needles," he told me. But since in jail he was also away from alcohol for the first time in years, it was impossible for me to know whether the episodes of rage were related to psychosis or to his alcohol con-sumption. Figuring out how much of his behavior related to alcohol versus psychosis – not to mention the interaction of the two, as peo-ple with chronic and severe alcohol abuse can also experience auditory hallucinations – was beyond my ability in this single assessment. I also knew it would be risky to return him unmedicated to his isolated com-munity where he had been in so much trouble before. Given his im-minent release, I started him on a long-acting injectable antipsychotic, requiring a monthly shot, with monitoring instructions for the nurse in his community. Whatever romanticized connection and confidence

I had felt with Jim was counteracted in this second encounter. With Joannsee, I felt my diagnosis was dim and uncertain, despite the need to "do something" to reduce the risk of his transition home.

My awe for the barren landscape and the parade of human nature that I encountered during my two trips to Baffin, now over a decade ago, gave me a strong sense of the artificial confines of urban academic psychiatry. In the small hotels and guest homes that housed the Nunavut communities' transient workers, I met people from all over the world – a disproportionate number of them from Cape Breton, my mother's family's home, and Newfoundland. Many of them were clearly incorrigible wanderers – cooks, nurses, teachers, construction workers, pilots, engineers, and geologists who traveled the globe with job skills that allowed them to alight for months at a time in the world's most remote settings. Some of them would fall in love with the strangeness of the place and stay. Others seemed to be running away from past lives.

When I was up north, I would think about Samuel Goldbloom, my paternal great-grandfather, who left the town of Naumiestis in Lithuania in 1880 with his brother to seek a new life in Canada. In the New World, Samuel was itinerant, living at various times in Montreal, Winnipeg, Vancouver, and Worcester, Massachusetts. But his son, my grandfather Alton, was born in Montreal and built his life and career there, so by the time I was born in Montreal, our family was part of the city's Jewish establishment. Whatever upheavals my great-grandfather and his family faced, they were better than the annihilation that the Jews of Naumiestis faced. When my sons visited Naumiestis several years ago, a city map included a Jewish Star of David that led them to nothing but a mass grave. My maternal grandmother, by contrast, left Russia as a teenager in 1913 and settled in Cape Breton Island, laying down loyal roots as a grateful immigrant. With the exception of Canada's Indigenous peoples, we are a nation of immigrants.

The Indigenous peoples with whom I worked and whom I saw in consultation in the North were equally fascinating in the contrasts they presented – enormous psychological strength in the face of great hard-ships and at the same time an existential frailty that all too frequently led to death. The mental health workers had the grim fatalism of war-time survivors. On each trip, almost every patient I saw had lost close relatives and friends to suicide, which occurs at ten to twenty times the rate among Canadians "down south." Among young Indigenous peo-ples age fifteen to twenty-four, the suicide rate is five hundred per one hundred thousand people, almost fifty times the rate for this age group nationally.[7] In the face of such demoralizing statistics, the community workers continue to plan and build, advocating for improvements in the social fabric of the communities: the infrastructure, the school and recreational programs, more mental health resources, support groups for abused women, opportunities for the young people to learn the ways of their elders, and arts and crafts programs that could generate income.

Life expectancy in Nunavut is ten years shorter than in the rest of the Canadian population; the infant mortality rate is four times higher; the lung cancer mortality rate is more than three times higher; the tuberculosis rate is twenty times higher; and the chlamydia rate is eighteen times higher. And that does not even begin to address the sui-cide and substance abuse issues. Given the vast socioeconomic forces affecting the health of Indigenous peoples, it was easy to feel when I was there that we were putting our thumbs in dikes. There were even times – unusual for me in my work – when I wondered if our presence did more harm than good, flying in and out, imposing Western ideas of psychiatric diagnosis and mental health on a people who had already endured enough from colonization and an uncertain future.

But the local mental health workers reassured me, making it clear that, for the most part, they treated those of our diagnostic assess-ments and plans that they found culturally insensitive with politeness and healthy skepticism. They also genuinely appreciated our efforts to provide floridly psychotic patients with medications that sometimes prevented our having to disorient them even more by flying them out of their community for treatment, and to give depressed patients pills that roused them from apparent stupor within weeks to rejoin their families and friends. We had less to offer when it came to the tidal wave of addiction and abuse that plagued all the communities. Over time I accepted that the successful community programs in these areas were a natural outgrowth of the Inuit history and culture and owed little to "down south" notions of recovery.

For other psychiatrists who repeated their Baffin Island trips many times, extended contacts with specific communities and workers led to good working relationships with the local experts, exchanging different areas of knowledge – the psychiatrists' expertise in the predictable manifestations of mental illness and its treatment, the local workers' awareness of the ways the Inuit expressed distress and the psychiatric illnesses that afflicted the families of the patients we saw together. Some good things were achieved.

Occasionally I hear sweeping dismissals of programs such as the Baffin consultation trips, and I think of a story a colleague told me. She was asked to see a sixteen-year-old girl who had started drinking and sniffing glue after the death of two of her cousins. The social worker quietly asked my colleague if she would see the girl alone, a change in protocol because they usually met patients together.

"I think she has something she needs to speak to a stranger about," the worker said. "She can't tell me because I know her mother."

"Do you know what it is?" My colleague wondered if the worker had heard something from the girl's mother.

"No. But I have a sense there is something. You leave tomorrow. You can take her story with you."

Sure enough, with prompting, and in the soft, lilting English of the Inuit, the girl told the psychiatrist that one of the two young male cousins who had died drunk in a snowmobile accident had sexually abused her. She said that she had told no one and did not wish to, now that he was dead.

"Can you help me go down south? I could stay with my aunt who lives in Ottawa. I can't stay here anymore. Everyone dies." She sat silently in front of my colleague, waiting for her to respond, twisting a braided leather bracelet round and round on her wrist.

The psychiatrist had been on too many consultation trips to promise anything. We had all learned that "down south" was no answer, although the times we were asked to prescribe it were countless.

My colleague left the room and, without disclosing the details, asked the worker outside what she thought of the girl's request. Given that the girl's abuser had died and posed no risk to anyone anymore, there seemed no reason to encourage the girl to make her secret known.

The worker surprised her. "I think she should go. Her aunt is a good person. She will make sure she goes to school. And keep her away from alcohol. I will speak to our nurse and see if we can fly her out next week."

My colleague never found out what happened to the girl, but the circumstances of that one encounter in a distant terrain and across cultures had allowed a girl in need to trust a stranger.

DESPITE THE INTERMITTENT successes of those consultations in the North and my fascination with the locales, psychiatric outreach trips were an astonishingly expensive way to provide mental health care. Because of the tiny number of passengers who fly north, the plane fares are astronomical – typically more than from North America to Europe – and the costs of the spartan hotels and largely imported foods reflect the high prices of flying supplies in and of constructing and maintaining buildings with electricity and plumbing in an inhospitable climate. Our absence was also costly to our home hospitals in Toronto. And the trips meant time away from family. Our sons were young when I made many of them.

It was therefore hard to argue when new technologies made it possible for us to consult with patients at the local mental health agencies via teleconferencing at a fraction of these costs. Still, I was left with a sense of loss. I don't know if it is only nostalgia and self-interest, but immersing myself in those communities, even for short periods, enriched my understanding of the patients; I can't get it back in the exchange of images on two screens, despite the practical superiority.

The telepsychiatry suite at our hospital is a far cry from the stark natural beauty of Baffin Island or Kenora. It's in the basement of a building adjacent to the one that houses my office. My commute to northern Ontario is now about five minutes, depending on how quickly the elevator comes. The suite features three windowless rooms extending off the telepsychiatry coordinator's cramped central office, each room equipped with a table with chairs and a flat-screen television monitor with a camera on top. The zoom on the camera lens allows me to set it so that the patient has only a head-and-shoulders view of me on their screen. In the coordinator's office is a large and detailed map of Ontario, with multiple pins stuck in each of the many communities we reach. Decor is absent, and technology is prominent.

Today, as I walk in, I am greeted by Achira Saad, the coordinator. "*Bonjour, Docteur*," she says to me in her continental French. "You will be in room one for the afternoon."

I sit down and review the referral form from a family physician in Kenora. Looking up at the flat-screen a few feet away from me, I am startled to see the head and shoulders of an older man. I am even more startled to realize that it is me. (I am reminded that one morning recently, as Nancy and I were both at our bathroom mirror, I commented to her, "I am really going gray." Her response was "No, you're not. You *are* gray.") This is the image of me that the patient will see on a TV screen in Kenora.

Soon Achira logs on to the telemedicine suite where the patient and his health worker are waiting. Kenora is a small city of about fifteen thousand people located on Lake of the Woods in northwestern Ontario, close to the provincial border with Manitoba. About 15 percent of its population is Indigenous, equally First Nations (who used to be called Indians) and Métis (the descendants of Indigenous and

European parents). It also serves as a hub for a number of more remote Indigenous communities.

Today's patient, Ken Eskola, is a fifty-eight-year-old miner. Fifteen years ago, he had a massive cardiac arrest underground and is now working a desk job for the same employer. Things are tough financially, as he is no longer eligible for some of the bonuses he used to get. Nevertheless, he's proud of the land and equipment he owns, proud that he was able to support his stepdaughter through architecture school. Ken has been married for the last twenty years to a woman a few years older than him, and he has two stepchildren from her first marriage, including a stepson with schizophrenia who lives with them. But neither Ken's dramatic heart attack and resuscitation underground nor the challenges of his stepson's illness explain why he is sitting in the televideo studio with his community worker.

Years ago, Ken acquired hepatitis C from a tattoo on his forearm done at a dodgy studio.[8] Treatment of the disease with interferon, an antiviral drug, was successful but was associated with the onset of depression, a commonly noted side effect. Compounding this were problems in his personal life, including his father's death, financial difficulties, and a number of family tensions.

On the screen, beside Ken, I see his community case manager, Moira Russell, sitting off to the side. I've seen other patients with whom this worker is involved, and I'm reassured by her presence; while the local GP will receive my typed report, hearing her perspective and giving her my immediate feedback will enhance the consultation.

I introduce myself to Ken and ask if he has ever taken part in a televideo assessment before. He shakes his head and swigs his coffee. I explain that it may feel weird to be talking to a TV set and having the TV talk back to him, but that as long as he can see and hear me clearly, he'll likely get used to it within a few minutes. I ask if he is comfortable with Moira sitting in on the assessment. He nods. We spend the next few minutes talking about the technology, the weather in Kenora, and his views on the current baseball season. He tells me that the season looks bleak for the Toronto team whose cap he wears. This seems to be all that is needed to overcome the foreign nature of the encounter and get into the substance of the consultation. Ken now talks directly to me on the screen, rather than looking over at Moira. The beginnings of trust. The remaining forty-five minutes pass more smoothly.

He quickly tells me that he's been depressed and withdrawn from friends and family. Looking away from Moira, and in response to my specific question, he says, "I just haven't been interested in sex for the past couple of months, Doc. I think it's my age, and to be honest, I've been worried about pushing it since my heart attack, but my wife thinks it's my mood." I recall from his referral form that three weeks earlier his family doctor increased his venlafaxine antidepressant dose from 75 to 150 mg. He tells me he enjoys things more recently and his concentration and memory are getting better. As for his energy, when the GP reduced the dose of metoprolol, his blood pressure medication, by 50 percent, Ken noticed a big improvement.

"We had sex this week, Doc, for the first time in months." I make a note that the venlafaxine has not adversely affected his sexual function, and that his sexual desire is returning. Ken and his wife are lucky, because this can be a side effect, although there are antidepressants that are worse.

Ken's family doctor requested this televideo consultation a month ago, but it is obvious to me that the changes he subsequently implemented on his own have already paid off for Ken. Although he is not yet out of the woods, the forest is much less dense than four weeks earlier.

Work-related injury and illness are not new to Ken. More than a dozen years ago, he broke his shoulder in the mine, was prescribed opiates for pain control, and became addicted to OxyContin. Eventually, after spending far too much money buying these pills on the street, he took methadone treatment. Methadone is a synthetic opiate-like drug that can save the lives of people addicted to heroin, morphine, codeine, and related substances. It is given daily as a carefully dosed liquid to reduce or eliminate the craving for illegal or abused drugs and to prevent the consequences (criminal behavior, infections from shared needles, poverty, etc.). Ken took it for two years, attending a local clinic and gradually reducing the dose until he discontinued it; he has never returned to opiate abuse. His success, which I have seen in many other patients, to my mind supports the role of such clinics, which periodically engender political backlash and not-in-my-backyard community reaction. These negative responses reflect a larger community ambivalence as to whether drug addicts deserve treatment or punishment.

Today, within the constraints of time, I offer some suggestions that will help him gain further yardage in his recovery. It's clear that the family tensions he described to me would benefit from an approach at that level, and Moira indicates she has some training in that area and would be happy to meet with the family. Then Ken mentions casually that over a year earlier, he had been taking venlafaxine at a dose of 300 mg per day, and he had both benefited from it and tolerated it. He had lowered the dose on his own a year ago because he was feeling better. I take what Ken has just told me based on his experience and knowledge and dress it up as a recommendation to the GP: his dose should be increased to the level that was previously effective. Ken is comfortable going back to what worked for him before, as well as trying to sort out some of the problems within his family. I offer to meet with him again on televideo in three months to check on his progress. I remind him that by then he'll have a better sense of how this year's baseball season is going to play out.

He agrees and adds, "Thanks, Doc. This wasn't so bad."

After saying good-bye, I hit the disconnect button on the remote control, and the image of Ken half rising from his chair to leave freezes for a couple of seconds before the screen goes black.

It's hardly an atom-splitting set of recommendations, but primary care clinicians are reassured to know that another set of eyes has viewed the problems they are grappling with, that they are on course with their management, and that there is further help available if needed at the other end of a secure video link.

WHEREAS KEN NEEDED SOME time to get used to seeing himself and me on a TV screen, my younger patients are completely at ease with it, and sometimes even have another electronic device on the go at the same time. When my next patient, Sarah Robitaille, a seventeen-year-old girl, appears on the screen, she seems totally at ease and is already using the remote to adjust the camera settings at her end. Her mother, Elaine, who has joined us for the interview with Sarah's permission, appears more befuddled by the technology.

The consultation note from the family doctor in Sudbury simply says, "Patient and her mother believe she has Asperger's disorder. Please assess."

Asperger's is a neurodevelopmental disorder, thought to be more common in males. It is characterized by lack of interest in social relationships, a lack of social awareness, a rigid focus on a few highly specific interests and activities (think battleships or car engines), and a general inflexibility in terms of routines and rules. It was originally described in 1944 by Hans Asperger, an Austrian pediatrician. He had observed four children with normal intelligence who were physically awkward and lacking in social skills and empathy.[9] He described them as suffering from "autistic psychopathy," a personality disorder defined primarily by social isolation.

Asperger's descriptions were similar to those of his fellow Austrian Leo Kanner, who while working as a psychiatrist at Johns Hopkins Hospital in the United States, described eleven patients with profound developmental delays (particularly language), social withdrawal, and poor motor coordination. Kanner labeled his patients as suffering from "early infantile autism." Asperger's patients, while displaying similar social deficits, did not have the dramatic intellectual and physical delays noted by Kanner.[10] For decades, it appeared that neither physician knew of the other's work, presumably as a result of the disrupted communication between inter-national academic medical circles wrought by the Second World War. Recent research by Steve Silberman has challenged that assumption.[11]

Kanner's groundbreaking work on autism was widely disseminated among psychiatrists and pediatricians, facilitated by his use of English. In contrast, Asperger's syndrome did not receive much attention outside Germany until the British child psychiatrist Lorna Wing published a case series and review in 1981, reintroducing the condition to medical attention.[12] Wing's interest was personal as well as professional. When her daughter, Susie, was six months old, they were seated on a train next to another woman who also had a six-month-old. Wing noticed the other baby pointing at things out the window, checking back each time to make sure his mother was watching. Susie, however, was oblivious to outside stimuli. Wing later recounted that at the time, "A cold chill settled over me and I became very worried."[13] It was not until Susie was three, however, that she was diagnosed with Asperger's, a condition that Wing had learned almost nothing about during her medical training. Wing went on to become a leading psychiatric researcher whose work on Asperger's brought it to the attention of physicians and the public.

The *DSM-5* no longer lists Asperger's as a discrete diagnosis but includes it within the broader category of autistic spectrum disorders where subtypes are separated primarily by intellectual function. The decision was attributed to the lack of any clearly distinguishing features between children diagnosed with Asperger's and children of normal intelligence with other autism spectrum diagnoses, such as so-called high-functioning autism, with which Asperger's was historically lumped together.

For the moment, however, such classifications and changes in diagnostic categories are of little interest to Sarah and her mother. They know what they know, and they have clearly already done their homework, since they have told their doctor about their concern. I therefore begin by asking them what made them concerned about Asperger's disorder in the first place.

As Elaine hesitates, Sarah blurts out, not looking into the camera, "People think I'm weird."

"Do you feel weird?" I ask.

At first she seems puzzled by the question. After some consideration, she says, "I never get the jokes at school. When Mark tells me something is funny, I usually think it's silly."

Elaine explains that Mark is Sarah's only friend, which concerns her, not because he's a bad kid but because the teachers have told her that he and Sarah talk only to each other in school.

I ask Sarah what else gets in the way of connecting with her schoolmates.

"They just want to 'hang' all the time, or go to the mall. The girls all talk about diets or celebrities, and they spend money on clothes and makeup and nail polish. It's not productive. It's like they don't care that the clothes are made in sweatshops. They're so frivolous."

I make a note about her "old-lady" vocabulary. I also note that despite her stated contempt for the girls at her school, Sarah's voice retains its atonal quality and her face remains expressionless.

"How do you and Mark spend your time?" I ask.

"When Mark comes to my house after school, we do homework or math club stuff or play League of Legends."

I ask Sarah to take me through a typical day. Elaine sighs as Sarah articulates a schedule punctuated by start and stop times and a preoccupation with Egyptology – for which there is not much raw material in Sudbury.

"My mother restricts me to an hour before breakfast on the British Museum website," Sarah tells me in a moderately annoyed tone. "There's a lot of information out there."

I am getting a clear picture of why they are wondering about Asperger's syndrome. In order to find out about some of the early signs of this syndrome, which can be evident in toddlers, I ask Elaine about Sarah's early childhood.

Elaine's presence is a huge help to me in this, since asking people to recall their own childhood development can be a wayward journey into unreliable memory, family mythology, and retrospective distortion. Emotion can color memory recall, selectively filtering out memories that don't fit with the mood. There is also evidence from experimental psychology of the capacity of the human mind to create memories of events that never happened.

Elaine tells me that Sarah learned to walk and talk at the usual ages and was reading before she started kindergarten. From an early age, however, she often made unusual and highly repetitive hand movements, especially when she was nervous about something. When Elaine tells me that she has to constantly remind Sarah to look at people when she speaks to them, Sarah says, "What counts is what I'm saying, not where I'm looking."

When Sarah was five, she became fascinated with all things Egyptian. By the time she visited the Royal Ontario Museum in Toronto at age eight, she knew more detail about their Egyptian collection than the tour guide did. Unlike the young girls in her class, who were generally social and interactive, Sarah spent her time poring over books and traveling through websites about her favorite topic. Artistically talented, these days she produces complex drawings, geometric and elaborate variations on the theme of building structures. She tells me she would like to work in "industrial architecture." Elaine struggles to keep up with her daughter and to set limits on how many hours Sarah spends on these pursuits each day.

At this time, I ask Elaine to step out of the studio so I can speak with Sarah on her own for a bit.

"I thought you might find it easier to talk about some things without your mother here," I explain to Sarah once her mother has left. "Things like the other kids at school – or boyfriends," I add.

"Fine," she replies somewhat dismissively. She seems much less concerned about confidentiality than I am.

She tells me that apart from Mark there are two girls at school with whom she communicates, mostly by text and mostly about schoolwork.

"Any romantic interests?" I ask.

She stares at the camera for a moment, then says, "No."

As part of my general assessment, I ask her whether she uses any street drugs or alcohol. I barely finish the question when she responds in a loud voice, "Do you think I'm an idiot?"

When I explain that I ask everyone this, she is not impressed or convinced.

"Really?" she asks. "I can't believe you asked me that, or that you'd even think I would drink or take drugs."

I feel this seventeen-year-old has swatted me across the nose with a rolled-up newspaper – or a furled papyrus.

When Elaine rejoins us, I tell them that I concur that the likely diagnosis is Asperger's disorder. In an ideal world, for a more reliable diagnostic process Sarah and Elaine would both need to complete lengthy questionnaires about Sarah's social relationships, behavior, and psychoeducational performance. The more pressing issue today is what kind of help, if any, they want.

They both seem relieved by this confirmation of what they believed to be true based on their extensive reading and visiting "Aspie" websites. But as Sarah contemplates going to university next year, she wonders what it will be like to live apart from a mother who is so attuned to her. We talk about Asperger's online supports, about student accessibility services on campus, and about the likelihood Sarah will encounter other students facing similar challenges. I recall another young woman with Asperger's I saw in my office for consultation, who brought with her for support a friend her age she had met in an online group. The friend joined us, dressed entirely in black, with a black tuque covering her forehead and featuring an Intel logo. When I asked the friend if she also had Asperger's, she looked at me disparagingly for a moment and said, "Apparently."

I ask Sarah and Elaine if they have further questions.

Elaine asks, "I gather from my reading that doctors don't really know what causes Asperger's?"

Sarah looks bored.

I nod my head in agreement and then say loudly, "You're right, we don't," unsure whether they will have been able to interpret my gesture from their screen.

Actually, far from knowing what one thing causes Asperger's, these days we suspect too many possible causes to provide parents with any clearer answers. Asperger's and other autism variants have been shown to run in families and in twins, pointing to both genetic and perhaps environmental factors. Brain-imaging studies have shown differences in both the structure and the function of brains of children diagnosed with Asperger's in comparison to children who do not have the diagnosis, with scientists postulating that the differences may be caused by abnormal embryonic neuronal development.[14] But better too many possible explanations than the destructive dogmatism of the 1960s German American child psychiatrist Bruno Bettelheim, who popularized the notion of autism as the product of a "refrigerator mother" (a mother lacking in maternal warmth).[15]

I wonder if Elaine blames herself and, in case she does, hasten to reassure her. I review the current research and theories with both of them, and finish by saying, "My sense is that it's been extremely helpful for you, Sarah, to have a mother who understands both what you're good at and what is tough for you."

Sarah looks up for a moment and stares at the screen. She takes her mother's arm proprietarily. "That's entirely correct, Dr. Goldbloom." Her tone is simultaneously dismissive and pleased.

Sarah has clearly decided that today's assessment is complete. I therefore tie up loose ends quickly, letting them know I will be in touch with Sarah's family doctor about how to access supporting psychoeducational assessments that will be helpful to her as she pursues higher education and independent living.

AFTER I FINISH DICTATING my notes of the telepsychiatry sessions, I wonder if I should call my parents from the office or wait until I get home. Remembering my trips to Baffin Island has evoked memories of childhood summer holidays spent on Cape Breton, the island off the tip of Nova Scotia and the place that my mother and father-in-law come from, even though they left it as young adults. Both would probably say they think of it as home, despite spending more than sixty years living elsewhere. The two of them also share a comfort level with life's grittiness – its poverty, its misfortune, its lack of significant education for many – that my father has never had, despite his long exposure to patients in Montreal's more deprived neighborhoods. Some of my mother's toughness, her insistence on her children working hard and striving, of their not dwelling on failure or emotional hurts, comes from having seen in her childhood community what it meant for other children to live in poverty without any clear means of escape.

Every summer as a child I left behind the urbanity of Montreal and my father's family for the more rough-and-tumble spontaneity of my mother's extended family in Sydney and New Waterford, the coal-mining town where she was born. Sydney is a city of just over thirty thousand people, making it the largest community in Cape Breton. New Waterford, by contrast, is a town of about nine thousand built around several coal mines, the last of which closed in 2001. It was incorporated in 1913, the year my maternal grandmother arrived from Russia as a young girl. A handful of Jewish families moved there from Europe in the remaining years before the doors to immigration and salvation from the impending Holocaust closed. The families include Nancy's paternal grandfather, whose store, as I mentioned earlier, was immediately adjacent to my grandmother's on the main street.

It would be an overstatement to claim that my childhood summers gave me the ability to connect with the patients I meet on consultation trips or during my telepsychiatry afternoons, yet that early exposure to people from different places and backgrounds from mine fueled my curiosity and made me comfortable with people outside my usual contexts. It has stood me in good stead in psychiatry, where success in diagnosis and treatment requires an ability to traverse the distances that inevitably exist between any two people.

I decide to wait to get home before calling my parents. On the drive, I can't stop my thoughts drifting back to my mother. She is a legendary persuader, as dogged in getting her grandchildren to eat food they would otherwise refuse as she is in cowing CEOs to support charitable causes. I have on occasion described her as the chief saleswoman in the opportunity store of life, managing to package everything as "once in a lifetime."

I have proved particularly susceptible to her saleswomanship over the years. When our family moved from Montreal to Halifax, she informed me as an impressionable thirteen-year-old of the upcoming transition. She sat me down to tell me she had "fabulous news": we were moving to Nova Scotia, and soon. Before I could even begin to process this first-ever uprooting from a comfortable life and friends in Montreal, she proceeded to curtain number two: "And I have even better news." Since she had already made the first bulletin sound incredibly positive, I was impatient to find out what else I had won in this bonanza. She explained that I had been accepted for high school at "the finest school in Canada east of Montreal," the Halifax Grammar School, with the dark implication that only one out of every ten thousand applicants was accepted; I was agog at my good fortune. "And there's one other thing," she added. "Your father and I can't move there until the middle of October. But so you don't miss out on the beginning of the school year, we have found *the nicest* family in *all of* Nova Scotia and they have agreed to let you live with them for six weeks." I felt I had won the lottery. She had effectively primed me with such positive expectation that it was perhaps inevitable that both the welcoming family in Nova Scotia and the new school fulfilled the promotional pitch. A quarter century later, I often watched her work this same magic on our boys, bending the truth or, if necessary, snapping it in two to make a sale on a life experience, whether it was taking sailing lessons or eating a foreign vegetable.

My memories of her mingle with those I heard today from my videoconferenced patients when I asked about their childhoods and their family histories. In any therapeutic relationship – even with thousands of miles between us and contact made possible only by the fiber-optic cables linking us underground – there are always essential similarities. However different their cultural, ethnic, and economic backgrounds, doctor and patient are both children of parents, similarly caught in intense relationship dynamics and affected by our parents' psychological makeup in ways that we cannot understand fully. Arriving home, I realize I don't want to call my parents. It's an uncomfortable sensation. I am tired. Too tired to convey successfully that I am not worried, not affected by the waiting. I know, though, that for my parents, I must.

Nancy is home when I open the door. I walk through to our family room, my favorite room in the house, two walls of windows perched over one of the city's ravines. She is at her computer, reading up on one of her cases.

She looks up and scans my face. "How was your day?'

"Long."

"Have you talked to your parents?"

I pause for a second too long. It was easier for me to use televideo technology to explore the suffering of people in northern Ontario today than it is to pick up the phone to my family who are geographically the same distance away.

"Why don't I start supper?" she says. "You change, and then we'll eat."

It's oddly comforting to be told what to do, a rare experience for me. I head upstairs, knowing I will be ready to call my parents after some food and an exchange of patient stories with Nancy over dinner.

6

Emergencies I

My BlackBerry vibrates against my hip as I drive from my squash game to the hospital. I have a Bluetooth-enabled car, but the research evidence is clear and compelling: talking on a hands-free phone is as dangerous as talking on a handheld one, the risk deriving from cognitive distraction, not lack of manual dexterity. I look for an empty parking spot as I barrel down Huron Street. Pulling over, I fumble to dislodge my phone from its holster before the call diverts to voice mail. I feel nostalgia for the pager I used to carry twenty-four hours a day. It was less intrusive and easier to silence, and even ignore. Smartphones and tablets have made pagers extinct, but for my generation of doctors, beeping of any kind – a van backing up, a particularly noisy crosswalk – induces a startle response, cueing us that a patient requires something, possibly urgently.

"David, it's Tish," the voice at the other end says. "I just wanted to give you a heads-up. Georges is back, brought in last night by police. He's restless and asking for you. No one here this morning speaks good enough French to settle him, and he isn't answering us in English. We tried the phone interpreter service earlier but it just agitated him. How long will you be?"

The voice belongs to Letitia Marshall, a psychiatric emergency nurse known to everyone as Tish. She hails from Cape Breton Island, a member of the small but vibrant black community there. In a six-degrees-of-separation moment early in our work together, Tish and I discovered that she had shopped frequently in my grandmother's clothing store in New Waterford. Tish exemplifies the Canadian stereotype of Cape Bretoners as fun-loving and direct; she is always ready for a laugh and never coats her descriptions of patients in judgmental jargon. Quite apart from liking her, I trust her clinical instincts.

My patient, Georges Mulumba, is a francophone Congolese refugee who fled that country's impending civil war triggered by the Rwandan genocide in 1994. He and his family left early enough that none of them witnessed its madness or became its victims. Georges has been my patient since shortly after he moved to Toronto; these days I usually see him for outpatient appointments in my office. As soon as I hear the news from Tish, I feel a stab of guilt that after Georges missed his last appointment with me, I didn't follow up to find out what had happened. My excuse at the time was that it's tricky to reach him. Georges lives in a rooming house and doesn't have his own phone. He's been on disability support for over a decade, taking English-language courses and hoping one day to work as an auto mechanic as he did in the Democratic Republic of Congo. I had made a mental note to follow up with his community worker if he missed his next appointment. In retrospect I should have known that even one missed appointment is a bad sign for Georges and checked up on him sooner. Tish's telling me that he isn't responding to questions in English is another bad sign. Although he hasn't yet mastered English, he speaks it in a rudimentary way – except when he becomes psychotic.

It is a coincidence, for better or worse, that he has been brought to the ER on a day I am covering a shift there for a colleague. I call Tish and ask her to tell him that I will see him as soon as I have met with the psychiatry residents from last night to complete our handover rounds. I am counting on the fact that our hospital is a familiar place to Georges from multiple previous admissions; its routines and structure, such as our morning teaching rounds, usually soothe him. I also suggest she order him something to eat, no meat, and tell him I want him to eat it before we talk. Knowing Georges, I suspect that he has had little to eat for several days, which will not help whatever psychiatric symptoms brought him to police attention last night. When he is ill, he gets paranoid about food. Red meat is usually the first food group struck from his diminishing options.

As I head from the parking lot, after arriving at the hospital, I feel a surge of energy. Unlike some of my colleagues, I like working ER shifts. When I first came to this hospital twenty years ago, I was "awarded" the Friday afternoon ER shift – the period when all hell tended to break loose as my colleagues left for the weekend. I have not had a regular shift for a number of years – my travel as chair of the Mental Health Commission has made it impossible – but I pick up shifts on occasion, filling in for grateful colleagues when they are ill or on holiday. Today I am covering for a colleague who has taken his young family to Disney World. Having been there myself when our boys were young, I would happily opt for a morning of psychiatric emergencies over another ride on the Tower of Terror, where a free-fall elevator ride took several years off my life.

There is something about the intensity and surprise of the ER environment that keeps drawing me back. It is probably the same irresistible rubbernecking I exhibit when I see a police car or a fire truck and want to – need to – know exactly what is going on. It is also very different work from my more scheduled and in-depth office assessments. In the ER, my job is to decide in the shortest possible time whether a patient is safe to leave or needs admission to the hospital and, if the latter, whether the patient comes in voluntarily or involuntarily. It is also my job to determine and negotiate with the patient, equally swiftly if possible, the immediate next steps in treatment, whether taking place in the hospital or consisting of a referral to some type of outpatient service. Going more slowly means other equally urgent patients have to wait. The risk, of course, is that patients may experience my attention as superficial and excessively outcome-focused, and certainly in cases of involuntary admission, inconsistent with what they want. The reality is that it can be hard to convey consistent empathy when I meet ten different people during a single shift. Most people's image of encountering a psychiatrist doesn't include the acuity and demands of an emergency room setting. The ER brings out the pragmatism in me, ever conscious of a crowded waiting room instead of sequential and scheduled outpatient appointments.

Today the traffic and demands of the ER satisfy a purpose for me, keeping me sufficiently occupied that I will have little time to think about anything other than the patients.

THE EMERGENCY ROOM OF the hospital where I work is the city's busiest psychiatric emergency service and operates twenty-four/seven. We are the city's only such service not located inside a general hospital emergency room; unlike in the general hospitals, here people with psychiatric illness are our clinical priority. Situated on the ground floor of the hospital, the emergency department features a sign on the door that says EMERGENCY in an array of languages that reflects Toronto's diverse population. The greeting is a bit of a tease because we can't provide immediate assistance that is as linguistically and culturally sensitive as the sign suggests, but we can usually access an interpreter of some sort, by telephone at a minimum, as evidenced by Tish's efforts this morning on Georges' behalf.

Patients find their way to our emergency room in all sorts of ways. Sometimes, particularly if they know a doctor in the hospital or have been a patient in the past, they come by themselves, out of desperation and a belief that we can help them. Sometimes family members and friends bring them, not knowing what else to do. Sometimes a family physician sends them directly to us from an appointment, or a community therapist sends or brings them down because of concern about suicidality or, more rarely, aggression or psychosis. Not infrequently they are brought by police, who have been called by frightened family members or neighbors, or even passersby if the patient's behavior is sufficiently bizarre to attract the attention of strangers. For reasons that may range from lack of familiarity with the medical system to limited access as a result of immigration policy, to fear of legal consequences, recent immigrants from diverse ethnoracial communities are reluctant to seek psychiatric help voluntarily.[1] By the time members of this group come to the ER, the crisis and the chaos are often more severe.

Of all the city's emergency rooms, ours is the favorite of police officers. While all the city's general hospitals accept psychiatric patients, police officers can spend many hours sitting in an ER waiting room while staff deal with people who are bleeding, having a heart attack, or facing other dire physical problems. Triage can often move people with mental illness to the bottom of a priority list. At a uniquely psychiatric ER like ours, a mentally ill person arriving accompanied by police becomes an instant priority. We work efficiently to transfer the patient to the most appropriate therapeutic environment and allow the police to return promptly to their other duties.

The physical space of the emergency department is neither attractive nor welcoming, the result of a design mandate aimed at minimizing expense and maximizing safety. Its spare, bland atmosphere is a bit like that of an airport departure gate that oscillates between emptiness and overcrowding multiple times a day. I'd be hard-pressed to describe it as soothing. When traffic is heavy, it can feel very cramped, especially for people in distress.[2]

I enter via a locked side door inaccessible to patients. It leads into a small hallway and a second locked door leading directly into the ER. When the first door closes behind me, I feel like I am in one of those decompression chambers of a submarine or a spaceship. As I open the inner locked door, the noise of people talking in the ER confronts me. The first space I enter is a long hallway leading to a large waiting room with a television encased in Plexiglas. Bench seats for patients are bolted to the floor so they can't be thrown. The waiting room has its own entry for patients, across from the hospital elevators. People waiting for a ride to an upper floor can casually peer through a window into the waiting room and get a sense of how busy it is, exposing the people coming for help. It's an accidental fishbowl, and it isn't ideal.

Along the length of the hallway is a series of individual interview rooms where the assessments happen; these offer some privacy but are also built for safety. The desks are bolted to the floor, the chairs are too heavy to pick up, the doors open both ways to prevent barricading, there is a panic button in every room, and each room has closed-circuit television monitoring.

About a decade ago, I argued unsuccessfully against the construction of what is now a triage room and waiting area outside the ER, positioned equidistant from the security office and ER on the ground floor. The triage room is a small glassed-in cubicle where nurses conduct a brief assessment to gauge clinical urgency before showing people into the ER waiting room. People await their screening on a very public bench, just outside the triage room, amid ground-floor traffic flow. It looks like the penalty box of a hockey game or a Pilgrim stockade minus the arm and leg restraints. If I were one of our patients, I would hate this exposure to every passerby. But it was built in a spirit of retrofitting into available space rather than of form following function.

In contrast to the overexposed triage and waiting areas, the ER resembles a rabbit warren. In addition to the interview rooms along the hallway, there is a negative-pressure room for containing someone with a highly infectious disease. On the other side of the hallway, there is a cramped nursing station lined with banks of computers. At the back of the station is a windowless conference room where doctors and staff meet for rounds. In addition, behind the conference room is a short-stay area, where as many as eight people who need up to seventy-two hours of further assessment and treatment can be admitted, each to an individual bedroom. It's a place where crises sometimes resolve, where alcohol wears off, where diagnostic uncertainties are explored and sometimes resolved, and where community resources can be rallied. Patients spend an average of thirty hours there prior to discharge or transfer to an inpatient unit.

I walk to the conference room at the back where the psychiatric residents from the previous shift wait, hoping to sign over their patients quickly so they can go home to sleep. On the large whiteboard that takes up most of one wall are blocks of writing in multicolored marker inks: the cell phone number of the staff psychiatrist on call, mnemonics for recalling symptom clusters, and a grid divided into four columns, crisscrossed by three rows. Each of the columns identifies risk factors under the headings *Predisposing*, *Precipitating*, *Perpetuating*, and *Protective*. The rows also identify risk factors but from different perspectives and have their own headings: *Biological*, *Psychological*, *Sociocultural*. Each box of the grid contains a list representing the resident's theoretical speculation on how genetic risk, psychological state, social environment, and culture might explain why the patient is now in the ER, ill, or in crisis. The boxes under *Protective* contain the strengths and supports – family, job, friends – that may help the patient pull through. I see that in the *Predisposing/Sociocultural* box, the resident has written "immigration, isolation from family and culture, poverty" and surmise that this is an analysis of Georges' current situation.

I resist an urge to erase the whole thing; the boxes aren't inaccurate exactly, just formulaic if you know the person whose situation is being fitted into this tidy schema. The positive aspect of the boxes is that they force people to think broadly about determinants of illness as well as an individual's strengths; their downside is the fill-in-the-blanks aspect and lack of weighting of the most important variables. I teach residents that predisposing and precipitating factors are less amenable to intervention – since they have already happened – but factors that perpetuate an illness and can be modified are our responsibility. When

I have had too much coffee and/or the ER is unusually slow, I wax political and argue that it is also the profession's responsibility to advocate for policies such as supported housing, employment opportunities, and income assistance that have been demonstrated to improve the quality of life and functioning of people with mental illness. My serious point is that whatever we do in the ER on a given day, if we fail to persuade the larger community to address the greater forces at play that lead to an individual patient's need for the emergency room, we will be more likely to see those patients again. Depending on the resident's political stripes, my comments are met with enthusiasm or disinterest.

The ER is staffed by a rotation of psychiatrists and psychiatric residents, a number of nurses, two social workers, a pharmacist, a primary care physician, a ward clerk, and a program assistant (PA), who in an earlier era would have been called an orderly. The archaic term captures the need for order in the midst of the chaos of psychiatric distress and disease. It is also true that some of the PAs are burly young males with the muscular capacity to contain visitors to the ER whose disorders render them aggressive.

Emergency psychiatrists are considered by their colleagues to be the "surgeons" of psychiatry. In contrast to the more intellectual internists or child-friendly pediatricians, surgeons – regardless of gender – are seen as the "action men" or "cowboys" of medicine and are endlessly lampooned by their colleagues as cheerful brutes who lack subtlety and enjoy the fix-it nature of their branch of medicine. Like any generalization, there is some truth here; in my experience, emergency psychiatrists like cutting into a psychological problem to open it up to inspection. The goal of the incision, similar to that of the operation, is then to open the wound, evacuate any infected, necrotic, or cancerous tissue, take care of any potential leaks, and cleanse in preparation for closing. It is an encounter at a ninety-degree angle to the trajectory of the patient's life and difficulties. Emergency room psychiatrists are a different breed from the long-term psychotherapists who come to mind when many people think of psychiatrists. The latter have endless patience and are satisfied by their patients' more incremental progress. Psychiatry as a profession, of course, needs both as it tries to help those in crisis or grappling with a chronic illness – or both.

BECAUSE WE ARE A teaching hospital, my shift begins with the hand-over from eager but fatigued residents who have been on call for the previous seventeen hours. After they tell us about the patients kept overnight, we will divvy up the patients to be seen. Today there are two residents, Niraj Mehta and Jennifer McClintock, describing their cases. A third resident would have gone home at eleven last night. It is now the residents' job to present concise summaries of the night's clinical encounters, including their diagnostic conclusion and a treatment plan. Paul Kurdyak, the other attending psychiatrist, and I listen and try to imagine what the encounter was like, looking for gaps, as much as for evidence that justifies the diagnosis and treatment, and identifying issues and themes that can be used as a segue into teaching material. Paul was my resident more than a decade ago, and despite completing a PhD and establishing himself as a highly regarded academic, he remains committed to clinical work in the ER. He is very good at it. He is calm in the presence of chaos, practical, and smart. He also happens to be an excellent squash player to whom I lose with discouraging frequency.

Jennifer, a woman in her late twenties, looks pale and tired. Her dark hair is scraped back into a short ponytail, and behind a pair of severe but fashionable black glasses the skin under her eyes looks bruised, a reminder that she has been up all night. She tells me about a young woman, Luana Rabinowitz, with bipolar disorder. Luana was brought to the ER in the early hours of the morning by police who, after receiving a noise complaint, found her wandering the residential neighborhood near her condominium building, without shoes and half naked, singing loudly. She agreed quite happily to accompany the police to the ER in their car, but almost immediately after her arrival here and the policemen's departure, her euphoria switched to extreme irritability. She argued with the hospital staff who tried to persuade her to put on a hospital gown and to usher her into an interview room. When she tried to scratch and bite one of the PAs, a so-called Code White was called (color codes announced over the public address system in hospitals signal various types of emergencies; Code White usually refers to physical aggression).

Jennifer tells me, "We had to give her loxapine [an antipsychotic] and lorazepam [a sedative] or she would have ended up in restraints. She was given the choice of taking them orally or our giving them to her IM [intramuscularly]. It was touch and go for a minute, but she took the meds by mouth. Then I put her on a Form 1 to keep in the ER."

Medication is administered against a person's will only when his or her explosive and aggressive behavior makes it likely that someone will get hurt. I ask Jennifer to explain her rationale for forcing the medication on Luana and keeping her in the hospital against her will.

Jennifer races through the symptoms and pertinent negatives – symptoms that are missing – that justify the diagnosis and point to the risks that led to her judgment regarding Luana. I try to focus on what she is saying: "Speech pressured; affect labile, alternating between euphoric and irritable, disinhibited; thought form characterized by flight of ideas and loose associations; thought content revealed grandiose delusions re a future career as an opera singer despite no previous training or experience." The phrases are as familiar as one of my favorite piano concertos, but there's no melody. Try as I might, Jennifer's description, despite its comprehensiveness and detail, leaves me with no visual image or sense of this person.

There is an exercise I used to do with terrified medical students when I worked in the Acute Care Unit of the hospital, where the most severely psychiatrically ill patients often spend their first few days after coming to the emergency room. It is a high-voltage setting of intense symptomatology, with people who are floridly psychotic and agitated or profoundly withdrawn and suicidal. I would ask each medical student to go to a patient and chat with him for sixty seconds about anything *except* his symptoms, treatment, or diagnosis. They could talk about the weather, sports, politics, food, or anything else. And then, when the students returned to the nursing station, I would ask them, "What's wrong with that person?" They would initially sputter that they couldn't say, because they hadn't asked any of the questions from their preparatory reading on psychiatric interviewing. But then I would ask them to simply describe what they saw, heard, and felt in the encounter, and to their own surprise, their observational powers led them to presumptive hypotheses. They would notice people's hygiene, patterns of thinking and speaking, interaction style, mood, and perspectives regardless of the subject being discussed. To be sure, they couldn't make a diagnosis in a sixty-second chat about the weather, but they learned that in such encounters they are observing clinical phenomena and unconsciously formulating possibilities that must be confirmed or rejected. And it begins in the first seconds of the encounter. I think of an anecdote author Malcolm Gladwell related about Thomas Hoving, former director of the Metropolitan Museum of Art in New York, who had the ability to recognize in an instant that an ancient Greek statue was not genuine without being able to articulate exactly why.[3]

I am not sure what's preventing Jennifer from making Luana real for us – probably a combination of fatigue and a desire to get through her handover efficiently so she can get home to sleep. I don't suggest the medical student exercise to her, as she would immediately intuit that I am disappointed by her report. She is too tired and has worked too hard to hear criticism right now. Conveying my concern about her ability to describe the flavor of a person and her distress to other health professionals, even when exhausted – an indispensable clinical skill in psychiatry – can wait.

When Jennifer finishes her report, Tish corroborates the resident's concern for Luana and the need for the actions that were taken. "The night shift passed on that she was in a real state when she got here, demanding to be seen in the middle of the night by the head of the hospital." She looks over sympathetically at Jennifer.

"I gather poor Jennifer and Iris, one of the night nurses, got the brunt of it. She was okay initially with the male staff, flirty, joking, but when Iris tried to get her to put on a gown, she started shouting and wouldn't go into the interview room. Iris told me that as soon as Jennifer tried to talk to her, she started raging, swearing, insulting her appearance, her weight, telling her she'd never get a man dressing the way she does. And then when Jennifer told her she was behaving inappropriately – very calmly and politely, Iris said – she completely lost control, wild, bouncing off the walls, scratching Tim, a PA, and pushing Iris against the wall. She's going to get hurt or end up in jail if she leaves."

In plain words that contrast with Jennifer's more technical description, Tish has described the interpersonal chaos that Luana wrought and the clinical alarm bell that it triggered for the ER staff, leading to the decision to detain and chemically restrain her.

Tish looks over at Jennifer. "Iris said Jennifer was a trooper. She really thought Luana would end up in restraints. But she obviously got the message that Jennifer meant what she said and took the medication."

The ER has several sets of so-called mechanical restraints that would have been used to tie Luana to a stretcher. They are fastened to the stretcher's frame and then around the wrists and ankles. There are strict protocols about their application, monitoring, and removal. A recent hospital task force on minimization of seclusion and restraint has dramatically reduced their use through extensive staff training in the prevention and management of aggressive behavior, and better monitoring and review of the use of restraints on any patient. In Luana's case, only the fact that she responded to the sedative medication to an extent that she stopped trying to assault the ER staff permitted her to remain physically unrestrained. Not that Luana was appreciative of this relative freedom, nor would I expect her to be. Psychiatrists and mental health staff who want to be uniformly liked or receive unadulterated gratitude from their patients don't work in emergency and acute care settings.

Jennifer seems unresponsive to Tish's praise. Maybe Luana's insults have upset and antagonized her, and she is trying to keep a lock on her emotions; maybe she is simply too exhausted to be pleased. I make a mental note to follow up with her after she has had a good night's sleep to make sure she is okay and to suggest some ways she can enrich her descriptions of patients so that her audience feels they are hearing about a person rather than a case report.

I ask about Luana's history. Jennifer looks down at her notes.

"A year ago she was diagnosed with a manic episode and was hospitalized voluntarily at St. Mike's [a psychiatric unit at another hospital in the city]. She stopped taking her medications on her own six months later with no immediate consequences. I contacted the crisis worker at St. Mike's, who faxed over the last available clinical note. It looks as though she had no active symptoms when she was discharged. There was also a final outpatient assessment that documented her mood as 'euthymic' [neither manic nor depressed]. She was supposed to return in a month, but there was no other visit documented. That was ten months ago."

Despite the tension between Jennifer and Luana, Jennifer had been conscientious in obtaining relevant clinical information about the patient.

"Do we know when she started to become symptomatic again?"

"Yes. The police sent one of their teams to her apartment building. The superintendent told them that Luana works at a popular clothing chain as a manager and was living with a close female friend. A couple of weeks ago, she became elated in a way her roommate had never seen before. She stopped sleeping and initiated several one-night stands, which really bothered the roommate as Luana brought a series of strange men back to their apartment. Apparently the roommate moved out suddenly, after trying to convince Luana to get help. The superintendent told the police that Luana said some terrible things to the roommate, who is Korean. Racist comments, which surprised the superintendent, as it wasn't like Luana at all. He told the officer she was a great tenant before all of this."

From Jennifer and Tish's descriptions, it sounds as if Luana knows which buttons to push: the verbal invective hurled at her roommate and individual nurses and doctors targeted their physical features, dress, and race. Here the staff has to withstand it and contextualize it in terms of illness to avoid a hostile or punitive response. The same wouldn't happen out on the street.

The ER waiting room is now empty; Jennifer and Niraj admitted or discharged everyone from the day and night before, and the whiteboard in the nursing station is blank, a tabula rasa that will be filled before the end of the shift. I prefer to start the day this way – encountering patients directly and freshly rather than sifting through the impressions and decisions of others.

Although the waiting room is empty, the short-stay unit behind the ER is not. This morning, there are five patients there, one of whom is Georges, awaiting their daily reevaluation. I thank Jennifer and Niraj and bid them good-bye, taking Jennifer aside as she gathers her belongings to tell her to book in to see me for a brief chat next week, if she has time. She is surprised; it's not the usual routine. I simply tell her that I want to talk more about managing responses to patients who are hostile and insulting. She's tired enough that I can tell if I weren't her senior, she would respond that she doesn't need any more discussion about Luana. Instead she gives an almost imperceptible shrug and thanks me for taking the time for more teaching, saying she will book in with Simone. I find myself wondering if she will.

As she and Niraj head off, I suggest to the team that I see Georges and Luana while the other three patients are divided between Paul and Barry Low, the freshly arrived first-year resident who is assigned for an ER day shift.

I ENTER GEORGES' DARKENED room. If our waiting room is spare, the bedrooms of the short-stay unit are positively spartan – just a hospital bed with side rails and dim overhead lighting. The absence of any furnishings makes the normal-size room seem huge.

Georges lies curled up on the bed with the covers pulled over his head. A sealed juice container that Tish had offered him after he refused any food sits on the floor in a corner. I have seen Georges like this before. A few years ago, the man running his boarding home called me, concerned that Georges, who is normally gregarious, had stopped speaking to anyone and was holed up in his room. At that time, I was able to visit him in his dark room, where a row of glass bottles filled with urine stood in one corner, and persuade him to get in my car and come to the hospital with me.

It's sad to see Georges in the grips of another episode, because when he is well, he has a million-dollar smile, is charming and friendly, and works hard to make use of the English he has acquired at night school. I attended his citizenship ceremony five years ago, his final step in the journey from refugee to landed immigrant to citizen. I have a picture of him from that day, obtained with his permission, on my BlackBerry, clutching his certificate and smiling in delight.

"*Bonjour, Georges. C'est Dr. Goldbloom.*"

He stirs slightly under the sheets but does not reveal his face.

In French, I tell him both what I know and what I can guess – that he is afraid to eat, that he is afraid of other people, that he doesn't feel safe anywhere. It's a monologue because Georges does not – cannot? – respond, but I continue on the assumption that he can hear me and that the familiar sound of my voice in his first language may be reassuring to him.

"Georges, I'm glad you are here in the hospital. You know this is a safe place and that our job is to take care of you. You and I have been through this before. These fears tell me that your illness is back. I need you to trust me to help you get well again, as we have done together in the past."

The covers remain over his face; I can't tell if he is taking in what I am saying, but he remains calm.

"Georges, we need to keep you in the hospital, to get you eating again, and to sort out what has caused your relapse. It's clear that you are not coping well at home. I'm worried you will become even sicker if we don't get you treatment."

No answer.

"Georges, I'm going to call Henri." Henri Mulumba, Georges' brother, lives in Belgium, part of the Congolese diaspora there. At times, Henri has provided substitute consent for treatment when Georges has been too ill to participate in decision making.

"You remember we all agreed last year that when you are too ill to make decisions, I'll ask Henri to help us. If you can't talk with me and decide what to do, I will need to fill out the legal forms that say you are too ill to decide. Then the rights adviser will come, as she did last time, to talk to you about whether you want to speak with a lawyer."

Still no response.

Georges is a veteran of our province's mental health legislation. He has been admitted to hospital about ten times, always preceded by a period of paranoia that leads to his not eating or drinking. When ill, he refuses to come to the hospital on his own, but once he's brought here by others and admitted as an involuntary patient, he rarely protests. A very few times he has lashed out physically at staff, his delusions persuading him that they are trying to hurt him, but he is always remorseful later.

It's not the fact that Georges refuses to come to the hospital when he is ill that gives me the legal right to say he is incapable of making his own treatment decisions. Patients often disagree with medical recommendations, for what presumably are – at least some of the time – perfectly good reasons. Neither does agreeing with one's doctor's recommendations guarantee that a patient is capable. If a patient is just being generically agreeable with no understanding of the treatment proposed, and of its benefits and risks, he or she would not meet the criteria for capacity to consent to treatment that exist in most countries with mental health legislation.

My assessment today of Georges' incapacity rests on my knowledge, derived from seeing him in this state before, that his illness and its symptoms drive his resistance: for example, an unwillingness to take medication because he fears it is poisoned. It is much easier for me to make this assessment than it would be for a psychiatrist meeting him for the first time. For that reason, I always document as part of my assessment that when he is well, Georges tells me that he trusts me and Henri to make the right decisions in terms of hospitalization and medication and to care for him if he becomes sick again.

In the past when the rights adviser, a representative from the province's patient advocate's office, arrived to ensure that Georges' rights were being observed and to inquire whether he wished to challenge his doctors' decisions, Georges, unlike Daryl, never wanted to make an appeal. I have not been able to learn from him when he is well whether this is because he knows deep down that he needs to be hospitalized, or whether his mental state prevents him from organizing his thoughts enough to challenge my assessment. He knows from experience that as soon as he is well enough to make decisions, I rescind the incapacity finding and hand back decision making to him, but this has historically taken weeks to months.

"Georges, please have some orange juice." I pick up the container and hold it out to him.

"You need the fluid. Look – it's sealed. No one can touch it without your knowing." I remember from past admissions that sealed lids have reassured him that there's been no tampering.

I decide to stay with him. My brain tracks back to his last several admissions, calculating how long it took each time for Georges to emerge from the fog of psychosis. After a few minutes he slowly comes out from under his bedcover, peels back the foil on the juice container, and drains its contents. He makes brief eye contact with me but remains silent. Based on experience, I doubt that there is more to be gained from this encounter. More may overwhelm and agitate him. When Georges hallucinates and hears multiple chattering voices in his head, I need to keep things clear and simple for him.

"*Je reviens plus tard ce matin, Georges, et nous allons parler.*"

Georges' illness, which presented not long after he left the DR Congo, has plagued him intermittently over the past two decades. When I first met him in 1998, the boarding home staff had brought him to the ER after he refused to eat and drink for days. He believed that religious people of an unknown faith were poisoning his food and following him in the street. He thought that things said on television could trigger headaches, and he admitted that he heard multiple voices inside his head telling him not to eat and instructing him to go to specific places at precise times. He ended up being admitted to the ACU where he and I first met. Our ability to communicate in French, which seemed to provide Georges with a sense of connection to me, led to my becoming his outpatient psychiatrist.

Over the years he has had numerous repetitions of this psychotic state. Early on, these occurred frequently after he discontinued his pills, but they have become fewer since he was stabilized on injectable long-acting antipsychotic medication. Instead of having to swallow a pill, which requires a daily decision, he now gets an injection once every four weeks. The monthly injections make him physically slightly stiff and slow, but they have greatly improved his ability to engage with other people, to take courses, and to do even simple things like eat. He has never expressed interest in discussing the nature of his illness, but he dutifully shows up for outpatient appointments and is happy to share details of his life, such as the English-language course he is perpetually enrolled in, meeting with Congolese friends to play cards, and news of his family in Europe. The most he will acknowledge about his symptoms when he is well is "*C'est une maladie.*" Compared to the late 1990s, his episodes of illness are far less frequent and his hospitalizations are rare, with gaps between them as long as six years. Nevertheless, he has experienced relapses even while on stable doses of medications, and when his illness takes hold, his understanding of it melts in the heat of psychosis, and his motivation to take the medication dissipates, causing a swift spiral down into his darkest place.

GEORGES' PSYCHIATRIC DIAGNOSIS is schizophrenia, arguably the most feared diagnosis in psychiatry, given its pejorative public reputation, our lack of curative treatments, and its frequently devastating social and economic consequences. The name itself derives from the Greek for "split mind," an origin that explains the illness' frequent misinterpretation as split personality à la *The Three Faces of Eve* or *Dr. Jekyll and Mr. Hyde.* A more accurate description of what the name tries to capture might be fractured consciousness. In psychiatric terms, schizophrenia refers to a condition of chronic or recurring psychosis, with psychosis defined as the experience of delusions (fixed, false beliefs despite evidence to the contrary), hallucinations (perceptions in the five senses – hearing, sight, taste, smell, and touch – in the absence of an external stimulus), and the chaotic thought, speech, and behavior to which these experiences lead their sufferers.

Twenty percent of patients who are diagnosed with psychosis will have only a single episode (known as a brief psychotic episode) in their lifetimes.[4] For a patient to be diagnosed with schizophrenia, he or she must have experienced psychosis for a period of longer than six months. A shorter period, somewhere between a month and six months, would be labeled as a schizophreniform presentation, allowing the psychiatrist time to rule out other potential causes for the psychosis, as well as to establish that the patient's symptoms are either not going away or, having done so briefly, will return. When it's less than a month of symptoms, it's called a brief psychotic disorder, a more neutral descriptive phrase without long-term implications. Of course, there are other psychiatric and nonpsychiatric things to think about when someone presents with psychotic symptoms; the symptoms could be the result of a mood disorder, such as severe depression or bipolar disorder, or illicit drug or alcohol use, or the consequences of a variety of medical illnesses or medical treatments (such as high doses of steroids).

The German psychiatrist Emil Kraepelin conceptualized the modern psychiatric model of schizophrenia, using the label of "dementia praecox" (premature dementia) to describe a deteriorating illness that began in adolescence and young adulthood. As a young doctor whose clinical career started in the Munich asylum, Kraepelin described the "demented, unclean, half-agitated, and fully agitated patients" who were now his responsibility, and their lack of treatment. Instead, they "would run around, yell, get into fights with each other, collect rocks, smoke and chatter." He noticed the impact of this neglect on the patients. "The tendency to violence was very widespread; there was scarcely a daily rounds in which someone didn't report a fight, window breaking or destroying tableware. Often enough I had to suture or bind up the wounds that arose in this way."[5]

He became convinced that the answers to these mysterious disorders lay in studying the natural history or progression of psychiatric illness. His conviction led him to probe patients' individual case histories to cull core signs of each disorder, rather than simply focusing on their immediate presentation or looking at brain tissue under the microscope – the diagnostic practices of the time.[6]

Kraepelin and his team filled out cards on each patient, recording their clinical observations and placing them in so-called diagnosis boxes. After interviewing the patient and obtaining more history, they would enter any revisions on the cards. At the time of discharge, the diagnosis would again be recorded. This process allowed Kraepelin to get an overview of the patients' hospitalizations and the rationales for those diagnoses that later turned out to be inaccurate. He insisted that his trainees avoid clinical jargon in their notes and simply describe in plain language what they observed.

Kraepelin also followed patients from institution to institution, recording the evolution of their illnesses, their remissions, relapses, and (rarely) recoveries, in files that he kept for research purposes.[7] As someone who has lived through generations of electronic health documentation initiatives, none of which has resulted in a single electronic record becoming universally available to any of the multiple healthcare professionals providing care to a single patient, I am full of admiration for Kraepelin's insistence on the importance of this task.

Kraepelin's description of dementia praecox or schizophrenia as a psychotic disorder that had its onset in adolescence and followed a uniformly deteriorating or "degenerating" course that would end in dementia understandably generated a sense of hopelessness for individuals, families, and clinicians alike. When a Cape Breton cousin of mine was hospitalized at the main asylum for Nova Scotia in the 1940s with psychotic symptoms, his sister told me the family received a phone call from the treating physician telling them to give up all hope for their brother's future. My cousin's illness turned out to be bipolar disorder, and although he had future episodes, he was never institutionalized. He worked steadily at his family's gas station and led a reasonably satisfying social life.

Kraepelin was not only determined but also prolific, producing nine editions of his *Textbook of Psychiatry* in addition to his clinical and research commitments. Reportedly the motivation for his first book, published in 1883 and the precursor for his more comprehensive textbook, was to earn money to allow him to marry.[8]

Kraepelin's protégé, Eugen Bleuler, noted in 1908 that many patients who otherwise fit the diagnosis of dementia praecox developed the illness later than adolescence and that Kraepelin's dire prognosis of inevitable eventual dementia failed to accurately describe many patients with otherwise classic presentations. In recognition of these departures from Kraepelin's original definition, Bleuler coined the term "schizophrenia" as a better fit for a disease with varied age of onset and no symptoms of a dementing illness even after years of symptoms.[9]

Although drawing from Kraepelin and Bleuler's work, contemporary researchers have approached schizophrenia from the opposite direction. The modern scientific lens envisions a variety of physiological pathways leading to the diagnosis, some influenced by environmental stressors, such as living in an urban area, immigration, obstetrical complications, and a birth date during late winter or early spring (hypothesized to be linked to the impact of the influenza virus on fetal neurological development) that, in conjunction with genetic vulnerability, may lead to the clinical symptoms we call schizophrenia.

The experiences of patients with schizophrenia are equally complex. One of contemporary psychiatry's best thinkers and most widely respected basic science researchers of psychosis, Shitij Kapur, the executive dean and head of the Institute of Psychiatry, Psychology & Neuroscience at King's College, London, has suggested that psychosis compromises the brain's ability to assign salience (that is, what is important or conspicuous) appropriately to stimuli such as environmental events and internal experiences. From a neuroscience perspective, salience represents the brain's prioritizing of attention and its decisions regarding the importance of a specific action as a means of reward or punishment. A psychotic brain's failure to assess accurately the relative contributions of stimuli such as a person's voice or a roadside billboard to cause benefit or harm results in those stimuli being abnormally interpreted in the form of delusions and hallucinations. For example, if I see an advertisement on the subway platform that shows someone in uniform, my gaze will flick over it and then move away. A person with psychosis may find her attention locked on the ad, convinced it is telling her that police or soldiers are following her.

Kapur, an old friend and colleague, is slender and surprisingly youthful for someone in his position. He describes the stages of psychosis in a manner that only a patient or a clinician with intimate knowledge of the phenomenon can, as "a stage of heightened awareness and emotionality combined with a sense of anxiety and impasse, a drive to 'make sense' of the situation, and then usually relief and a 'new awareness' as the delusion crystallizes and the hallucinations emerge . . . Once the symptoms are manifest, delusions are essentially disorders of inferential logic, as most delusional beliefs are not impossible, just highly improbable."[10]

Kapur's theory of misinterpreted salience explains the destructive impact of the core belief at the center of Georges' illness. When Georges is psychotic, he is convinced that religious men of unknown faith are pursuing and threatening him. He interprets everything that happens to him in the light of this belief. Since he doesn't know who these men are or what faith they represent, everyone he sees is potentially a member of the group. If strangers make eye contact with him, what may be a social courtesy becomes a malign threat – as does the failure to make eye contact by other individuals. A conversation between two strangers as he passes may include words that by coincidence are relevant to some aspect of Georges' life, thus confirming his core belief. And if they don't, then Georges must worry that messages are coded to conceal their content about him. He can't win because everything, benign or otherwise, reinforces his core belief. So he minimizes the risk, first by isolating himself and then by not eating.

Kapur's research may also explain some of the factors that contribute to the disability experienced by patients with psychosis in their lives. An individual's inability to respond in a socially normal way to day-to-day stimuli will alienate the vast majority of people. This majority includes potential employers, landlords, romantic partners, friends, and even family. As a result, schizophrenia's sufferers generally struggle in their social relationships and in their ability to work. Given that an estimated 1 percent of the population is affected – an astonishingly high proportion given the relatively tiny amount of money devoted to its research and treatment in comparison to less prevalent disorders – this presents a huge social and economic burden to society, quite apart from the devastating impact on individuals with the disease.[11]

While Kapur's theories shed light on the cognitive processes of schizophrenia, we have made scant progress as to determining its cause. Research over the past thirty years has focused on a number of potential culprits, most prominently the possibility of malfunction among the chemicals that act as messengers (neurotransmitters) between cells in the central nervous system (CNS), genetic vulnerabilities, and potential environmental agents. Dopamine has been the most widely investigated neurotransmitter. Kapur describes it as the "wind of the psychotic fire." It has also been identified as a mediator of reward, reinforcement, and salience, and dopamine receptors are known to be central in how antipsychotic medications affect the brain. Despite these overlapping findings, however, our understanding of how levels of dopamine and its transmission among different networks and structures within the brain relate specifically to psychosis and schizophrenia remains crude.[12]

Other neurotransmitters such as glutamate, thought to be responsible for excitement and stimulation within the CNS, GABA (gamma-aminobutyric acid), which in contrast serves to inhibit or dampen CNS responses, and acetylcholine, famous in neuroscience circles as the neurotransmitter that responds to nicotine, have all been suggested as playing a part in the development of schizophrenia. In probability, all these neurotransmitters are relevant to some degree, but the cascading effect of a malfunction in any of their neurological pathways will make identification of their specific contributions extraordinarily difficult, rather like multiple pebbles hitting the surface of a lake simultaneously so that the ensuing ripples create overlapping circles.

Despite a well-established finding over many decades that schizophrenia can run in families, studies looking at genetic causes for schizophrenia – like the neurotransmitter studies – currently continue to resemble the proverbial search for a needle in a haystack. Identical twins, who share 100 percent of their DNA, do not always share the disease, something that should occur if the illness were entirely genetically determined. They do, however, share it at a rate significantly higher than the 1 percent of the population diagnosed with schizophrenia; if one such twin develops schizophrenia, there is about a 50 percent chance the other twin will as well. By contrast, nonidentical twins share much less genetic material, and the rate of a nonidentical twin of a person with schizophrenia developing it drops to just 5 to 10 percent – which is still five to ten times higher than the rate for the general population.

On the other hand, since more than half of sufferers have no family history of the illness, it is clear that genes do not provide the sole explanation for the development of schizophrenia. We now know that genes can spontaneously mutate or change, challenging the more popular linear view of genes and destiny. As a result, environmental factors are assumed – but not proved – to have as much relevance as genes to the development of schizophrenia.[13] Georges had a maternal aunt who had had some kind of debilitating psychiatric illness in the DR Congo, but the details were never clear, cloaked in the secrecy that all too often accompanies these diseases.

Newspaper and media reports often feature the headline "Gene Found for . . ." The fine print reveals that this breathless summary of a research study overlooks that this gene accounts not for the disease itself but rather for a small percentage of the risk of developing the disease. Even more often, the exciting results have not been independently confirmed by another research laboratory. While there are diseases with single gene markers, like cystic fibrosis, the vast majority of all heritable diseases feature multiple genetic influences. Nevertheless, entrepreneurs in health care have seized an opportunity to have worried people spit into a test tube for high-cost DNA analysis to tell them of the myriad diseases they are at risk for. It's a daunting and demoralizing list, but for most disorders in psychiatry and medicine in general, genetics reflect risk, not destiny.

After a century of "Let's get an X-ray just to be sure," in which ever more sophisticated diagnostic-imaging technologies have provided physicians with answers to many of the causes of illness, psychiatrists and neuroscientists hope that our newfound ability to obtain images of the brain from which mental illness emanates will similarly help us to understand, classify, prevent, predict, and treat psychiatric disorders. Unfortunately, despite extraordinary advances in the technology and application of brain imaging, we still can't say, "I've reviewed the scans; I'm afraid you've definitely got schizophrenia." It's not unusual, however, for someone like Georges to have a CT scan or an MRI at one point in the trajectory of his illness, despite how typical his symptoms are of schizophrenia, because we would hate to miss something in his brain that horribly mimics the illness and could be treated in a different way. I've been careful in this regard, especially with young people at the onset of a psychotic illness, but I don't remember ever being surprised by scan results. It's not only the doctors who seek this reassurance; it's patients and families as well. But brain scans rarely lead to answers for patients who present with psychotic symptoms. Georges' scan report included that three-word mantra of health: "within normal limits." Except that Georges' brain was ill.

That being said, neuroimaging research has already made differences to treatment and patients' quality of life, including some pioneering studies done at the hospital where I work, which demonstrated that much smaller doses of medications than were traditionally used resulted in significant levels of brain dopamine receptor blocking (a desired therapeutic effect). The clinical result of these smaller doses was fewer uncomfortable and disabling side effects for the patients on them.

Unfortunately, Georges continues to experience medication-related side effects, which contribute to his decision to stop his medications completely when he becomes more symptomatic and starts to believe that they may have been tampered with. In addition to missing his last appointment with me, Georges missed his last three appointments with the nurse at our injectable medication clinic and the needles that accompanied them, leaving him vulnerable to the resurgence of his illness. He did not return calls from her inquiring about him and he dropped off the radar – until he came onto the police radar the night before. I have no doubt her calls became incorporated into his delusions. I am struck by how profoundly these delusions isolate him, including from the treatment that is his best hope of relief.

Last night, the police picked him up at an intersection where he had been trying to direct traffic. Thankfully, Georges is known to the police from previous apprehensions for refusing to leave a coffee shop or walking into traffic; they also know he is never combative or resistant but almost always silent.

I GO TO THE NURSING STATION to make sure there is a bed arranged for Georges in the ACU. As Tish looks through the messages on the desk to see if the ACU staff have confirmed when he can go upstairs, she casually lobs a curve ball into my well-constructed psychological defenses.

"How is your mother?" she asks. "She is such an amazing woman."

My mother is known throughout Cape Breton and most of Nova Scotia as the woman who almost single-handedly raised money for the creation of Pier 21, originally a local museum to honor the site where millions of immigrants first touched Canadian soil as they got off boats to find a new life. It is now a national museum honoring all immigrants to Canada.

I hear myself telling Tish that my mother is fine. Once the words are out of my mouth, I am paralyzed, unsure whether to explain or simply to leave them there, putting a distance between me and this kind woman who has known me for almost a decade.

Before I can decide whether to change my story, Tish tells me that now Georges is settled, Luana is the most urgent patient to be seen. First, however, Tish and I agree that I should call Henri because I need to catch him during daylight hours in Belgium.

I am fortunate. Henri responds immediately to the cell phone number I have for him. We speak in French. He is deeply apologetic on his brother's behalf. I know from my previous contact with Henri and other family members that they do not fully understand Georges' illness (and to be fair to them, who does?) and are ashamed at the havoc he causes when ill.

I reassure Henri that we are happy to help Georges, and more important, that we do not expect Henri to fly to Toronto. He has a family and a job, and dropping everything to come to see his brother, despite what has historically been a close relationship between the two men, is simply not always feasible. I review with Henri my proposed treatment plan for Georges: admission, restart antipsychotic medication, make sure he is eating and drinking, and reconnect him with his community treatment team. We have had this discussion many times before.

There is a moment of silence on the other end of the phone after Henri agrees to the plan.

"Doctor, is there a way we can force him to take the medication once he leaves the hospital? He always tells me he will take it when he is well, but then when he starts to have symptoms and the voices tell him he cannot trust the people who give him the medicine, he changes his mind. I hope I am doing the right thing by pushing this, but I cannot bear hearing that he is ill again, and police are involved. The medicine must be better than this, than the handcuffs, and being tied up."

I explain that I am in the ER with more patients to see and will call him later in the week to talk as the answer to his question is complicated.

"Thank you, Doctor, for looking after Georges. I know he trusts you. Even when he trusts no one else. Please tell him I want only the best for him. I just want him to be well. We all do – me, Sara, and the girls."

I make a note on Georges' chart confirming that he is incapable of consenting to treatment of his psychiatric disorder and that Georges and Henri both consent to Henri acting as his brother's substitute decision maker. I also note that since I cannot confirm that Georges is agreeing to hospitalization, and since discharging him to his home would clearly pose an immediate risk to his safety given his inability to eat and drink, he meets criteria to be hospitalized as an involuntary patient. I fill out the legal papers and ask Tish to make sure the paperwork is faxed to the Patient Advocate's Office so that they know Georges is in the hospital. The trust that both Georges and Henri have in me feels like a weight at times. A shared language seems a flimsy bond in the face of my repeated failures to keep Georges well.

I return to Georges' room to give him the forms notifying him of these decisions. While I explain each form, all of which he is familiar with from previous admissions, he remains under the covers, not responding. I tell him that I am going to leave his copy of the forms on the window ledge near his bed. In previous episodes of illness, he has become paranoid about documents and destroyed them. One such episode set back his citizenship application several years.

"Georges, I've spoken with Henri on the telephone and he agrees with me that the best place for you right now is with us, in the hospital. Since I am not sure if you agree, I have asked Tish to call the rights adviser to come to talk with you. Henri asked me to tell you that he wants you to get well and be home as soon as possible. He can't come to see you right now because of work and the expense, but he said he and Sara and the girls send you their good thoughts."

When I mention his sister-in-law and nieces, Georges pulls himself up on the bed and nods at me. I consider staying to see if I can get him to eat some breakfast, but I make the calculation that Luana, my next patient, has waited long enough and that the wait is likely not helping her agitation. I will ask Tish if she has time to sit with Georges for a while and encourage him to take some food.

As I say good-bye to Georges, reminding him I will see him later in the ACU, and make my way back to the nursing station to pick up Luana's chart, Henri's question on the phone gives me pause; the pattern of relapse he describes for his brother is entirely accurate. After a period during which things have been progressing for Georges for anywhere between a few months to a couple of years, he will start to slip into paranoia and become increasingly focused on and unhappy with the medication's side effects. At those times we change medications and doses, or add medication to help with the side effects, but to date, none of these strategies has proved entirely satisfactory in persuading Georges to keep taking them.

It's a difficult thing. I cannot imagine tolerating the chronic physical discomfort that Georges feels on the medication, but I also see the chaos that emerges for him when he comes off it. And I feel for Henri. What is the role for a family member when a relative is ill and ambivalent about treatment? For a split second my brain runs ahead to my mother. What if the cancer is back and she has to choose between active treatment and palliative care? I can imagine my father's choice for her, but what about my mother's? What about me?

I give myself a mental slap for allowing my thoughts to wander at work and pick up Luana's chart to read about the events leading up to her arrival in the ER last night. It's hard to focus; my mind wanders back to Georges and Henri's question: Can I force Georges to take medication once he is out of the hospital? My own question is a bit different: Even if I can – by obtaining what's called a community treatment order – should I? Community treatment orders (CTOs), sometimes called assisted outpatient treatment, are available in many Western democracies. They mandate a patient to comply with outpatient treatment or to be brought by the police to the hospital for reassessment. It is intended to provide treatment in a less restrictive environment than a hospital while ensuring that treatment does get provided. What would doing so mean for my relationship with Georges and the trust he has in me, a trust that has got him through some grim times?

Community treatment orders in Ontario cannot be issued in a cavalier way. They are restricted to people who have experienced recurrent involuntary hospitalization and who have improved with treatment. They require consent of either the patient when capable of consent, or, if the patient is incapable, of a substitute decision maker, and their legitimacy can be challenged by the patient at a review board hearing. Contrary to popular belief, a CTO does not allow a health professional or anyone else to administer medication against a person's will. If the person refuses to comply with an order for medication within a CTO, however, he or she can be brought to hospital for psychiatric reassessment, which may or may not result in hospitalization.

Issues of restraint and involuntary treatment, the rights of doctors (and the influence of family members) to hospitalize and treat those citizens who have psychiatric illnesses that put them or others at risk of harm are at the heart of the antipathy felt by some people toward the psychiatric profession. These are the ethical questions that keep psychiatric trainees, at least the best ones, awake at night. The determination of what level of risk justifies taking away a patient's liberty is arguably a psychiatrist's gravest and most difficult task. In my view, it should always involve an intellectual and moral tussle on the part of the psychiatrist – is this patient's experience and behavior when ill likely to result in harm to him or her or to others, and is forced hospitalization the only way to prevent that harm, or is there a more collaborative or less intrusive option?

This dilemma is as old as the profession, as old as madness itself, and I am not sure we are any farther along today in achieving consensus as a global society. I know that conditions within hospitals are better, at least in much of the developed world, than they have ever been, but that is likely of little comfort to those who object on principle to the entire premise of forced hospitalization and treatment for patients with severe mental illness.

Psychiatrists have to justify their decisions to restrain and detain people at risk not only to themselves and to their colleagues, but also to the public. It can seem like a no-win at times. Patients who kill themselves or others while under the care of a psychiatrist undermine the public's confidence in our ability to care for those suffering from mental illness and to protect others from its worst consequences. Simultaneously, some of the public views psychiatrists' powers as symbolizing society's most reactionary and oppressive aspects. I have known psychiatrists (fortunately, not many) who have sought to avoid this catch-22 by applying a formula rather than approaching each patient's risk individually: choosing either to remove liberty when there is even a modicum of doubt about the patient's or others' safety, or choosing never to impinge upon it. To my mind those psychiatrists are avoiding one of our job's most challenging and uncomfortable aspects, and in doing so are betraying the trust of their patients and their families.

My opinion is obviously at odds with the view that psychiatrists enact society's abusive power structures, a perspective that was given voice in the second half of the twentieth century by the antipsychiatry movement that had as its bible the French sociologist Michel Foucault's famous 1961 work, *Madness and Civilization* (republished most recently in a posthumous translation in 2006 as *History of Madness*). Foucault saw modern psychiatry as a bastion of moral hypocrisy and social norms, with madness itself characterized as a cultural construct. In his view, psychiatrists were unwitting instruments of society's efforts to control the marginalized, nonconformist, and rebellious. Counterculture groups led by psychiatrist-writers such as Thomas Szasz and R. D. Laing built on Foucault's work to claim that psychiatrists did more harm than good, coercing rebellious citizens into conformity, often by violent and damaging means.

There is no doubt that in previous centuries the lack of any protective legislation meant that patients had no rights. As well, paternalistic attitudes led to women being locked away by their families for imagined illnesses such as promiscuity or "unfeminine" behavior.

But in today's world, the antipsychiatry movement has offered little that has been of practical help to patients like Georges who are suffering, are in danger, and are potentially dangerous, or to the growing number of mentally ill homeless citizens whose illnesses act as barriers to relationships, decent housing, and meaningful work. In recent years, the movement has received a new burst of energy from the considerable funds provided to it by the Church of Scientology, whose members dutifully picket every meeting of the American Psychiatric Association and whose celebrity members – of whom Tom Cruise is perhaps the best known – take advantage of their status to discourage people from taking psychiatric medication.

Even so, in 2011, a World Health Organization survey of 184 nations found that 40 percent had no mental health legislation,[14] which leaves people and their rights vulnerable to abuse. To my mind, however, the pendulum in developed nations has swung too far away from an ethic of care, a view that the state has responsibilities to provide help to its most vulnerable citizens. In this, my views have been shaped most recently by encounters across the country in my role as the chair of Canada's Mental Health Commission. As family after family reports being turned away, often reluctantly, by psychiatrists who say they cannot admit their relative for treatment until he actually threatens to hurt someone or himself or until appropriate inpatient resources are available, or who tell families for reasons of patient confidentiality that they cannot give any information about their relative despite his or her desperately ill condition, I find myself wondering how Foucault or Szasz would perceive these people's plight.

AS I READ THROUGH Luana's chart before meeting her, my thoughts move immediately away from theoretical questions regarding psychiatry's role in society, and whether or not to explain my mother's health status to Tish, to focus on the familiar notations describing Luana's psychiatric assessments overnight. Everything written lets me know that Luana presented in a way that points to a full-blown episode of mania. The notes also tell me she has a history of being physically aggressive. As I remove my tie in preparation for meeting her – part of my usual protocol when interviewing a potentially aggressive patient – I can feel that my defenses are comfortably back in place. Neckties, once a marker of male physician formality, are on the wane in hospitals for a variety of reasons – the evolution of every workday into "casual Fridays" attire, the evidence that neckties can serve as an excellent transport medium for infectious organisms, and their vulnerability to getting yanked in acute psychiatric settings.

Entering psychiatry, I found the need to anticipate physical aggression when on call to the emergency room foreign and disturbing. I didn't articulate my uneasiness; that would have been humiliating for my younger self. Today I am wiser and talk to inexperienced psychiatry residents about how to listen to and respond to that anxiety in a way that will protect both them and the patient, rather than distancing themselves completely from the person they are there to help – either by overusing security guards or restraints, or ignoring their instinctive anxiety, which can lead to dangerous clinical errors.

I enter Luana's darkened bedroom. The environmental scan of her surroundings as a physical reflection of her mental state, and the physical tension I feel in my muscles as I approach Luana, are so familiar to me I almost don't notice them anymore. Luana's room is a mess. The sheets are on the floor, and in the few hours she has been here, she has been generating artwork and taping it to the walls. I suspect the nurses were relieved she was so engaged. But Luana isn't here now.

I find her standing at a telephone next to the assessment unit's nursing station, pacing, yelling into the receiver, and crumpling papers furiously. I invite her into the glassed-in interview room, a former smoking room dating back to when that addiction was permitted (and even used as a "reward" for appropriate behavior) in the hospital. It's within sight of the nursing station and therefore a good place to interview potentially explosive people, while still affording acoustic privacy.

Luana is dressed in an open hospital gown, with her breasts barely concealed. It's more than she was wearing last night, having discarded the few clothes she was still wearing in the waiting room when she found the delay to be interminable. It was in one sense effective; she was seen immediately. She has long teased, streaked hair, most of it pulled back into a knot on the top of her head with locks falling onto her shoulders. It looks like a disheveled version of what was once a carefully coiffed hairstyle. There is evidence of makeup that is several days old. Black specks from heavy mascara have fallen onto her cheeks, and her eyelids are outlined in black à la Cleopatra. The rest of her face is blotchy with patches of heavy foundation interspersed with bare skin. She has kicked off the blue hospital slippers, and I can see chipped orange nail polish.

"Hi, I'm Dr. Goldbloom. I heard about you from the doctor you saw last night, but there's no substitute for hearing things directly from you. Can we talk for a little while?"

"Are you Jewish, Dr. Goldbloom? You know what? I am too! We *are* the chosen people. Ha! What's that Barbra Streisand song? *People, people who need people, are the luckiest people in the world.* I love the world. Do you? You should. You need to loosen up!" She speaks and sings quickly, a tempo that seems difficult to sustain, smiling and laughing as the sentences and phrases gush from her mouth.

Briefed by Jennifer and Tish on Luana's potential explosiveness, I realize I have to engage her in a friendly way to try to understand what is going on with her. This is a potential slippery slope given her seductiveness and disinhibition. I also know I am going to disappoint and upset her – because if she refuses to stay voluntarily in the hospital, I will likely have to detain her for an additional period of time against her will. Her short fuse has already led her to shove a nurse into a wall. What would happen to her outside the walls of the hospital?

"Luana, tell me how you got here. I want to know what's been going with you."

She laughs again and leans toward me so that her shirt falls open. "I bet you do, Doc. All the guys want to understand me. There was a hunk of a cop here with me last night, P. C. Fung. He was so sweet to me. And so handsome . . . And hung! Hung Fung!" Another peal of laughter.

"I shouldn't have said that, should I, Dr. Goldbloom? That was a bad thing to say! But it was true! And I told him I am going to come and find him as soon as I get out of here. You know what song those gentiles love? What's it called? 'Do You Hear What I Hear?' Ha! I'm allergic to shellfish. Do you need to know anything else? Is that a Timex? Aren't you a rich doctor?"

Luana's thoughts are going, as the Canadian humorist Stephen Leacock wrote, "madly off in all directions." I realize I am going to have to try to contain her expansive thinking if I am to complete the interview, and so I shift to asking short, very focused questions about the last few weeks. As she talks, Luana looks frequently through the glass wall at seeming distractions, although none are visible or audible. She starts to answer a question, speaking rapidly, and then finds herself lost within the maze of her own answer, all the while smiling coyly at me.

"Tell me about yourself, Dr. Goldbloom. Are you married? I bet you are, a nice doctor like you. And kids, do you have kids? I want kids. Ten. I think I'm pregnant."

Luana's jumping from subject to subject – linked only by a word or single idea or even a rhyme – is characteristic of mania and is called "flight of ideas" by psychiatrists, reflecting a similarly chaotic loosening of cognitive thought processes. So is her sexualization of all her encounters. This can lead some manic patients to engage in high-risk sex with strangers, without protection. When the mania has passed, these patients often experience devastating remorse. Reconstructing the events of a manic episode after it has subsided is a painful journey that I have taken with many patients.

Listening to Luana, I recall a patient in a severe manic episode whom I saw during my residency and who taught me about the enormous and sometimes irrevocable damage that psychiatric disorders can wreak on lives that were previously progressing according to plan. That woman had had impulsive sex with every man she could find in her condominium building and racked up enormous amounts of credit card debt that was well beyond her ability to repay. When the mania subsided, she was so humiliated by her own behavior (not to mention impoverished) that she had to move.

I don't want Luana to humiliate herself, even though the risk of that is imperceptible to her at that moment. And yet I have no crystal ball that allows me to predict with scientific confidence what will occur to her in the next few days if she leaves the hospital. I have to rely on what is known about her previous episode as well as my own extensive experience seeing individuals with a variety of bipolar disorder trajectories.

"Luana, I've reviewed your chart. You've been down this road before. Your bipolar disorder has made trouble for you, and you're manic now. I want to help you."

She moves closer to me, flipping her hair behind her shoulders.

"I'm fine, Dr. Goldbloom. I'm only a teeny-weeny bit manic. Maybe a quarter to a third manic. Not really manic at all. Just feeling fine. Really fantastic. I bet you wish you felt as fine as me. Call me Feinstein!"

"Luana, I think you should come into the hospital, so we can get you back on your mood stabilizer medication and feeling more like your normal self."

"That's so sweet of you, Dr. G, but I don't want to be in this hospital or any fucking hospital and I don't really like my medication. I put on fifteen pounds when I was taking it, which didn't look good at all. I look much better now, don't you think? You do think, right? I think I need a drink. Care to join me?"

She sits back in her chair and poses as if for a camera.

"I think, Dr. G, that I am just going to go home, and if I need anything, I'll call you, or maybe P. C. Fung. That would be fun . . ." She laughs loudly again, enjoying her rhyming couplets, a speech pattern that is also seen with mania, as is punning, and something called "clanging," where the person repeats words that sound alike. I am realizing that if Luana were to leave the ER now, the likelihood of her becoming dangerously entangled with male strangers is unacceptably high.

"I think you should just come home with me and take care of me there if you are so worried about me."

It's clear I am not getting very far. I remind Luana that she was apprehended by police last night. I also remind her that she was aggressive with staff last night in the ER, telling her that I don't think that she is someone who would normally behave in a way that others thought was unsafe or threatening. Her expression changes like a cloud passing in front of the sun.

"Well, fuck them, Dr. G, if that's what they told you. I told them I didn't want their help and that I was going home and that they should fucking keep their hands off me. And if you don't open that door and let me get the fuck out of here, then fuck you too!"

She is shouting now. One of the PAs, Dimitri Podolski, who has been watching from the nursing station, can now hear her through the Plexiglas door of the interview rooms; he and Tish rise from their chairs and briskly walk toward us but wait outside the room. I'm glad they're there, but it's a delicate balance between preserving everyone's safety and not making Luana feel ganged up on. I've worked with Dimitri for many years in the ER and the ACU; he is a no-nonsense guy who has good clinical instincts and a calm demeanor, coupled with a solid build.

I keep my voice quiet, firm, and slow. "I can't do that, Luana. I won't. You need to be in the hospital now to get your mania treated and to keep you safe. And the sooner that gets started, the sooner you'll be well and out of here. Are you willing to be here voluntarily and get some help?" This is a question I have to ask and must later document having asked.

"Fuck you!" she screams, racing out of the room, flipping over breakfast trays in the dining area, and pulling hard on the handle of the locked door leading out of the assessment unit. Dimitri and Tish follow her but keep their distance. I also follow her to try to talk with her more, but the more I do, the more loudly she sings a medley of Carole King songs (which I happen to like, but not under these circumstances). Fortunately, she becomes preoccupied with her singing and allows Tish to escort her back to the room and to bring her a second breakfast.

For the moment, Luana and I have gone as far as we can in an exploration of options. Based on admittedly limited information, I have to make that fundamental binary decision of the ER: stay or go. She stays. Allowing a patient like Luana to experience the same shame and financial ruin as my former patient in the name of idealized human autonomy and resistance to paternalism seems to me cruel and ignorant.

Fifteen minutes later, Luana stares stonily at me as I hand her the legal document (the so-called Form 3 that allows me to detain her in the hospital for a period of two weeks after her initial Form 1 assessment). I advise her of her new status and let her know that a rights adviser will come to see her within twenty-four hours to explain her legal options. She does not take her eyes off mine as she tears the paper into many pieces.

Luana's mood is caustic and irritable as she glares at me through the nursing station glass while I write the clinical note that will justify her involuntary detention. The encounter, which began in a friendly tone, has ended badly, although not with the physical combativeness that characterized her arrival at the hospital. Is the part of her that acknowledges the mania more accepting of the verdict? Has the medication numbed some of the sting of her anger? These questions cycle through my mind, but I am confident that my decision to detain her is correct.

One of emergency psychiatry's most important tasks is the prevention and containment of violence, whether self-inflicted or directed toward others. This assessment occurs frequently in situations where violence has not actually been committed but simply imagined, predicted, or threatened. In this sense, psychiatry is distinct from other medical specialties where patients who are medically ill, and whose illnesses entail clear concrete risks if untreated, may be restrained if they are perceived to be at risk – a delirious, demented, or unconscious patient who cannot give consent; a child who does not understand the seriousness of illness – reasons that tend to be more palatable to society. Only psychiatry limits the freedom of apparently physically well patients because of their beliefs, thoughts, and feelings.

Despite media sensationalism and popular culture stereotypes that fan public perceptions of severely mentally ill individuals as unpredictably and uniformly violent, only 5 percent of all violent crimes are committed by people with psychiatric illness. However, it is the case that emergency psychiatry, and its closest sibling, acute care psychiatry, have to grapple with the issue of restraint (physical, chemical, and environmental) in seeking to prevent the relatively small number of acts of violence that patients commit. Of all the lightning rods that excite the public's suspicion of psychiatry, its use of detention and restraint is the most criticized, apart, arguably, from electroconvulsive therapy. It constitutes an outrage for some people that Luana, an adult woman, living alone, and most of the time functioning well, was forced last night to take medication she didn't want to take in order to avoid being placed in restraints, and that today I told her that I will not allow her to leave the hospital until I believe she can be safely discharged without the risk of hurting or simply embarrassing herself.

I would like to think that we are approaching the end of an era when seclusion and restraint are part of the routine landscape of emergency and inpatient psychiatric care. More emphasis on verbal de-escalation, with which Jennifer had some success with Luana last night, talking her down from her heights of rage and fear to accept medication; the pharmacological treatment of agitation that is referred to as "chemical restraint," such as the combination of loxapine and lorazepam that Jennifer used to sedate and settle Luana; and collaborating with known patients about what helps them to settle, in advance of their becoming agitated – all these are making a difference. For example, assigning Luana to older female staff member like Tish, to whom she responded with neither seductiveness nor competitiveness, may help her stay calm. Having assisted countless times in placing people who are extremely psychotic and agitated into physical restraints, I know it is frightening for all involved – the patient, staff, and observers. I hope ultimately we will find a better way.

The extent to which people feel degraded and dehumanized by restraint is palpable, even when it is clinically necessary. Their paranoid fears are likely to be reinforced by the reality of restraints. On the other hand, I have seen too many patients for whom a central symptom of their illness is the fear that no one, including doctors and nurses, can be trusted, and they must defend themselves by force if necessary. I therefore do not believe a psychiatry emergency room without restraint will be achieved in my professional lifetime. I cannot envision how we could have persuaded Luana to remain with us without medication or the legal power to detain and restrain her in the face of her manic sense of invincibility and explosive aggression.

Most of the morning has passed, and the bulk of the shift lies ahead after a break for an early lunch. Since it's already eleven fifteen and I am starting to feel hungry, I ask Tish if this is a good time for me to take a break. She waves me off, telling me to take my time and that she will have the next patient ready to be seen in forty-five minutes.

Only later that night will I have time to wonder if my ability to move on so easily from thinking about the two patients whose liberties I have just taken away reflects professional experience or callous distractedness, or both. Whichever it is, a requirement of emergency work is to be satisfied with knowing not as much as possible but rather as much as is necessary to make critical decisions.

7

Emergencies II

WEDNESDAY AFTERNOON

Entering the ER via the staff-only side door after my lunch break, I scan the waiting room and see half a dozen new faces. In one corner is a group of three black men, the younger of whom I immediately guess is the patient – a tall, thin man with dreadlocks, dressed in dirty pants, part of a suit that has seen better days, and a too-large T-shirt that envelops his skinny torso. He is wearing sandals, one of which has a loose strap. He stares fixedly at the wall ahead of him, his fingers playing with a string bracelet tied around his left wrist, and ignores his two older companions, who talk quietly across him to each other.

A few seats away from this trio is a middle-aged white woman with shoulder-length dark hair, dressed tidily in a skirt and blouse and low-heeled pumps, who types busily on a cell phone. She is alone. Across the room from her is another black man, perhaps in his mid-forties, who is dressed in clean black jeans and a striped sweater. He looks sweaty and fidgets incessantly with his watch. He is accompanied by a man of a similar age, who leans toward him occasionally, murmuring quietly. Almost unconsciously I register the new arrivals' relative states of agitation and attention, together with their grooming and hygiene, assuming that at least two of them will come to me this afternoon for their emergency psychiatric assessments. The emergency room setting requires rapid scanning and processing, monitoring for both meaningful details and one's own internal responses.

I enter the nursing station, where the chatter ranges from figuring out how to find inpatient beds for everyone who needs them to weekend social plans.

"Who is the most urgent person for me?" I ask Tish, who is just about to head off for her lunch.

"Allan Walcott," she replies, pointing at the young black man flanked by his two older companions. "He's really sick. Hasn't spoken in two weeks."

I check Allan's previous clinical record. Just twenty years old, he was admitted six months ago to the hospital's Early Psychosis Unit, which focuses on young people experiencing their first episode of possible schizophrenia. Before his previous admission, he had felt increasingly that strangers were laughing at him on the street and monitoring him with cameras. He heard snatches of conversation from people he didn't know and believed they were saying disparaging things about him. His worried father had contacted a community mental health agency, and a youth worker eventually persuaded Allan to be assessed by our First Episode Psychosis outpatient program. He had been admitted to the hospital directly from the clinic. In the hospital for a six-week stay, Allan improved. His hallucinations and delusions melted away with the first antipsychotic medication he tried. He remained aloof, however, described in nursing notes as "isolative . . . difficult to engage." He had dropped out of community college almost a year earlier and wasn't prepared to consider returning or looking at work options. So although the heat of his psychosis had subsided, the charred framework of his life had not been rebuilt.

After he was released, he continued taking his antipsychotic medication as an outpatient and attended appointments regularly in the

First Episode Psychosis outpatient clinic. Two months later, for un-known reasons, he stopped taking the medication. He then returned to live with his mother in the Caribbean. According to the clinic notes in his chart, Allan's relatives hoped that if they sent him away from the bad influences of urban life and surrounded him by multiple genera-tions of his family, he would heal.

THE PHENOMENON OF PSYCHOSIS is mental illness' most mysterious and frightening aspect – for laypeople, for medical students, and for health care professionals. Even psychiatrists have difficulty accepting the trickery that psychosis inflicts on its victims. Someone who was previously well now believes herself to be receiving omens and mes-sages from various technological devices, hears voices commanding her to actions that may be entirely uncharacteristic and bizarre, and loses track of hygiene and becomes unable to manage time to an extent that she appears eccentric and disorganized. It is an unnerving and sobering experience for everyone involved.

Science has come closer each decade to understanding how the psychotic brain works. And we now understand some of the contexts of psychosis, among them reactions to prescription and illegal drugs, excessive alcohol intake, delirium (a catchall medical term that refers to patients who experience impaired consciousness from a variety of possible causes), dementia, and certain congenital diseases, such as the genetically linked velocardiofacial syndrome (a disorder that includes cleft palate, heart defects, a characteristic facial appearance, and a risk of psychosis). But there is much still to be learned about cause and precise brain mechanisms.

As is often the case in medicine, a measure of luck has advanced treatment of psychosis well ahead of our understanding of it. The golden age of discovery of drugs for people with psychiatric illness began in earnest after the Second World War. Medicines intended for other uses demonstrated unanticipated benefits for people with

schizophrenia and mood disorders. Chlorpromazine, initially investigated as a surgical anesthetic, was the first such medication to be
widely used with psychiatric patients. Between 1954 and 1975, about
forty other antipsychotic medications with similar molecular structures
were introduced worldwide. All these drugs appeared to soothe psychotic symptoms to an extent that had previously been inconceivable.
But there was a high price. Many patients developed drug-induced
Parkinsonism, with slowing of movements, tremors, and a reduction
in facial expressiveness that was sometimes confused with the effects
of the illness itself. Longer-term use led to a condition called tardive
dyskinesia, characterized by involuntary, tic-like facial and body movements. And, of course, like all drugs in medicine, they didn't work for
everybody.

Clozapine, another antipsychotic drug, was synthesized in 1958
and tested on patients in the 1960s. After reports emerged of complete
obliteration of white blood cells in a number of patients on this medication, it was understandably withdrawn. More than a decade later, it
gradually returned to clinical use with rigorous blood monitoring, and
solid evidence began to accumulate that it helped people with psychosis who were not helped by other antipsychotic medications – the first
drug in this class to distinguish itself in this way. Further, it appeared
to reduce suicidal thinking in psychotic patients, a group known to be
at high risk.[1] Clozapine has been a godsend to many, including a relative of mine with a psychotic illness, where conventional antipsychotics
were not effective or not tolerable.

In the late 1980s and early 1990s, a new wave of antipsychotics
– the so-called second generation or atypicals – hit the market. They
soon almost completely supplanted the drugs that preceded them, with
their promises of fewer side effects, better responses, and even an ability to treat not only hallucinations and delusions but also social withdrawal and lack of motivation. There was a groundswell of enthusiasm
for risperidone, olanzapine, and quetiapine – the "big three" of this
new generation – as well as a plethora of positive research reports on

their benefits funded by the pharmaceutical industry. But the bloom came off the rose, as independently funded research revealed no clinical advantage to the atypicals over the old drugs from the 1950s and 1960s. They showed no more success targeting the less florid but still debilitating symptoms associated with psychotic disorders: isolation, dulling of emotions, and inactivity. The newer studies also identified a different but equally worrying set of side effects, including weight gain, high cholesterol, and a vulnerability to diabetes.

Even when these medications are successful at ameliorating active psychosis, patients are often resistant to taking them or stop once they start. Not surprisingly, the serious side effects, especially weight gain, are frequently cited. The reasons people do or don't take antipsychotic medications are complicated, and part of any psychiatrist's job is to find out what motivates his patients in this regard.

TODAY, I WILL NEED to find out if Allan has discontinued his medication again and, if so, why. I will also need to explore with him whether he is willing and able to reconsider his decision. I peer through the glass of the nursing station to where Allan sits calmly and silently with two men, whom Tish has told me are his father and his community worker. I see in Tish's notes that his recent trip to the Caribbean ended when he threatened his mother with a knife.

As I step out to the waiting room, I monitor my gut instincts regarding safety as I recall a previous incident with a psychotic patient. I know my caution is inflected by assumptions and fears of which I am not proud. But I also know the literature: black individuals (and non-Western immigrant groups) have higher rates of contact with psychiatric emergency services than their white counterparts, and higher rates of compulsory admission, if not forcible restraint.[2] The reasons for this overrepresentation of immigrants and blacks are complex. They include the fact that among non-Western immigrant groups, blacks are statistically more likely to experience psychosis. And because members of these groups face multiple barriers in our society, they often do not have easy access to the health-care system, leading to worsening of their symptoms before help is provided. It is also true that since psychiatric assessments are still largely subjective, the biases and even racism of health-care professionals may contribute.[3]

Since there are other patients and families in the room at that moment, I decide to take Allan and his companions to one of the interviewing rooms, although I would prefer to remain in the waiting area, which is a safe, open space with seats bolted to the floor and sight lines to the nursing station and the security office. As I approach, I am reassured to note that Allan is not pacing, agitated, accusatory, or threatening – that is, he shows no signs of potential impending violence. We should be okay in one of the side rooms, all of which are equipped with video cameras.

"Hello, Allan. I'm Dr. Goldbloom," I say as I extend my hand (with younger patients, I tend to be more informal and use their first names). Allan shakes it but doesn't make eye contact or speak. I press on. "I'm one of the psychiatrists working in the ER today, and I'm here to help you in whatever way I can. Please follow me. Would you like your father and worker to come with us?"

Allan doesn't respond, but his companions stand up, somehow moving Allan with them, without any overt evidence of physical contact.

Once we are all settled in the sparsely furnished interview room, I turn once again to Allan. I have taken the chair closest to the door in case I need to make a swift exit. Rule 1 of the emergency-preparedness lore handed down from psychiatric resident to resident states: Never position a potentially violent patient between you and the door.

"Allan, can you tell me why you're here today?"

When Allan remains silent, I turn to his father and youth worker to learn the story.

"Doctor, we are at our wits' end with this boy," his father begins in a soft lilting voice that gives away his island origins. "Two months ago, his mother called me in a state, and no wonder. This boy here took a knife to her throat for seven hours. No reason, no why to it, she says. The police came but couldn't do nothing with him for hours. Finally, he stood down and they took him to the local hospital. My boy, he was lucky. The police at home, they don't mess around. His mother's brother knows the commissioner and called him at home, tells him what's going on. The commissioner talks to the police and the hospital. They treated my boy with kid gloves and he returned home to his mother after a week with some medication."

Allan stares ahead, showing no signs he is listening to his father's account. At the same time, he seems calm and undisturbed by what must have been a traumatic series of events.

"His mother called me yesterday to say the doctors at home thought he would be better off here. She said she can't manage him anymore, that he needs his father, and she was putting him on the plane. I picked him up from the airport a few hours ago." He hands me a sheaf of documents, which I scan quickly. The most useful contains a few lines from the Caribbean hospital stating the final diagnosis (schizophrenia) and the medications Allan has received.

"Do you know if Allan was taking the medications after he left the hospital?"

"His mother tells me he did at first, but then she finds all kinds of pills in his room when she's packing him up to send him here."

"How had Allan been doing in the hospital?" I ask.

"Doctor, the strange thing is that although his mother tells me the boy is better than before he went into hospital, she says he hasn't said a word to anyone for two weeks – not her, not his uncle or cousins, not his doctors there. He stopped talking to everyone. I asked his worker from before" – he nods at his companion – "to come to the airport with me to get him. The boy likes him. But the boy hasn't said a word to either of us since he came out of the doors at the airport. Don't know how he made it through Customs."

It is clear to me from Allan's gaze on us and his body language that he is listening and following everything we say.

I fall back onto a technique that is sometimes successful with people who are selectively mute. "I know you're not able to speak right now and I'm sure there's a reason for it," I say to Allan. "Can you at least tell me why you're not speaking?"

Allan slowly opens his mouth, gazes unblinkingly at me, and says, "Because I don't want to." He then resumes his silence and looks away.

His father appears stunned by this utterance; I feel as if I have pulled a cheap parlor trick, which in a way I have. I continue to ask Allan yes-or-no questions, and he continues to reply silently by nodding or shaking his head. By means of this slow one-sided dialogue, I determine that something is indeed terribly wrong; he still feels people are laughing at him and taunting him. He concedes he doesn't feel safe on the streets and acknowledges that his previous stay in our hospital was a positive one. He is willing to come back in and to get some help without requiring an involuntary admission. Fortunately, a bed is available on the inpatient unit where he had been before; the staff and surroundings will be familiar to him.

Everybody seems relieved – Allan, his father, his worker, and me. My relief stems from the fact that although Allan is ill, he is not violent or threatening. He is able to acknowledge his distress and accept our help. I hope this means a smoother course of engagement and treatment. While the last admission resolved his hallucinations and delusions with medications, maybe this time once his symptoms subside, he will be more able to take part actively in looking at school and work options. We all like to think magically that once adversity is behind us, it won't return, but experience – including illness relapse – is the best teacher.

I return to the nursing station to write up the history and admission orders, happy that things have worked out but uncomfortably aware that initially I may have given off a palpable vibe of apprehension and assumption. I am not sure this is something I thought about until I heard a colleague of mine who has expertise in issues of race and psychosis talk several years ago about microepisodes of racism – such as the white person who tenses up on a first encounter – and how they may affect young black men. As I listened to him I thought about family stories from almost a century earlier when my grandfather, a well-trained pediatrician, found out he could not be appointed to the medical staff of the Montreal General Hospital because he was a Jew; when my mother, a physical education graduate of McGill, received a letter from the school board in Montreal indicating that she would not be hired as a gym teacher as a Jew; when as a twelve-year-old I was told that I could not join a Montreal tennis club because they had already accepted "too many Jews." I also know that not all expressions of anti-Semitism or racism are as overt. Some, like my apprehension, are subtle – from assumptions without evidence to body language.

I TURN TO THE WHITEBOARD and erase Allan's name, a ritual that appeals to my need to signal achievement and progress to myself and to others – a need first identified in me on a second-grade report card by an astute teacher and unchanged in the subsequent half century and beyond. The closing scenes of a particular detective show that I liked more than a decade ago, *Homicide: Life on the Street*, always featured the detectives erasing the names of solved cases off a similar whiteboard. I romanticize myself as a bit of a detective in the ER, using interview techniques and clues to understand what is going on with my patients. The nurses know that I like the challenge and are quick to hand me the chart for my next case as soon as Allan goes upstairs.

It turns out to be the woman I had noticed earlier in the waiting room typing avidly on her cell phone.

"Sofia Turra. She's afraid of flying," Phil Silveira, one of the nurses, tells me, reading from his triage report. "She's a thirty-seven-year-old municipal administrator, living with her husband and three young children. Her parents came over from Italy when she was a child but returned there last year to enjoy their retirement. I think that's part of the problem."

Sofia sits nervously in the waiting room, which has started to fill, surreptitiously wiping tears away. I infer from her tense demeanor and anxious scanning of the incoming patients that she is not a regular to the ER.

I introduce myself and take her to an interviewing room. My antennae that respond to people with psychosis in this setting are dormant; she is clearly very upset but not in a way that makes me hypervigilant.

Sofia explains that five weeks ago she booked a plane trip to Italy for herself and her family to visit her parents. The flight is in a few days. Shortly after she made the reservations, she became anxious and tearful, ruminating about the flight and reading constantly online about aviation safety.

"Did you see the article in the paper last month about the commercial jet that lost a chunk of fuselage over the ocean?" she asks me. "The jet had to make an emergency landing. I know it's crazy, but I can't stop thinking about it. My husband keeps telling me that these cases are rare, and that everyone survived, thank God, but I can't stop thinking about it. If he tells me once more that the most dangerous part of the flight is the drive to the airport, I am going to scream at him!"

I respond that I did read the article, but I make no attempt to reassure her. She has already heard all the rational arguments as to why this event should not deter her from flying, and they have simply added to her sense of herself as irrational and weak.

"Now I can't get it out of my head. It's like a dark cloud that has taken over everything. I can't enjoy things, I can't concentrate at work, and worst of all I can't sleep. I just lie there tossing and turning, trying to think of a way I can get out of the flight." She twists the rings on her fingers so forcefully I worry she may hurt herself.

"So what was the final straw that made you decide to come here today?" I ask.

"I feel so ashamed and embarrassed. I was so desperate last week that I went to my family doctor. She gave me an antianxiety pill, I think it's called Ativan, to take twice a day. It has definitely helped, my husband thinks so too, but I can feel it wearing off between doses. Now I keep wondering what will happen if it wears off in the middle of the flight. Part of me thinks that I should just cancel the flight altogether and have everyone go without me, but I know that would be letting everyone down. This morning my husband and I had a bad fight about it. Then on the subway on my way to work, I saw an ad for your hospital with that redheaded woman from TV talking about her daughter getting help for anxiety. I got off at the next stop and came right here. It's so stupid to let my anxiety spoil this for everyone."

I am correct in assessing Sofia as new to the ER. She has never talked with a psychiatrist or other mental health professional before. She had never taken a psychotropic medication until two weeks ago. She doesn't have any history of drug or alcohol misuse. She had, at least on superficial scrutiny, a happy childhood, free of any particular trauma; she has a good job and a stable marriage – although her children and husband are getting increasingly fed up with her worry and indecision.

I try to decipher what underlies her anxiety about this particular flight. After all, there have been a few media reports of plane crashes in the past few years, some with much less happy outcomes than the one she has just described to me.

"Have you ever been on a plane before?"

"Yes, many times."

"When was the last time?"

"Five years ago."

"What happened?"

"Nothing much. There was some turbulence."

"Did you think you were going to crash? Did you think you were going to die?"

"I suppose I did." She dissolves into tears. "Since then I've made our family take driving holidays. Sometimes we've driven ridiculous distances – all so I don't have to get back on a plane. I know even though they're fed up with me, my husband and the kids would understand if

I canceled now. What's stopping me is my parents. They aren't getting any younger. What if they need my help or, God forbid, one of them dies? I need to be able to fly over there. And I want to see them before that happens."

Sofia wipes her eyes. While she talks about her parents, I suddenly picture my father, older, proud, and alone. My parents have been an indivisible unit for more than sixty-five years, leaving their children free from any sense of obligation to look after them or to provide companionship, their lives seemingly busier than ours. If my mother . . . I realize that I have not heard Sofia's last few statements, and I force myself to focus on what she is saying.

I know that superimposed on Sofia's long-standing avoidance is an acute anxiety response triggered by a single frightening event and the possibility of its recurrence. I also know that the best and most curative thing for her anxiety would be to get aboard the plane. She knows it too. But anxiety overwhelms that knowledge and pushes her toward canceling the trip – the other cure, at least in the moment, for her anxiety.

We talk for a while, and she becomes more relaxed. It is easy to engage with her, and she has moments when she can even laugh at her predicament. She is also extremely competent in many domains in her life; however, in the midst of her anxiety, she feels good at nothing and a burden to others. We consider strategies to get her to the boarding ramp, and we discuss what medications will keep her calm enough to get on the plane and endure the flight.

I know that in the eyes of some, medicating anxiety is seen as a cop-out on the part of both the patient and the health professional, that somehow the "root causes" need to be mined, exposed, and fixed through extensive therapy and exercises. Medication in this context is also perceived as a conversion of normal human experience into an illness of which the pharmaceutical industry greedily takes advantage. But Sofia has only a few days until her scheduled departure, not enough time for a course of exposure and response prevention, which is an essential feature of cognitive behavioral therapy (CBT) for anxiety and the therapeutic gold standard for her predicament. What's more, taking the trip – assuming it's uneventful – will be the best treatment of all.

So how to get her there?

"Sofia, my suggestion is for me to prescribe you clonazepam. It's a longer-acting antianxiety pill, one you can be confident will get you through the whole flight without having to worry about its wearing off. It will even get you through an airport delay. It's a powerful medication and will relieve your anxiety effectively for the duration of the plane trip."

The tension in her face starts to dissipate. This is why she came today, missing a morning of work – the hope that we would help her find a way out of the predicament that has escalated day by day to an extent that is now causing significant distress and conflict for her and family.

"My prediction is that once you complete the return leg of your trip, and you have the experience of having mastered your fear of flying, your need for the pills will disappear, and you will be able to discontinue them with a tapering schedule. If for any reason I am wrong and your anxiety doesn't go away, I suggest seeing a psychologist for some targeted cognitive behavioral therapy."

In her relief, Sofia starts to talk about her anxiety. "You know, Dr. Goldbloom, when I look back, I think I've always struggled with anxiety, just never this bad. But it's always been there, lurking and shadowing me. When I was a little girl, I was always afraid of someone coming into our house after my parents went to sleep. My mother used to have to stay with me until I fell asleep, until I was a teenager. When I had friends stay over, I would tell her not to come in; I was too embarrassed for them to know. And later, when I was in high school, I never went on the school ski days or the trips to Quebec City because I was so afraid of breaking a bone or something bad happening. So many things I missed out on. If the phone rang when I was home alone, I always thought it was terrible news – the police calling to tell me my parents were killed in a car crash. My parents never pushed me; they just fig-ured I'd grow out of it. And they were immigrants; I am not sure they saw the point of the trips as long as I was getting good marks. I'm glad my husband pushes our kids to do stuff even when they don't want to at first. We're a good pair; I do the worrying for both of us. They all snowboard and do sports. And they love traveling, which is a big part of why this is so hard. I've always imagined the worst, but it hasn't gotten in the way like this before. I've always found a work-around, like the IT guy at work says. And it's not necessarily a bad thing to be concerned or careful."

She's right. Her anxiety has not been insurmountable before, and she and her husband sound like they do make a good team. She has built a good professional and family life for herself. But now, after many years of adapting to and coping with her worry, it stands as a roadblock between her and her parents. We talk a bit more about cognitive be-havioral therapy, the idea of which clearly intrigues Sofia. I provide her with the names of some private clinics where I know she can be seen quickly. Fortunately, she has extended health coverage insurance through her work that she believes will pay for six sessions of private therapy. It won't be what most therapists consider a full course, even in these days of more abbreviated psychotherapy models, but it may be enough to help her significantly. Even in Canada, an international poster child for universal access to health care, wait lists for publicly funded psychotherapy are long, whereas private therapists provide im-mediate access for those who can afford them. The fact that our pro-vincial health plans pay physicians to provide a multitude of medical treatments but do not cover the majority of health-care professionals who provide psychotherapies well supported by research strikes me as evidence of the residual stigma that clings to mental health treatments. In Australia and the United Kingdom, public funding of psychologist-provided cognitive behavioral therapy has begun, a trend I hope will spread as governments see the benefits for people and the potential reduction in health-care costs.

For now, Sofia appears relieved, and I am grateful for both the psychic pain relief that medications can provide and her insurance coverage. I brief her on the potential side effects of clonazepam, with particular reference to not mixing it with alcohol (a well-known form of airport support for anxious fliers) and not driving if she feels slowed or sedated while taking the medication.

More than twenty years earlier, a distant cousin of mine, a young woman in her twenties, was brutally murdered in Toronto. I accompanied her father to the morgue to identify her body. In preparing him for this horrendous parental task, I loaded him up with antianxiety medications. They did not numb the pain – which haunted him for the rest of his life – but they allowed him to get through an ordeal. I saw this at the time as the psychic equivalent of Demerol for someone passing a kidney stone, but I also recognized that physical pain had a higher order of social legitimacy and acceptability when it came to pain relief.

It's strange: with my cousin's father, I had put myself squarely in the physician role the way I knew my father would have if he had been available for the task. In that role, there was no room for me to falter, to feel squeamish, or to experience pain. I had a job to do and I did it. At the same time, I was aware that I could be initiating a journey of benzodiazepine (the Valium family) use that could be endless without appropriate monitoring. Some people start these medications and never stop them. But for many people, occasional use makes a huge difference in getting through difficult situations; just knowing that they have a pill if they need it can reduce anxiety.

Sofia leaves the ER with a prescription, an explanation, and an expectation – that she will survive the flight, that her anxiety will disappear or can be treated, and that her need for antianxiety medications will similarly evaporate. I hope all three aspects of the intervention will be helpful, and recall the words of one of my teachers at McGill, Pierre Dongier, from many years earlier – that the goal in research is to minimize a treatment's placebo effect (a positive response to an inactive medical intervention), whereas the goal in clinical practice is to maximize the placebo effect.

I discuss Sofia's case briefly with Sunil Mehta, one of the other ER nurses. He tells me about a friend of his who hasn't flown since 9/11 ("Maybe I should bring her to see you, Dr. G"), and then I sit down to write up the notes. The conversion of the ER charting in our hospital a couple of years ago from multipage sheets, which required a stiff ballpoint to make an impression down to the third page, to single-page sheets has been a boon. It allows me to use my favorite Waterman Phileas fountain pen and to display a calligraphy that is both highly recognizable and legible. When staff or students comment on it, I tell them I was sick the day they gave the lecture in medical school on how to screw up your handwriting. But clinical documentation throughout the rest of the hospital in inpatient and outpatient settings is exclusively electronic, so my pen-and-ink days will soon be part of hospital history. The whiteboard is filling up faster than I can erase names. Barry Low, the resident working the day shift, and Paul Kurdyak, the other staff psychiatrist, have completed work in the back and are now helping with the influx. In a few hours, a team of three residents will arrive for evening and night call, and they will look at the whiteboard to see how many cases have been left for them by the day shift. I know they won't see the names of the patients for whom assessment and "disposition" are already taken care of; an immature part of me wants them to know that it could have been much worse for them.

THE NEXT PATIENT, MOHAMMED Dibaba, is the other black man I noticed on my way back from lunch. A tall, balding, fine-featured man, he is still sitting in the waiting room with his cousin Abdul, to whom he bears a striking resemblance. As I peer out through the glass and see the two men sitting on the bench, Tish, who is back from lunch, says, "The guy on the left, he's from Ethiopia."

Once again I leave the fishbowl nursing station to meet someone new. As with Allan, here a concerned family member may prove vital in trying to figure out what is going on.

"Hello, Mr. Dibaba. I'm Dr. Goldbloom. I'm a psychiatrist here in the emergency room. Tish, the nurse, tells me you're from Ethiopia."

"Yes, Doctor, but I have been to Canada before. I was here in 1990 because of the war. Abdul brought me here. But I went back. And now I am here again."

"How can I help you?"

"I can't sleep, Doctor."

Despite this promising beginning, Mohammed is not able to provide much detail about his sleep problems. But he tells me that he has had psychiatric treatment before.

"In 1982, Doctor, I was in Somalia. A refugee. They put me in the hospital twice and gave me shock treatments."

"Did it help?"

"I believe so, Doctor. I don't know."

He speaks softly in reasonably fluent English and has beautiful manners, waiting courteously for me to finish my questions and apologizing frequently for not being able to provide me with the level of detail I am asking for. He has an air of bewilderment about him as though he is not quite sure what has happened to him and why he is here. He repeats the same phrases: "I am sorry, Doctor, I am not being much help." "I am sorry, Doctor, I do not want to waste your valuable time." "Doctor, I am sorry, I am very tired. I cannot sleep."

I wonder what barriers there are to getting more of the story. Is it the huge culture shift from rural Ethiopia to downtown Toronto, even though he has lived here before? Is it the difficulty of the journey itself? Did something horrible happen to him in Ethiopia? Did whatever affected him in Somalia in 1982 recur? Mohammed is preoccupied with his inability to sleep and hasn't mentioned any other difficulties.

I turn to Abdul and ask what he thinks might be happening. He explains his perception with the same old-fashioned courtesy as his cousin.

"Doctor, my cousin was fine when he arrived in Toronto, but within two or three days he began to change. He slept during the day but was up all night, and when he was outside he was fearful and told me that strangers were talking about him. He said he could hear them, even though we were in my car at the time with the windows up. I told him it made no sense and he agreed, but he kept saying he could still hear people saying things."

I turn back to Mohammed. "Mr. Dibaba, what did you hear people saying about you?"

He looks uncertain. "Doctor, I don't remember. Abdul told me no one was saying anything, but I heard them. Maybe if I could sleep I would remember."

"Are you hearing them now?" It is essential for me to understand if Mohammed is having auditory hallucinations right now, and whether he is receiving instructions from these voices that might put him or us at risk.

He shakes his head. "No, Doctor. Not now. But in the car on our way here, I heard someone saying I owed Abdul money. But I don't, do I, Cousin?"

Abdul reassures him but shoots me a look as if to say, *You see.*

When I ask about anything that might have happened in Ethiopia, Abdul replies that while there Mohammed chewed khat, a drug unfamiliar to me, daily. When I ask Mohammed about it, he tells me that he hasn't chewed it since his arrival. Finally, Abdul adds that Mohammed has no place to stay and cannot stay with him any longer.

"Doctor, my wife and I have very little space in our apartment as it is. My wife's parents arrive next week for a visit. I am very sorry not to be able to help Mohammed, but he needs somewhere to live. We have friends he could stay with but not like this . . ." He shrugs.

Abdul explains that Mohammed has no money and his Ontario health insurance card has expired, although he is a Canadian citizen as a consequence of his long stay here in the 1990s.

I excuse myself to look up khat online. In the twenty-first century, seeking such information requires only a couple of seconds; in fact, a Google search locates more than eight million related websites in 0.16 of a second, including video footage of people chewing and talking about khat. I learn that it is a plant that may have originated in Ethiopia. It is a stimulant when chewed, releasing chemicals with amphetamine-like properties. Lethargy, depression, nightmares, and tremors are listed among the withdrawal symptoms, and khat-induced psychosis has been described, and associated in one British study with a high recurrence rate. It offers a likely explanation for Mohammed's symptoms, but I have learned over the years not to go too quickly with my initial assumption. In doing so I may miss other contributing factors or indeed an entirely different diagnosis as a result of failing to do due diligence in at least screening for other possible causes.

When I ask if Mohammed has sought other help, Abdul mentions that last week Mohammed was assessed in Amharic by his Ethiopian family physician in Toronto, who has known him since 1990.

"Mr. Dibaba, may I speak to your doctor? Since he knows you well, it may help us understand what is happening."

Mohammed nods. "Yes, Doctor. I told him I couldn't sleep and he gave me pills. But they don't work; I still don't sleep."

As he talks, Mohammed continues to fidget with his watch, an old Timex with a worn brown leather strap, moving it up and down his forearm and scratching the skin underneath it. The skin shows some superficial scratches that look as if they were made by his nails.

I go to the nursing station and call the general practitioner in his office, hoping to get a more nuanced, culturally and historically informed perspective on Mohammed. A helpful receptionist puts me through to him immediately.

"Do you remember this patient?" I ask the doctor.

"Of course I do. I saw him last week. I used to see him when he lived here before."

"What did you think was going on with him?"

"He's crazy! He kept pacing up and down in the waiting room. He drove my receptionist and the other patients nuts. He just kept telling me he couldn't sleep. Over and over again. I gave him some Ativan and Risperdal samples. He wasn't like that before."

By now, I have the sense that this doctor has a busy office, that his encounter with Mohammed was brief, and that he will not be able to provide much more information. Mohammed's symptoms, while loosely defined and of uncertain origin, are interfering with his sleep, his sense of safety, and his behavior with both family and strangers.

I go back to the waiting room and sit down beside Mohammed. "Would you like to come into the hospital so we can help you get some sleep and understand what is going on?" I ask.

"Yes, that would be nice, Doctor. If you have room for me."

I assure him that we do have room and that we will monitor his sleep and try to understand better what is disrupting it – whether it is khat withdrawal or whatever problem led to his intensive treatment in Somalia two decades earlier. There is no substitute, when attempting to reach an accurate and comprehensive diagnosis, for the opportunity to observe a patient closely over a period of time and get to know him.

"Mr. Dibaba, I would also recommend we provide you with a medication that should help quiet the voices you have been hearing in your head and also help you sleep. I am not sure if the voices relate to your no longer using khat, or to some other brain illness, but I do think you would benefit from medication. The one I am going to suggest is similar to the one your family doctor prescribed for you, but I am hoping it will be more effective."

I outline for both Mohammed and Abdul the common side effects and potential risks of the atypical antipsychotic I propose. It is clear to me that although Mohammed is befuddled by his experience, both he and Abdul agree that what is happening to him is abnormal and likely illness related, and that they understand the goals and risks of using medication.

Abdul shakes my hand, clearly relieved. "Thank you, Doctor. This is a good plan."

I admit Mohammed to "the back" for further observation and prescribe a more sedating antipsychotic at bedtime.

In the ER, there are two choices: admit or discharge. Whatever uncertainty clouds the clinical picture, whatever myriad explanations account for the distress, this essential decision must be made. Admission has many permutations: voluntary/involuntary, capable/incapable of making treatment decisions, routine/continuous observation, treatment/watchful waiting. Discharge does too: against medical advice/ agreed upon, to family doctor follow-up/to psychiatric outpatient services/to community agencies/to shelters/to nothing, with meds/without meds. For every patient admitted, there is a cascade of imposed events, good and bad, reflecting the rules and regulations of the hospital and its culture. What is routine in the life of clinicians – admitting someone to the hospital – is often a nodal point in the patient's life in terms of needing help, support, and shelter. For every patient discharged, there is the curiosity about what will unfold subsequently and the worry of not knowing.

Discharging patients from the ER is one of those aspects of psychiatric practice that require a high tolerance for ambiguity. While the ambiguities of diagnosis and disposition remain aspects of psychiatry that bother some doctors (and patients and families and lawyers and philosophers), the reality is that the entire field of medicine is riddled with ambiguities. Watching two radiologists disagree over the findings on an MRI or two pathologists arguing over the interpretation of a microscopic tissue specimen provides some comfort to those of us bereft of diagnostic laboratory tests. Throughout medicine, listening to patients and taking a careful history is still the best route to diagnosis and a plan of treatment.

A FINAL PATIENT AWAITS before the afternoon shift ends. I look for her in the waiting room but cannot find her.

"She's gone to put money in her parking meter and maybe get a coffee," Phil informs me.

"Should we be worried?" I ask.

"She's not suicidal. She just doesn't want to get a parking ticket."

So far I know she is both responsible and able to afford a car. She returns, apologizing for the delay. Apart from her unhealthy pallor and the dark circles under her eyes, Mimi Harvey resembles the smartly dressed, poised, professional young women who attend the talks I give to the downtown law firms and investment banks on behalf of my hospital. She is dressed in tailored clothes that hang loosely, suggesting she has lost weight since she bought them.

After I introduce myself, Mimi tells me that she is thirty-five, married to an investment banker, and the mother of a two-year-old son.

When I ask why she is here today, she tells me she feels depressed.

"When did it start?" I ask.

"I really think it began three years ago. I left my job at a big architectural firm here to move to England. Andrew, my husband, was transferred to the London office of his company. I think things went off the rails after that. We had a great setup; his firm put us up in an apartment off Sloane Square and he was making great money. But I didn't know anybody there, and I didn't have anything to do. I got pregnant almost right away, which was wonderful and seemed to make up for not having my friends and family around. I'd spend hours in my local Waterstones, buying book after book about pregnancy and parenting. And I met a couple of other expats at my pregnancy yoga class who I'd have tea with after class.

"But then after Michael was born two years ago, things went downhill fast. My mother came over for the birth and first month, so that was fine, but after she left, I wasn't getting out at all and I felt miserable at home. A couple of the mums from my yoga class tried to get me to meet up with them a couple of times, but I didn't return their calls and they stopped trying. I would try to take Michael out in his stroller, but I felt like it always started to rain as soon as I managed to get out of the house. The gray skies day after day really got to me. There are only so many trips you can make to the Victoria and Albert Museum with a baby. He'd always start to cry somewhere I couldn't find a place to stop and feed him, and I'd feel like people were looking at me, disapproving of my having him there disturbing everyone."

I make a mental note of Mimi's slow, deliberate, even speech pattern. It's as though she is describing another person. She includes a level of detail in her account that makes me wonder about an obsessional personality style.

"Andrew tried to introduce me to some of the women at his firm and to the other partners' wives, but I'd lost my confidence somehow. I felt frumpy and stupid around the women bankers, who either didn't have children or had nannies who seemed to do absolutely everything for them, and the wives who had children all seemed to know each other. One of them invited me round for coffee with a group of them, but they had all been to the same schools, their husbands had all been to the same schools, and I didn't get the jokes. And the English are tricky. They seem friendly, but if you are not one of them, it's hard to feel accepted.

"Anyway, it just got worse and worse. I would call Andrew every five minutes once six o'clock rolled around to see when he was coming home, and if he was late for any reason, I would be in tears and screaming at him by the time he got home. And the worst part was, I felt like a caricature – some shrewish wife with no life who loses it with her husband because he went to the pub after work with a few of his colleagues. I didn't recognize myself. I had been one of those women who always thought I would juggle parenting with a big job, who'd been a bit dismissive of women who stayed home."

She pauses to take a breath. I guess that she hasn't talked to anyone like this for months, probably more. It's as though a dam has broken, releasing a novel's worth of words that surprise her.

"Andrew felt that I was too far away from my family and applied for a transfer back to Canada. He said if I did want to go back to work, this would make it easier. I didn't know what I wanted at that point. I couldn't imagine leaving Michael with anyone else, but I thought things would get better when we moved back to Toronto a year ago. They didn't. I still feel lost. I don't know who I am anymore. Andrew and I want more children, but we both agree I couldn't manage another right now. I can barely get out of bed in the morning."

"Have you felt like this before? Before Michael's birth."

She nods. "I have, actually. That made it worse, the feeling that I was sliding down into a morass I'd gotten out of eight years ago. At that time I'd just broken up the only really serious relationship I had before Andrew. I couldn't eat. I couldn't sleep. I wasn't concentrating at work. I ended up seeing a psychiatrist in a private office in midtown; she told me I was depressed and put me on Prozac. I saw her weekly for about eight months. It really helped, and I got back in gear. It made a huge difference to my work."

When I ask if she returned to the psychiatrist after coming back to Toronto, she replies that she did, and the doctor recommended she go on a medication similar to Prozac, or fluoxetine, called sertraline, which has demonstrated minimal risk to mothers who are breast-feeding. Even so, Mimi was reluctant, feeling even a low risk was not acceptable. Ironically, the psychiatrist then went on maternity leave, and Mimi had no further contact with her.

She is now fighting tears. I have a sense Mimi is not comfortable crying in front of others, even a doctor in a psychiatric emergency room.

"I can't believe I'm here. I am not that person who ends up in a psychiatric hospital. I am sure I don't seem so to you right now, Dr. Goldbloom, but I have always been a self-starter. I have always looked after myself. I've supported myself financially since university, at least until we went to England. I can't believe how poorly I am functioning. It's not me; this is not who I am. I would never have thought I would be someone who couldn't cope with a child. I don't recognize myself."

Without comment I hand her a box of tissues, since her crying is now impossible to ignore. She blows her nose.

"What are your days like?" I ask.

"I feel overwhelmed all the time. I wake up in the morning, and I am tired. I can't even imagine getting through what needs to get done. I make all these lists of the things that I need to get done, but they just pile up on the kitchen counter. They haunt me. They're part of the reason I don't want to get out of bed: just thinking of all the things that I have to get done but am letting slide. Andrew must think I am pathetic. He comes home and I haven't done the grocery shopping, or called the plumber about our shower, or made dinner. Sometimes I haven't even showered. Even Michael, who is such a lovely boy, doesn't make me happy. All I can think of when he wants to play with me is how much I have to do around the house or how we will make a mess that then I'll have to clean up. I don't see any way out of this."

"Before we look at that, I need to ask you some questions," I tell her. "First of all, have you been feeling so depressed you've thought of killing yourself?"

"Oh, no," she says, "but I do sometimes think that Andrew and Michael would be better off without me. I'm a burden to them both."

"What about unusual experiences, or feelings that may not be entirely rational – a sense that other people are trying to harm you or Michael? Or a belief that Michael himself is damaged in some way despite his pediatrician saying he's fine?"

She cuts me off. "I'm not psychotic, if that's what you are asking me. Part of the reason I am here is that I know how bad my depression can get, and I don't want anything like that happening to me and harming Michael and Andrew."

I confirm with Mimi that she did not experience any psychotic symptoms during her initial depression, before moving on.

"How has all of this affected you sexually?" I ask.

She averts her gaze. "Andrew and I have had sex maybe four times since Michael was born." She puts her head in her hands and talks to the floor. "I know, I know it's crazy. It's not a marriage, but Michael's still in our room at night, and I am always exhausted. Andrew doesn't say much, but I am worried I am driving him away. Sometimes I imagine he's interested in the women in his office. He says of course not, but I wouldn't blame him. It's not as though I am any fun to be around."

"Tell me why you feel the baby still needs to be in your room at night?"

She explains that even though Michael is eating solid foods, he still wakes in the middle of the night to breast-feed and sometimes also breast-feeds during the day.

"It's just so much easier than getting out of bed and going to a different room to bring him into bed with us."

I have to contain my immediate reaction as a parent that it is "weird" that a mother is breast-feeding a walking, talking, and solids-eating two-year-old child. My sense of alienation dates me; my younger colleagues tell me that the most recent dictum on the subject is to continue breast-feeding until a child reaches two, advice that poses a challenge for women who work outside the home. But since Mimi is clearly exhausted, part of me wants to use my authority as a physician to give her permission to stop breast-feeding.

Instead, as neutrally as possible, I ask why she is continuing to breast-feed.

"I was the youngest in my family, and my mother breast-fed me until I was three. She was a bit of a hippie, and ahead of her time in a way. She wanted us to all eat natural foods, no white flour, no pop, no Kraft Dinners. She had a vegetable garden and made our clothes. At the time, it was embarrassing; I was so jealous of my friends who got to take Oreos to school in their lunches, but now I really admire what she was trying to do. My older sister is just like her," Mimi explains. "She has three children, and she breast-fed all of them until they started kindergarten. And she made all their food herself once they were ready for solids. I don't think she ever had a jar of baby food in the house. I had a lot of time to think and read about what kind of parent I wanted to be, and I realized that I want to be like my mother and sister in that sense – making sure Michael isn't exposed to lots of processed foods and chemicals while he's still growing."

For a moment, I am distracted again by my own thoughts, this time by memories of getting married at the tender age of twenty-two, which was already a year older than my parents were when they got married. More than thirty-five years later, I remain happily in love with my wife but am amazed at what "young idiots" we were when we made the decision to marry. As I watch people who have waited longer, I am struck by how careful they are about choosing their partners, how much more conscious calculation and appraisal is involved, and how much they educate themselves and worry about the best parenting approaches and skills for their children. In addition, Mimi has a layer of perfectionism that has not proved helpful to her.

As I probe further, it becomes clear to me that Mimi knows intellectually that despite her own childhood experience, the major benefits of breast-feeding in terms of physical health and bonding have passed. But Michael is in a routine and so is she. It is pleasurable for him but not for her; her sleep is disrupted nightly. In the midst of her depression, her pervasive sense of inadequacy as a person compels her to continue to provide to her son the one thing that no one else can.

I review her symptoms with her; her experiences, like those of Anya and Frederick, fit precisely with the diagnosis of depression. In the midst of her unique family and background, she shows a pattern of suffering indistinguishable from that of millions of other people.

I ask what she wants to do, while also recognizing that part of why she is here is that she wants to be told what to do. It's tricky. It would be easy for me to fall into the old-fashioned male physician role: telling women what to do with their bodies. Mimi has all the intellectual machinery and experience to figure this out on her own. Her depression, however, has completely undermined her ability to trust her instincts or her decisions. And she is in pain in a way that threatens to hurt her child (and, I suspect, has already hurt her marriage).

I emphasize that she is clearly trying to do the right thing for Michael, but that at twenty-three months, having a depressed, nonfunctioning mother is worse than relinquishing the breast. I add that

Michael will protest loudly because he is used to it, but screaming his head off is one of the few quivers in his behavioral bow when things don't go as he likes.

"You don't have to feel this way," I say. "Mount Sinai Hospital down the street has an outpatient clinic that specializes in women with depression in pregnancy and postpartum, or you could reconnect with the psychiatrist you saw before."

She nods slowly, her eyes welling with tears again. "I suppose you're right; that makes sense. It's pathetic; I can't even figure this out on my own."

"If everybody could figure it out on their own, people like me would be out of business."

She tells me that she thinks the suggestions offered are reasonable, thanks me politely, and says that she will follow up. As she leaves the ER, I wonder if she will.

I hope that I've struck an appropriate balance – providing her with practical support and recommendations while not overriding her beliefs or undermining her faith in her parenting decisions. I can hear my mother's voice commenting critically; she is a believer in strict parenting that promotes childhood autonomy and self-reliance, and her idealized recollections of our childhood had us going to bed at seven thirty each night without resistance, tying our shoelaces by age three, and writing thank-you notes by age six.

POSTPARTUM DEPRESSION IS A scourge that affects women worldwide.[4] I am deeply relieved by Mimi's immediate and persuasive denial of suicidal thoughts; I know the importance of asking mothers directly about suicide because they may be ashamed of such thoughts and try to hide them. I was also relieved that Mimi showed no evidence of having lost touch with reality despite the length and impact of her depression.

As I was posing Mimi those grim questions, my mind had been pulled back to a terrible case that shocked Toronto more than a decade ago: a young, accomplished professional woman, reportedly similar to Mimi in many aspects, jumped in front of a train with her baby. The story had been the subject of much discussion among colleagues as she had been seen by health-care professionals who apparently underestimated the severity of her illness.

It can be hard to tease out postpartum depression from its more benign relative, postpartum blues, and difficult to persuade the much smaller percentage of mothers who are psychotic and frightened to disclose their symptoms. Many women who experience postpartum depression have been psychiatrically well until the postpartum period brings darkness, for reasons that are still not fully understood, despite decades of theorizing and studies. And their friends and family have heard of or experienced the baby blues and may not understand the difference between the tears and transient mood swings that many women experience within the first couple of weeks of delivering but that resolve on their own with support and rest,[5] and the tidal wave of postpartum depression that may bring psychosis in its wake and render a formerly functioning woman a wreck.

About 13 percent of women are estimated to struggle with postpartum depression, uncomplicated by psychotic symptoms.[6] Postpartum psychosis is fortunately much more rare, occurring in approximately 0.1 percent of deliveries and among women who are far more likely to have a prior history of psychosis or a personal or family history of bipolar disorder.[7] Postpartum psychosis arrives swiftly, usually within a month of the baby's birth, with a mother giving birth for the first time at greater risk than a mother who has had previous pregnancies. Both postpartum depression and psychosis are potentially lethal. Suicide has been identified as the leading cause of maternal deaths in the UK, and the rates in other countries that record such statistics are similar.

A fact that frequently gets overlooked is that paternal postpartum depression affects up to a quarter of fathers within six months of their child's birth.[8] I had not asked Mimi in any real depth about how Andrew was doing; the timing of emergency room assessments doesn't permit the thoroughness of an outpatient consult and relationship, but I find myself wondering how he is dealing with the triad of a demanding job, a depressed wife, and a sex life curtailed by a breast-feeding infant for the past two years. Once Mimi's depression has been treated, they might benefit from a referral for couples therapy to help get their relationship back on track.

I WIPE MIMI'S NAME off the whiteboard as the evening crew of three residents arrives, warily eyeing the list of unseen patients. I tell them I have no cases in progress to hand over, that they will be starting fresh with new patients (much as I did eight hours ago). This is visibly cold comfort to them. They have a sleepless night ahead, doubtless punctuated by the arrival of people in more disarray and distress than those who visit during the day. The night is when intoxicated, homeless, and suicidal people are more likely to appear. I wish them a good shift, wondering whether their definition of a good shift will be different from mine.

Today has been a good shift for me; Georges is safely admitted, and given the steady stream of patients requiring assessment and treatment, I have not had more than a couple of minutes to think about my mother. Once, as Sofia, the patient with the flight phobia, talked about her fear of not seeing her elderly mother again, I felt a jab of what it would mean not to see my mother again. And again with Mimi as she talked about her two-year-old being better off without her, I thought about the richness, the fun, and the support my mother has brought to my life. In each case, the feelings left almost as quickly as they arrived, but I was conscious of them shooting through me all the same.

As I sign off all my notes, I am struck for a moment by how satisfying I have found the day's work. Much of psychiatric care is a journey shared by patient and doctor across time, unraveling a story, monitoring symptoms as they evolve, dealing with crises and life events as they come up, and developing a therapeutic relationship that deepens as the months and years pass. Such lengthy relationships can be rich and rewarding for both patient and psychiatrist. In contrast, emergency room encounters provide snapshots of people's lives. The heat of these encounters appeals to me – their immediacy, their challenge, the help that can be provided when people are feeling or behaving their worst.

Some psychiatrists choose to retreat from regular contact with patients who have a potential for violence, self-inflicted or externally focused. For those of us who like emergency psychiatry, preventing the type of harm that sometimes ends lives lends our work acuity and drama that are, in some ways, close to those occurring in other acute care areas of medicine, such as the Intensive Care Unit or operating room. The stakes are often life-and-death; each statement and gesture matters, potentially paving the way to a good or bad outcome; instincts shaped by experience and training frequently guide the physician's responses.

As I pass by the triage desk, I see a young woman accompanied by an older man speaking urgently to the triage worker. I suspect that even if other, better routes to psychiatric care are developed (as they should be), the need for emergency psychiatric care will always be there – and it is important that the door always be open.

8

Restraint

THURSDAY MORNING

After I drop my computer bag, overcoat, and squash gear in my office, my first task on Thursday is to wipe the overnight slate – checking voice mail for messages that came in after I left the ER yesterday and email ungoverned by the working hours of my time zone. It is a Sisyphean task to empty my electronic in-box, since it silts up with an unpredictable rhythm throughout the day. But it gives me some cooldown time from squash and helps me set some priorities for the day. Almost an hour passes quickly, time that in the pre-email phase of my career might have been spent handwriting or dictating letters or working on academic manuscripts.

Leaving the quiet of my office, my first stop is the Acute Care Unit, to visit Georges. I know from experience that it eases his fear and disorientation in the hospital to see familiar faces, and that our relationship is part of what helps him accept the need for treatment.

I access the locked stairwell at the end of the hallway outside my office with a special key – another reminder of the limits to liberty in the hospital. Descending the three flights of stairs that see very little traffic apart from staff racing to a Code White, I reflect on the fact that this morning's squash game was my third loss of the week, this time to a player I usually beat handily. My game is definitely off. Neither the fear of injury nor the effects of age account for the slump. Squash is a head game, and I was playing mechanically rather than monitoring my opponent's position and placing winning shots that carom off the side wall of the court before grazing the front wall and dropping to the floor.

I arrive at the reinforced and locked door of the ACU. This door has been broken a number of times since the unit was constructed in 1993, kicked open by people whose psychotic fury and fear fueled desperation. The Plexiglas window affords a view inside – partly so that the door isn't advertently opened as someone is barreling toward it trying to leave. It is also festooned with warning signs: AWOL RISK and HIGH AWOL RISK. AWOL, an acronym for "absent without leave," usually refers to soldiers who are missing from their posts, with or without intention of deserting. In my experience, patients who have left the ACU unauthorized have every intention of deserting the hospital.

Despite its contemporary design and light, the ACU is a stubborn legacy of the nineteenth-century psychiatric hospitals with their rows of locked wards where patients with chronic psychiatric illnesses languished for years, receiving little in the way of active treatment. It is hard to know whether these asylums constituted progress over what came before. Despite the growth in small-scale asylums, private madhouses, and hospitals catering to the mentally ill during the 1700s, it continued to fall primarily to families to look after their severely mentally ill relatives.[1] As late as 1817, an Irish member of Parliament told of his mentally ill constituents whose relatives had chained them in holes in the ground until they died.[2] Those mentally ill individuals lucky or unlucky enough not to have relatives to shelter them found themselves in workhouses or poorhouses where they might be shackled to the floor or walls with iron restraints.[3]

The dominance of large institutions throughout Europe and North America to house the mentally ill evolved in the 1800s. Two well-known paintings of the period – William Hogarth's 1733 depiction of the massive London asylum Bedlam in his finale to his series of eight paintings *A Rake's Progress*, and Goya's *Madhouse of Zaragoza*, painted between 1793 and 1819 – portray inmates clothed only in rags, chained, and housed in filthy conditions. Both paintings reflect the harsh reality that the staff in the historic asylums of Western Europe saw themselves as having a primarily custodial function, with little belief or interest in the institutions' ability to treat or cure their inhabitants.[4] Chaining the more unruly inhabitants was seen as necessary for the safety of staff and other inmates.

Soon, however, the intellectual sea change ushered in by the Enlightenment, with its emphasis on human reason as a guide for both individual and societal organization, was to elicit a new enthusiasm for the power of science to better the lives of human beings, even its most benighted examples. Alienists or, as they were soon to be called, psychiatrists, began to think of the asylum as a place where insanity could be tamed by therapies based on rational principles. By the early 1800s, proponents of "moral treatment" called for regimens for those in the asylums based on routine, schedules, empathy, and kindly communication to manage behavior that had previously been dealt with by force and physical restraints.

One of the movement's leaders, Philippe Pinel (1745–1826), a psychiatrist from relatively humble origins in southwestern France, was a well-known attendee of the revolutionary Parisian salons of the 1780s, drinking in his companions' Enlightenment philosophies and reformist fervor.[5] After the revolution, he became director of the Bicêtre asylum (where the Marquis de Sade was later incarcerated) and subsequently the Salpêtrière, where he became famous for abolishing the chains that had previously been used on patients seen as unmanageable. Like his fellow proponents of moral treatment in the United States and Britain, Pinel argued that restraints could be rendered unnecessary if patients were provided with distractions, skills, and a measure of control. Patients were seen as worthy of respect and capable of practicing self-control and taking part in community social activities.[6] While these measures were extraordinarily paternalistic by today's standards, with Pinel writing that some coercion was reassuring to patients and inspired trust and respect for their physician, moral treatment was radical for the times in suggesting that even psychiatric patients had inalienable rights to humane treatment.

Although Pinel's theories were informed by the conversations of the salons, his interest in moral treatment and his motivation to better the lot of the mentally ill was initially personal. A friend had died by suicide in 1783 after becoming "insane through excessive love of glory," presumably what we would now call a manic episode. Pinel, frustrated by the ineffectiveness of "pharmaceutic preparations," explored other therapeutic approaches.

In his *Treatise on Insanity*, published in 1801, Pinel condemned the usual treatment of patients, "where the domestics and keepers are permitted to use any violence that wanton caprice, or the most sanguinary cruelty, may dictate."[7] He contrasted the effects of this punitive approach with the moral treatment for which he advocated, and protested the practice of abandoning patients to the care of untrained and unsupervised individuals: "In the lunatic infirmary, which is insulated from the body of the hospital, and which is not subject to the control of the governor, it has frequently happened that lunatics, who were perfectly composed and in a fair way to recovery, have, in consequence of the silly raillery and rude brutality of their attendants, relapsed into the opposite condition of violent agitation and fury."[8]

Pinel and his protégé, Jean-Étienne Esquirol, put patients and physicians to work together in structured activities such as military exercises, wood chopping, and art classes, with patients intentionally isolated from the perceived pressures of the outside world. Like most new treatments in medicine, moral treatment was overvalued by its first practitioners and seen as curative; however, it quickly became obvious it would not entirely eradicate the need for restraint of agitated and violent patients. Pinel resorted to straitjackets and seclusion when needed.

But he and his followers helped to direct psychiatric practice to a place where restraint is today seen as a last resort, to be used only to protect patients, staff, and family members, rather than as a "treatment."

The use of restraint – in all its forms, including seclusion (the so-called padded cell or, as it is known in prisons, solitary confinement) – reemerged as a political issue just over a century later in Michel Foucault's work. In Foucauldian theory, restraints – whether physically, in the form of manacles, or through constant observation and strict enforcement of schedules and behaviors – were simply society's method of regulating outliers and rebels.

Despite the widespread influence of Foucault's theories and almost seventy years of advances in psychiatric medications and the public's understanding of mental illness, we still need places where patients who are potentially violent (either to themselves or others) can be locked up. And in modern hospitals that place is the psychiatric ACU. Patients are kept in the ACU, often against their will, until they are assessed by their treatment team to be safe to handle the increased freedom available in the hospital's other units or the community. There is no whitewashing what this means: the patients in the ACU are incarcerated, whether one believes it is for their own protection or solely for the comfort of society. Having spent part of my career as the physician in charge of the ACU, I hold firmly to the former view: that patients are held for their own good.

THE ACU WAS MY FIRST clinical home when I came to this hospital in 1993. The fifth floor had just been renovated to convert it from outpatient offices to a twenty-three-bed general psychiatry inpatient unit and a six-bed ACU. In a building built in 1966, this floor had already had multiple lives as outpatient and inpatient facilities, and one of the maintenance men told me if we renovated it one more time, the whole building would fall down. Nevertheless, it was once again stripped to its joists, and a newly designed ACU was retrofitted into the available space. It was a significant step up from the cramped crisis unit that extended off the emergency room on the ground floor, which had previously housed the hospital's most acutely ill patients.

Two years later, when I became chief of staff and vice president of Medical Affairs of the hospital, I continued my ACU work. To my mind it was a good fit: the clinical head of the hospital having clinical responsibility for its most ill and high-risk patients. My father and father-in-law both continued frontline clinical care while serving as academic and administrative leaders, and they gave me powerful models for how it could be done. After the creation of CAMH in 1998, as its first physician-in-chief, I was the only person on the senior management team (largely senior administrators) with major clinical responsibilities. A sense of service was not my only motivator: I worked my uniquely dual status to my advantage when management meetings dragged on past my limited ability to tolerate them, legitimately excusing myself to see patients.

Today I am not alone in the hall facing the locked door of the ACU. A middle-aged woman wearing an elegant leather coat and a silk scarf has emerged from the bank of elevators. She takes out a pair of glasses to read the signs on the door. Then she waves a hand, trying to make eye contact with the nursing staff on the other side of the glass.

"Can I help you? I'm Dr. Goldbloom. I work here."

She turns away from the door to look at me, startled to find me behind her, but quickly recovers. "Thank you. I got a call this morning that my daughter is a patient here at the hospital and is asking for me. The woman at the information desk downstairs sent me up here. What is this ward? Why is the door locked?"

"This is the hospital's Acute Care Unit, where patients who need intensive monitoring and treatment are looked after."

She is visibly rattled. "Are the patients not allowed to leave? How long do they have to stay here?"

I don't want to provide false reassurance to this woman, but neither do I want her believing her daughter is lost to her. "It is locked for the patients' safety. Once they are more stable, they go to a more open unit or return home. Many people are treated here for only a couple of days or a week before they get transferred."

"Will they let me see my daughter?"

"Certainly, if she has asked to see you." This woman is lucky; I know how painful it can be for both patients and family members if the patient remains too ill to understand the need for hospitalization and blames her relatives or friends for being there. "Friends and family are encouraged to visit. It helps most patients, and often provides the staff with important information. Families can give a longer-term perspective and help put the patient's illness in context. You will be able to give her doctors and nurses – who have only seen her ill – a sense of what she's like when she's well."

The woman fumbles to put her glasses case in her purse.

"I want to see her. If she wants to see me, that is. I haven't seen much of her the past month. I kept phoning, but she just screamed at me the last few times we spoke. She wouldn't come to the house. My husband and I could tell something was terribly wrong. I was trying to persuade her to see a doctor, but she would hang up on me as soon as I suggested it. She was in the hospital last year, but she wouldn't let us visit her then. I am so relieved to know she's here, but, to be honest, I am scared to go in there. My husband didn't come with me; he tends to upset her."

I try to reassure her, hoping I don't sound patronizing. "Most people are scared, particularly if they haven't been to a unit like this before. And the reality is that the patients here are very ill. But the staff are very experienced at dealing with whatever comes up, and you can ask them anything."

A nurse comes to open the door. The woman gives me a tentative smile.

"Thank you, Doctor. I appreciate your taking the time to talk to me. I hope I haven't kept you from something; I'm sure you are very busy."

"I'm Luana Rabinowitz's mother," I hear her say to the nurse. I kick myself for not having noticed the resemblance to the manic young woman I saw yesterday in the ER. Even her voice is reminiscent of her daughter's. Now I understand the context of her worry. Before I can introduce myself as the doctor who decided her daughter should be kept here, she has followed the nurse through the door.

Our ACU, like the medical Intensive Care Unit (ICU) in a general hospital, houses the hospital's sickest patients. In our case, they include people who do not accept their need for treatment or hospitalization, people who have demonstrated by their behavior that they cannot keep themselves safe, and people believed to constitute a threat to the safety of others. While it may feel like jail to the patients who are there – and sometimes to visitors as well – it's still a hospital unit where people can expect the staff to try to understand them and help them. And what I told Luana's mother is true: most patients are in the ACU for less than a week before being transferred to other units that have unlocked doors and lower staff-to-patient ratios, or sent home as the intensity of their illness subsides.

There are a few patients who will not have such a brief stay, most commonly those who straddle the boundary between psychiatry and the penal system and who await beds in a forensic psychiatric unit.

Mentally ill people who have committed violent crimes are the hot potatoes of the medicolegal system. Many psychiatric facilities lack staff trained to manage violent offenders, and they also do not want their other patients exposed to the risks offenders may pose. The jails say, not unreasonably, that they cannot offer adequate treatment to inmates with significant mental illness. Nevertheless, our prisons are the last great asylums, warehousing many individuals whose mental illness has not been treated and who have come to the legal system's attention by breaking the law. Prisons house many more mentally ill offenders than do hospital psychiatric units. In the United States, Chicago's Cook County Jail has been characterized as "the nation's largest inpatient mental health facility." Psychiatric illnesses affect approximately one-third of the ten to twelve thousand inmates housed there at any given time.[9] But prison mental health systems around the world are understaffed and underresourced, with the result that mentally ill prisoners are particularly vulnerable to being victimized and rarely receive the treatment or the safety that a hospital environment can provide.

The solution in most developed countries has been to build separate psychiatric forensic units in large psychiatric hospitals. These are usually full to overflowing, with the result that patients may languish in prison for weeks to months awaiting beds. An infamous case in the Canadian penal system involved Ashley Smith, a teenager who died from self-strangulation in prison while being watched by guards who had been told not to intervene. Smith, who had initially been jailed at fifteen for throwing crab apples at a postal worker after a string of previous such offenses, had been buffeted between provinces and seventeen prisons and forensic psychiatric facilities in the last year of her life, the constant moves preventing her from receiving consistent treatment for a pattern of escalating self-harm and suicidal behavior. Images of her being transferred from one prison to another show prison staff duct-taping her into an airline seat. The managers of all the facilities were clearly at their wits' end as to what to do with this extraordinarily disturbed young woman whose reported diagnosis of borderline personality disorder (in addition to a learning disorder and ADHD) was likely exacerbated by solitary confinement for the majority of her incarcerations. While a psychiatric facility might not have been able to guarantee Ashley Smith's survival, staff members experienced in dealing with the chronic self-harm with which Smith struggled would have had a better chance over time to help her than a facility focused on security and correction.

I follow Luana's mother and the nurse into the ACU and make my way to the nursing station, which is separated from the rest of the unit by a long counter behind Plexiglas that reaches to the ceiling. When the unit was built in 1993, the same counter was there but the Plexiglas sheath was not. I worry that the increased fortification has diminished the spontaneous interaction between patients and staff, the see-through barrier protecting staff but potentially alienating and inflaming patients.

One of the nurses, Jose Flores, is busy at the computer, while on the other side of the Plexiglas a couple of patients pace. There is a common space: a small dining area, with chairs and tables bolted to the floor, and the TV viewing area, with a couple of sofas and armchairs. A row of six single rooms, with Plexiglas sliding doors and full-length curtains the patients can draw for privacy, faces the nursing stations. Each room has windows with a view of the city to the south.

The ACU tends to be intermittently quieter than our other units, without the bustle of people coming and going. There are relatively few visitors. Some of the six patients lie on their beds, heavily medicated. Others pace incessantly in the limited space, their psychotic agitation aggravated by close quarters, and sometimes by other patients or nicotine withdrawal. Today a couple of them are watching a daytime talk show on TV, and one is reading a book. Morning team rounds have already occurred, and the staff have dispersed, getting on with the day's work.

Rhonda Samuels, another ACU nurse, is seated at the dining table, deep in conversation with a young man of medium build dressed in baggy jeans and a sweater that seems the worse for wear. He looks frightened. I can't make out what either is saying, but the steadiness of Rhonda's tone and her calm demeanor seem to be sustaining the interaction.

Whereas the other units in this hospital look and sound far more like today's general hospital wards – more cluttered with furniture, activities, and the increased noise of chatter from up to twenty patients and their visitors – our ACU looks astonishingly like popular culture depictions of a psychiatric ward – bright, white, and spare, its shape angular and regimented. All entrances and exits are locked, as is the door within the ACU that leads into its nursing station. Video cameras provide a continuous feed from the bathroom and from a seclusion room where especially agitated patients can be placed as an alternative to mechanical restraints.

Even in the ACU the patients wear their own clothes if they have them, an effort to preserve their identity when so much else has been taken away – by the hospital environment or their illness, or both. But there are none of the cards, vases of flowers, or stuffed animals that people deliver as offerings to patients in general hospital wards. Even if they were brought in by visitors – which they rarely are – they have to pass the test of whether they can be used as a missile or an instrument of self-destruction. Nothing that can be used for harm is allowed. The cutlery is plastic and the plates are paper. Yet with all these precautions, a desperate, ingenious soul can find a way to end a life that has become intolerable. During my tenure as physician-in-chief, there were suicides on our inpatient units as there are in every hospital, despite our efforts to "suicideproof" the environment with shower rods designed to give way under the weight of someone trying to hang himself or herself, monitoring protocols, and so on.

The sense of outrage both within and outside the hospital when a psychiatric inpatient dies far outstrips the impact following the death of a medical patient. Patients die in medical ICUs all the time, the victims of their illnesses, and yet the ICU staff is rarely held responsible unless there is evidence of a gross medical error. In a psychiatric ACU, it is our failure if a patient who has suffered for decades from depression or bipolar illness and has a history of multiple serious suicide attempts manages to outwit staff to achieve what she sees as the sole answer to her intolerable pain while on our watch. I don't mean to act as an apologist, but the patients I encountered who managed to end their lives, ostensibly in full view of our staff, were superhumanly determined and ingenious, outmaneuvering any barrier or observation we put in place. Short of keeping someone in physical restraint indefinitely – a reductio ad absurdum of protection – there is no way I know of to guarantee the safety of a patient determined to die by suicide. Nonetheless, we try our best, looking for that indeterminate balance between safety and freedom, between privacy and monitoring. The design of the ACU reflects hours of painstaking attention to design details that attempt to offer a level of comfort while minimizing risk.

Woody Pinsent, a veteran nurse from Newfoundland who, despite years in Toronto, still speaks with the accent of his home province, greets me in the nursing station. He and I first worked together twenty years ago and I like his degree of comfort when talking with acutely and severely ill people. He knows how to engage them in conversation, but he also knows to listen to his gut when it tells him to be careful.

"I bet you're here to see Georges. We knew you'd be by. The team wants your advice about what to do about his meds."

Finding a computer terminal without an occupant, I look at the recent entries on Georges' electronic health record. He was calm during the evening and slept overnight but engaged little with the staff, not speaking at all. He has not eaten a thing or taken any fluids since being brought up from the ER. The ACU attending psychiatrist saw him late yesterday. The progress note reads,

> Patient seen and history reviewed. He is well known to CAMH for a long-standing diagnosis of schizophrenia, paranoid type, and has missed his last several depot injections. Collateral information obtained confirmed a characteristic pattern of relapse, with severe social withdrawal, suspiciousness, deterioration in self-care, not eating. Repeated efforts to engage patient in discussion of his symptoms, illness and treatment met with silence. In view of clear decompensation and inability to engage in dialogue, Dr. Goldbloom declared the patient incapable of consent to treatment; Rights Adviser has been notified and brother already contacted as substitute decision maker.

Georges' file tells me that the rights adviser paid a visit early this morning and Georges wouldn't speak with him either, which means there will be no appeal of the finding and treatment can begin with substitute consent.

I head toward Georges' room, a mere ten feet across from the nursing station, and knock on its closed sliding door.

Just as I am about to let myself in, the overhead public address system throughout the hospital announces, "Your attention, please. Code White, fifth floor, ACU. Code White, fifth floor, ACU."

Within seconds, a stream of people, including three security guards, enters the unit and gathers by the patient's room at the end of the row. Through the open door I see the patient whom I had noticed earlier sitting with Rhonda. Now he is rocking back and forth on his feet, shouting a volley of obscenities. The object of his wrath is Rhonda, who is now trapped at the window of his room. His hand is clenched in a fist, and he is shaking it in front of her face.

"Mike, you need to put your arm down," Rhonda says calmly, making eye contact with him. "Mike, I know you're upset, but I also know you don't want to hurt anyone. These staff members who just came to your door, they're here to help make sure that no one gets hurt."

The three security guards move to the front of the growing throng. Mike pauses for a moment, looking confused. He doesn't say anything but brings his fist closer to his own body. He keeps rocking.

Behind me at the nursing station, Jose draws up two syringes filled with medication, one a sedative and the other an antipsychotic. He already has some pills prepared in a small white paper cup, so that Mike can be offered the option of oral medication to help him calm down. A nurse from the adjacent general psychiatry unit brings an athletic bag that contains a set of restraints to just outside Mike's door. Finally, the seclusion room next door is unlocked and made ready. Thus, the five pathways used to calm an aggressive patient – verbal de-escalation, seclusion, physical restraint, chemical restraint, and mechanical restraint (with straps) – are all in place within a minute, although the direction this particular Code White will take remains unclear.

Nurses from other units move all patients and their visitors who are within the immediate vicinity of Mike's room away, escorting them back to their rooms or to the television area at the opposite end of the unit.

Jose moves toward Mike's room and hands the medication cup to Woody, who has inserted himself inside the door about two arm's lengths from Mike. Woody takes over the conversation, and Mike moves his attention from Rhonda to the door where Woody stands.

"Mike. You remember me. I'm Woody, the nurse in charge today. We met this morning. We were talking about the Toronto Maple Leafs and their lousy season. I agree with your nurse, Rhonda. We're here to help you settle down and to make sure no one gets hurt, especially you and Rhonda. I have some medication to help you calm down so we can talk about whatever it was that upset you. I'm going to hand you the medicine, and I want you to put it under your tongue. It's loxapine and lorazepam; you've had them both before and they helped you."

Woody slowly holds out the paper cup containing the medication. Mike takes the cup, and for a moment it looks as though he is going to take the medication. But after staring at the tablets for a moment, he throws them on the ground in front of Rhonda and once again brandishes his fist at her. Woody signals to the security guards to come in.

"Okay, Mike. We're going to move you toward your bed. This isn't a safe situation anymore for you or Rhonda. We're going to lay you down and give you some medication in a needle to help you settle."

As Woody talks, his voice invariably clear but low pitched, the three security guards and two nurses move swiftly to surround Mike. They each take one of his limbs, and one his head, while Woody continues to talk slowly, telling Mike what is happening to him at each step as he is lifted on to the bed.

"You fucking bastards!" Mike yells. "I'll sue every one of you. I'm calling the cops." He wriggles against the grips of five people, but not in a sustained way.

A nurse has taken the restraints out of the restraint bag, and she and a colleague apply one to each limb, strapping Mike to the bed so the injection can be given safely. As the restraints are secured, he becomes less agitated, even before getting any medication.

Woody continues to talk quietly and is now able to make eye contact as well. "Mike, no one's trying to hurt you. You're in hospital, remember. Our job is to help you feel better, more in control. As soon as you can get control of your behavior, we can get you out of the restraints. We're giving you the medication by needle to help you calm down and get back control. You're about to feel a sharp pinch in your right butt cheek. The medication will take a couple of minutes to work, but then you're going to feel a whole lot calmer. Once you're able to take control of your behavior again, we'll be able to take you out of the restraints. And then you and Rhonda and your doctor will go over what got you so upset. You're safe here in the hospital. You're here because you're ill. No one's going to hurt you. It's our job to look after you. One of our staff is going to be here with you the whole time in case you need anything. In a minute, when the restraints are completely fixed, I'm going to get you some ice chips to moisten your mouth; it looks dry to me."

Rhonda, finally free to move now that Mike is no longer blocking her exit, is in the nursing station. Through the Plexiglas I can see her drop onto a chair and put her head between her knees. One of the Code White team goes to her and suggests that the two of them leave the unit for a bit.

Woody also leaves Mike's room and asks the unit clerk to call the switchboard and announce that the code is over.

"Thanks, everyone," he says to the Code White team. "I think we're good here now. Well done. We'll debrief in a couple of minutes."

Moments later, the public address system offers the coda: "Your attention, please. Code White, fifth floor, ACU, all clear. Code White, fifth floor, ACU, all clear."

Across the unit, I can see Luana curled up at the head of her bed, with her mother seated beside her, cupping her daughter's hands in her own. They both look shocked. Despite all the rationales and justifications, there is something inescapably upsetting about a Code White for everyone involved – patients, visitors caught up in the code, and staff. It takes place in a hospital, where people are supposed to get care, support, and treatment. The Code White follows a set of policies and procedures, it relies on staff being well trained, and it is closely scrutinized by hospital authorities, but it nevertheless may close with a physical confrontation – albeit a controlled one aimed at avoiding a far worse outcome. Code Whites occur every week at my hospital because of the patients with moderate to severe mental illness treated here. I hope advances in psychiatric treatment and care can one day get us to a lower frequency, but I have not seen a significant decrease in my time there.

Staying calm during a Code White or during the events that can precipitate one is important for the staff as well as for the patient. There are jobs to be done – one person who knows the patient best to speak calmly with him or her while others monitor the safety of the environment, move other patients away, draw up medications for oral use or intramuscular injection, and prepare a stretcher with mechanical restraints if needed. Our security staff, who are well trained and tend to be on the beefy side, respond quickly to the Code White call, as do many of the clinical staff throughout the hospital. It's always reassuring to tell people they are not needed and send them away, as a large crowd can also be intimidating for patients. I still leave outpatients sitting in my office when a Code White is called, typically returning in less than five minutes because the situation is in hand.

Code Whites are not prolonged standoffs. While the staff tries to offer patients a choice of ways to calm down, sometimes the situation dictates that several people simultaneously rush the patient to prevent him or her from striking out. Time seems to slow down when you're holding the arm of someone who is trying to break free, swearing at you, and threatening you – but in reality it is often all over in less than a minute, almost always without injury to patients or staff. All staff members have mandatory training in Code White responses. The best leaders of Code Whites communicate clearly, unequivocally, and respectfully to patients what is going to happen each step of the way. For people who are confused, frightened, or angry, this clarity is crucial. The legal framework that permits the kind of institutional response entailed in a Code White is similar throughout the developed world. There are only two consistent legal rationales for using restraints: the patient is doing something that places him or her at imminent risk of bodily harm or something that puts another person at the same level of risk. Similarly, the use of medication in such circumstances, known as chemical restraint but in reality the beginning of a form of treatment, can be given without the consent of a patient or of the patient's substitute decision maker only for the same reasons. While the law seems clear, it can be tricky in practice; the health-care staff members have to predict at what point violence is inevitable without restraint, while intervening before it actually occurs. In Mike's case this happened when he threw the pills on the floor and raised his fist toward his nurse.

A recent World Health Organization study found that many countries still lack national mental health legislation to protect the rights of individuals with mental illness.[10] Without such laws, there is nothing to guarantee that psychiatric patients will not be restrained arbitrarily or unnecessarily. In addition, in a significant number of the countries that do have national mental health legislation, it has not been updated since the 1960s and does not include the same safeguards for patients as more recently passed laws. China notably passed its first mental health laws in May 2013, for the first time putting limits on the use of seclusion and restraint, forbidding involuntary psychiatric treatment as a punishment for individuals without a diagnosed psychiatric illness, and guaranteeing patients the right to communicate with the outside world.[11]

In countries with advanced mental health systems, the people with responsibility for carrying out the legislation – mental health workers and professionals in other fields that deal with mentally ill or potentially violent individuals – are usually trained in so-called de-escalation techniques, the goal of which is to avoid the use of physical force. They are also taught to recognize markers that indicate that de-escalation efforts have not been successful and that they will need to move swiftly to restrain the aggressive person. The three stages routinely described in de-escalation training are verbal engagement with the patient, an attempt to establish a collaborative relationship and, finally, verbal de-escalation from the agitated state. The focus is on helping the person perceived to be a threat to reestablish self-control. Both patients and staff are less likely to get hurt when physical confrontation is avoided.[12]

In Mike's case, Rhonda recognized that his increasing physical agitation was a signal that she was not going to be able to talk him down, and that she was at risk of being punched. She called out for help, and her colleagues sprang into action, activating a Code White. Woody took over as lead for the code, recognizing that Rhonda had reached the limit of her ability to appear unruffled. He tried once more to de-escalate the situation in the hope that the increased number of people might signal to Mike that it was contained. Once it became clear to Woody that he too was out of time to resolve things without force, he moved swiftly to get Rhonda out of Mike's range, and to subdue Mike as efficiently and nontraumatically as possible.

At all times Woody sounded calm and empathic to Mike's plight. He consistently predicted to Mike his ability to regain control of himself. Once it was clear Mike would not take the offered medications by mouth, the only alternative was to give them by injection to decrease his agitation. An agitated patient in physical restraints constitutes a potentially dangerous situation at multiple levels; paranoia may be reinforced by the experience of being restrained, and fighting against the restraints can lead to soft tissue injury. Finally, Woody promised Mike that he would have a chance to address the source of his initial upset as soon as he was out of restraints and able to conduct a conversation from a less stressful position. Unfortunately, in this case the use of restraints was necessary on a number of levels, but in my view the situation had been handled relatively well.

While I had been a few feet away the entire time, and ready to assist, this was not my Code White. I was an observer of a team working smoothly together, well choreographed and fluid. With the unit returned to calm, it's clear that I am not needed. I turn my attention to Georges.

I open the door to his room. Georges is sitting at the head of his bed, his arms around his drawn-up legs.

"*Comment ça va, Georges?*" I say, sitting down at the foot of the bed.

He nods noncommittally, but at least it's a response.

"I'm sorry you had to see that. You probably remember your own Code White, when you first got ill in Toronto, before you got to know us all. As I recall, you thought we were all trying to send you back to the Congo."

He nods again but doesn't respond verbally.

"How did you sleep last night? Have you eaten?"

Sleep has never been an issue for Georges, in and out of the hospital, psychotic or well. While some people with psychosis stop sleeping, that has never been part of Georges' pattern. In his case, my asking about his sleep is more of a social question, one that is unlikely to tell me much about how he is doing clinically, but it allows me to establish some normalcy for him and shows my interest in his well-being.

"I have not eaten." Eating, on the other hand, is an excellent bellwether for Georges' mental health.

"Can you tell me why?"

"I don't know."

"Is it not safe? Are you afraid of the food? Is anyone telling you not to eat?"

"Perhaps. Religious men. I see them on the street. They do not want me to eat."

"Do you hear them inside this room?"

"Yes. I think so."

"If you could eat, what would you like?"

"Maybe McChicken," Georges eventually offers.

He always requests this when his psychosis intensifies. He then eats the same thing twice a day for a couple of weeks before stopping eating altogether. The sequence has repeated itself with every relapse of his illness. I have no idea what it is about McChicken that establishes its safety for Georges, at least initially. In contrast to some of my patients over the years who have suffered from paranoia about being poisoned or who were obsessional about germs, who were reassured by food that was hermetically sealed, Georges' dietary choices when he is ill are less comprehensible. McChicken is acceptable but not Big Macs, and chicken sandwiches from other fast-food chains do not meet his standards for safety. Over the years, Georges' brand loyalty has caused some stress for staff trying to persuade him to resume eating, especially since there is no McDonald's near the hospital.

"Georges, do you know why this is happening to you again?"

"No."

"It's your illness, Georges. You and I have seen this before. Georges, you need some medication and food to get well again. The doctor and nurses here need to give you some pills as well as the injection you missed. This has always helped you get better."

"I don't know."

"I do know, Georges. Will you trust me?"

"Perhaps."

I return to the nursing station, where Woody is writing up the report of the Code White. He looks up and asks for an update on Georges.

"He's still psychotic, of course. Not eating and still paranoid. He thinks he is hearing the religious men again, even here," I say. "But I think he'll take meds – and at least he mentioned McChicken."

"I could get him one on my lunch break," Woody offers. "I'll head down to Dundas and Bathurst. There's a McDonald's there."

I thank him and suggest that if Georges starts eating, the team ask the hospital kitchen what they can do to get him food he'll eat. I explain that when Georges is in this state, he's not agitated but withdrawn. If the team can get him eating, coming out of his room, and talking a bit, they may be able to engage him in talking about his need for medication.

"I'd like to try to get it into him without a struggle. His brother in Belgium has provided substitute consent for treatment. Once he's back on his meds, he should be able to transfer out of ACU in a couple of days."

I add that it will be important to have one of his community workers come to see him.

"We need to reconnect him with them. And someone should call his landlord just to make sure there's no danger of his being evicted."

I hope that we're not too late; his landlord has known Georges for years and likes him. But you never know; sometimes when Georges is like this, the food he won't eat rots in the apartment and the other tenants complain.

Georges is fortunate in his landlord, who has put up with a tenant who, when ill, isolates himself for weeks at a time, keeps bottles of urine and rotting food in his room, and stops bathing. Georges' landlord sees his tenants, many of whom are down on their luck, as a vocation. Not all people with chronic mental illness are so lucky. For most landlords, providing spiritual support and housing to society's less fortunate, particularly those prone to unpredictable outbursts or bizarre housekeeping practices, is not part of the business plan. The latter, as a result, all too frequently end up in run-down flophouses or shelters, or on the street.

You don't need any health-care training to recognize the countless mentally ill individuals among the homeless huddled in dirty sleeping bags on city streets. It has been reported that up to 67 percent of people who are homeless have a history of mental illness.[13] In Canada, the world's largest research action project on mental illness and homelessness, funded to the tune of $110 million by the federal government, confirmed and expanded upon the findings of a previous study in New York City that demonstrated the value of providing housing before any other treatment. Participants who were randomized to "housing first," a form of immediate, stable, and rent-subsidized housing, mostly maintained a stable residence and experienced improvement in quality of life and their ability to function in their communities.[14] For those who were housed, it translated into less time spent in jails, shelters, and emergency rooms, all very expensive places to be.

But what Georges needs immediately from the ACU is the careful support, treatment, and monitoring that its high staff-to-patient ratio can provide. Beyond keeping track of his food and liquid intake, and making sure he gets his medication, they engage him in conversation that pulls him away from the internal world that preoccupies him. His illness endangers his physical health but doesn't threaten others. And if this episode mirrors the previous ones, within a matter of days his psychosis will start to recede, and his engagement with food and the world will resume incrementally. It's discouraging to see him ill again, but his capacity to recover has so far never let him down.

I leave electronic tracks of my visit by typing a note in his chart on the computer and then tell Woody my latest Newfoundland joke. Ten feet away from us, Mike is still in restraints and now deeply asleep from his injection. The restraints will be removed after he wakes up and is assessed by the nurses.

As I pass Luana's room on my way out, I see that she and her mother are now playing cards. I ask Jose, Luana's nurse this shift, if I should say hello.

"I wouldn't recommend it," he says. "She had difficulty falling asleep last night after she came up from the ER and was verbally abusive to a number of staff, stopping just short of triggering a Code White." He reports that today has been better after she met with doctors this morning and agreed to take medication.

"Seeing you might wind her up again," he says. "Maybe tomorrow, Dr. G. After she has had another good night's sleep. It was nice she was able to have a shower this morning, and now she is having a visit with her mother. Yesterday when she came up from the ER, we had to tell her mother she wasn't ready for a visit. When her mother tried to speak to her on the phone last night, she exploded at her, swearing and telling her she had to get her out of here. Today she's better, calmer. Happy to see her mother."

I am in awe of the power of sleep, even medication-induced, to calm the fury of mania. It takes the foot off the gas pedal, sometimes quickly, and I hope that will be the case for Luana. That's the beauty of the ACU from both a therapeutic and a learning perspective: sometimes a day or two can witness a huge difference.

I LEAVE THE ACU via the locked doors to the hallway. As they click behind me, I think of the decade of my professional life that happened within its confined space. I have had a number of conversations with ACU staff over the years about what it is that draws us to this work. There is no doubt the rewards can be great. A patient who is convinced on arrival that he is being kept in the hospital by a government conspiracy to silence him and that the hospital food is poisoned leaves after a couple of weeks with his wits about him, trusting us enough to accept that his delusions are the product of illness and agreeing to work with another hospital treatment team. A chronically depressed woman hospitalized after taking a bottle of antidepressants washed down with vodka is nursed back to a point where she is willing to entertain the possibility that she may have a future. These are reasons to come to work.

The pace of recovery in the ACU is as much a pull for those who like working here as the extent of recovery that can be achieved. Although people arrive in the throes of severe illness, the rapidity and extent of the improvement are often dramatic, much to the relief of the patient, the family, and the staff. With milder mental illnesses, improvement tends to be gradual or involve adapting to the reality of living with a chronic disease. Patients in the ACU are in great distress, but they're also in great need. Being able to provide calm, reassuring support and explanation in the midst of their fear, chaos, and uncertainty is the first step toward establishing the trust that is necessary for successful treatment. Medications are a critical factor in the pace of recovery, but they represent a tiny fraction of the time staff spend with patients.

IT WAS THE LOOMING SHADOW of my father-in-law, Nate, that inspired me to pursue the intensity and acuity of patients I found in the ACU. He regaled me with stories of his training sixty years earlier, when he was in charge of a ward of hundreds of patients in a Boston hospital. The treatment of schizophrenia at that time, in the pre-antipsychotic era, was based on psychoanalytic principles. At case conferences, treating physicians described the great progress patients were making. But Nate quickly learned to trust the clinical appraisal of the seasoned orderlies who spent far more time with the patients, who plainly confirmed that in spite of such heady evaluations of the impact of psychoanalytic interpretations, the patients were no better. Nate was a team leader who knew how to make people feel valued without a phony abandonment of hierarchy. He was never reluctant to call people on what he labeled "bullshit," both within our profession and beyond. And he clearly loved engaging with patients.

And yet I wasn't him. I was more conciliatory, more conflict-avoidant, more ingratiating. None of these qualities struck me as simply different when I was younger – just inferior. He had a toughness that was simply not in my DNA (except for that contributed by my mother, so there may have been something in the drinking water of New Waterford).

In one sense I resembled Nate closely. ACUs are not for the decision-averse. Clinicians need to be able to size up situations quickly, live with the inevitable ambiguity, take chances, and tolerate regrets.

They need to thrive on turnover and variety and be drawn to action and illness severity. The intensity can make for cohesive teams. The clinical encounters are memorable, especially for students, often with a social science background, who enter psychiatry skeptical that mental illness is more than a variant of normal. These students leave with much less doubt.

Working in the ACU suited me for a whole bunch of reasons. I liked the immediate reward when patients recovered quickly, both for them and for me. In addition to the speed of improvement, there was the severity of symptoms. It may seem odd that this would be alluring, but I didn't think my forte was in treating people who are derisively described as "the worried well." I don't agree with the pejorative use of the term; I don't believe people go to the effort of seeking psychiatric help for insignificant symptoms or idle intellectual curiosity. They do so because they are in distress even if they are still able to function. At the same time, I am drawn to the more acute and dramatic psychiatric diagnoses, as some internal medicine specialists prefer to work in intensive care settings rather than in clinics or on general medicine inpatient units peopled by the elderly and chronically ill. I also like the ACU because I have a low tolerance for being alone – at work or at home. Working with a team is, for me, much more fun than working on my own with a patient, more of a chance to teach, to learn, to connect, to lead.

But one has to be able to tolerate the losses – the suicides, the patients who leave only to be brought back by police within forty-eight hours of discharge, having snorted away their hard-won sanity on a crack cocaine binge. And the violence, threatened or actual. Not daily but often enough. Unlike most of the population of psychiatric patients who pose more of a risk to themselves than to others, the ACU patient population can be unpredictably aggressive. Some of the staff here have healed injuries and scars to show for the inevitable chances one takes with volatile people who are ill. Like any acute care team, the ACU group has its coping strategies: black humor and a camaraderie that comes from knowing that most people would think you are insane to do your job. I liked (and miss) those aspects too.

I have had times in ACU when I was really scared – the kind of nauseated scared as a scene seems to be unfolding in front of you and you're helpless to control it. I was standing in the middle of the ACU one day when a large, muscular man strode up to me. He had been admitted three days earlier in the midst of a psychosis triggered by illegal steroid use; he was competing in the local preliminaries of a Mr. Universe body-building contest. He believed in the thick of his illness that he was the product of genetic engineering by Dr. Josef Mengele, the infamous Nazi physician who committed medical atrocities. He was suspicious of me as a doctor and as a Jew. That morning, he jabbed his finger in my chest.

"I'm on to you, Doctor. I know *exactly* what you're up to."

I saw the PA perk up at the nursing station and get ready to move.

"Let me tell you something, Doctor. There will be letters about you. I know your game. I will send letters – to *Hustler*, *Penthouse*, *Mayfair*, and *Playboy*. Because let me tell you something, Dr. Rosenbloom. I REMEMBER YOUR NAME."

"That's right," I replied, relieved that his response to my perceived threat was a series of letters to men's skin magazines. "My name is R-O-S-E-N-B-L-O-O-M."

There was no Code White, just a brief encounter. It was repeated a few days later when, after his psychosis had resolved as quickly as it started, he once again strode across the floor of the ACU toward me. As he got near, he opened his arms. I tensed up, thinking, "Oh, shit," fearing that unlike three days earlier I might not get off with a warning letter. This guy easily could have decked me. Then he enveloped me in a huge bear hug (I almost disappeared among his many layers of well-defined muscle). He wanted to say good-bye and thanks.

Staff do burn out or choose to leave in order to see a dimension of mental health care different from the confined environment of the ACU, which lacks exposure to patients' longitudinal journey through illness and recovery. Those individuals tend to move into jobs in the community or even to leave mental health altogether.

I have noticed that in psychiatry the most difficult inpatient work tends to be done by the newest psychiatrists in a department. Bright young people fresh out of their residencies and looking for work will be offered the Acute Care Unit or inpatient beds as a foothold from which to climb their way into an academic center or a community hospital. Many of them leave these initial jobs as soon as they have paid their dues, moving on to less stressful and less high-risk work.

The ACU once consumed me in a different way from my outpatient clinical work now. Most evenings, I would call in for a rundown on how the patients I had seen that day were doing – because in the acute throes of their illnesses, dramatic changes for better or worse could occur within hours. Each morning at eight o'clock, our team would huddle to go over the latest clinical updates and to decide which patients we needed to see first.

It had felt good to be there today. To see Luana and Georges taking the first steps out of their psychotic isolation, and to reconnect with the staff with whom I used to share my working life. Today, it was the perfect distraction. But maybe – like squash – it is a younger person's game.

9

Off the Path

As I eat lunch and answer emails, I feel discombobulated, off balance. Something about my morning's visit to the ACU with its memories of my life ten years ago – arguably the time when my professional life was at its busiest, most focused, and most intense – has unsettled me in its contrast to the distractedness I feel this week. I can't reach beneath the sensation to the underlying emotion or, more accurately, I decide I have neither time nor inclination to probe more deeply.

My first appointment of the afternoon is with Mark Blair. I met him last week at an evening session for parents at one of Toronto's private schools, where I spoke about mental health, adolescence, and young adulthood. The evening was coordinated by my hospital's charitable foundation; the school made a donation to the hospital in thanks for the event. The purposes of these evenings are twofold – awareness-raising and fund-raising (an uphill battle for a psychiatric hospital compared to a children's hospital). The reality of modern hospitals is that they are permanently on campaigns for donor support.

Of the forty-odd presentations I do each year, a number are public awareness sessions for specific audiences – schools, workplaces, health-care facilities. They are not detailed academic presentations about a particular disorder. Instead, they are plain-language talks about the breadth and reality of mental illness, stigma, and hope. They address some of the challenges of entirely normal behavior as well as the reality of mental illness.

I try to ensure that they include a copresenter, usually a young person who can talk about his or her own illness and recovery. Usually these presentations have far more impact than mine, and it is important to me that I don't perpetuate the problem of physicians talking *for* their patients rather than *with* them. In the same way current medical practice tends to work best as a partnership between health-care professional and patient, so does fund-raising and research, albeit at a community rather than an individual level. The slogan "Nothing about us without us" has become the rallying cry for the active engagement of people with mental illness and their families in the design, implementation, delivery, and evaluation of mental health services, and I agree with that view.

Humor helps these evenings. I joke about my own adolescence and that of our sons (especially now it's over), which seems to defuse some of the anxiety in the room. I assure the parents in the audience that their sons and daughters will eventually recover the ability to communicate in complete sentences rather than grunts, sighs, and eye rolls, and that it is the job of teens to keep their parents on a need-to-know basis about their personal lives, citing my own highly fictionalized accounts of my teenage activities to my parents – who undoubtedly saw through the ruse.

Following the formal presentation, there is always an hour for discussion. Some parents raise their hands and ask questions, often courageously disclosing their own struggles or, without names, those of their children. Others take advantage of index cards on which they write their questions to preserve their anonymity. At one talk at a

Catholic high school for boys, I faced an audience of two hundred parents and a phalanx of priests in the back row, their arms crossed and their brows furrowed. Without prescreening them, I read aloud the first audience question submitted on an index card: "Should my wife and I tell our son about our own experience with premarital sex?" This was not, of course, fundamentally a psychiatric question, but as I lifted my eyes from the card after reading it aloud, my gaze met those of the priests. I paused.

"Well, honesty is the best policy," I said. "And it is much easier to tell the truth than to sustain a lie. However, if one of you says we did and the other says we didn't, what does that say about how memorable the experience was?"

The laugh allowed me to quickly move on to the next question.

The night I met Mark I was tired from a long day. Still, I had my usual surge of adrenaline as I looked out at the audience, so I don't think my fatigue was obvious. Afterward, as I returned to my table amid polite applause, I observed that the tall man seated beside me, wearing an obviously expensive gray suit, looked as tired as I felt. He was distracted by frequent texts on his wafer-thin smartphone. I assumed that he was in one of those financial jobs where his international colleagues cross all time zones, ensuring he will get minimal sleep, and that he was answering their business emails.

He looked up and saw me watching him. "My wife. Our fifteen-year-old is giving her a hard time. I may have to go."

I nodded sympathetically. "It can be a tough age."

"It certainly is for us. You made some good points tonight. Especially the one that mental illness affects every family at one time or another. I heard you talk a couple of years ago at the bank where I work. You were discussing psychiatric illness and how frequently it starts in teenagers."

He moved his chair closer to mine, seemingly having made some sort of decision. "My kid's a mess. We had to call the police last week after he'd punched a hole in the wall and threatened Jane, my wife.

He's been kicked out of his last three schools and we're not sure how long this one's going to last. He's skipped an entire semester to smoke dope with his buddies. Our house is a war zone. God knows what our neighbors think. Jane's taken a leave from her job. Every time I have to go out of town I'm a basket case, not knowing if everyone's going to be in one piece when I get back."

I murmured something about how sorry I was to hear about his son, but he barely stopped for breath. "And your lot. Can't say I have much good to say. The first shrink we saw said it was ADHD and put him on stimulants. The meds turned him into a skeleton who never slept. We've seen lots of other people – psychiatrists, therapists. Then we took him to our local emergency room one night when he was just out of control and they referred us to the psychiatrist he's seeing now. She initially thought it was all anxiety and suggested adding cognitive behavioral therapy and wanted us to go to family therapy. Sam wouldn't come to the family therapy but went to the CBT for a while. He said it was okay and helped a bit, but not enough, so then the psychiatrist wanted him to take Prozac, which maybe helped, maybe didn't, but Sam wouldn't continue to take it because it made him sweat all the time. This psychiatrist's the best of the lot, but even she says she can't rule out bipolar, especially since my wife's brother is a bad manic-depressive. She said we won't know for sure until Sam stops doing the drugs."

He gulped some wine.

"I don't mean to be rude, Goldbloom, but why can't your lot get your act together and give us some real answers? Jane and I can't make head or tail of all the different labels they give him, not to mention the meds. Jane's done a lot of reading, and she says even the psychiatrists don't really know what's going on with a kid like Sam . . . Is that true?"

As Mark's voice rose, people around the table began looking at us. I noticed that his wineglass was empty, having been refilled just a few minutes ago.

"It sounds really hard." I paused before saying anything else, realizing if I did that I was committed to at least another half hour before I could head home, but said it anyway. "How are you coping?"

Mark leaned back in his chair. "We're not, frankly," he says, then goes on to tell me that after they called 911 a week earlier, the police called Children's Aid, which he found humiliating.

Whatever worry, anger, or sense of ineptitude I had experienced as a parent didn't come anywhere near the intensity of what Mark was describing, but I recognized the feeling – of shame that as a parent you haven't behaved in the way you know you are supposed to, that your child is in trouble and you don't seem to be able to help. Beneath Mark's anger at a mental health system that had so far failed his son and him, it was easy to see that he was floundering and desperate.

"Why don't you come to see me in my office? We can talk more there about what's been going on, and I may be able to suggest some resources for you and your wife." I was careful not to say anything medical about his son. These parents were clearly confused enough by the multiple diagnoses their son had received, and they didn't need a helpful, albeit informed, stranger muddying the waters even more. I took my card out of my wallet and handed it to him, not sure if he would follow up.

He took it and looked at the printed contact information for a long minute before putting it in his jacket pocket. I sensed his ambivalence about having opened up to me.

"I may just do that. Jane keeps telling me I'll have a heart attack if I keep going like this, and that I need to talk to someone. I just don't see it helping. But thank you for the offer and for not just getting rid of me; this must happen to you all the time at these things."

He was right. I do get approached after these talks by people seeking clinical assessment and treatment, and I don't usually comply. But something worried me about Mark that I couldn't put my finger on, hence my offer. I know it takes a lot for a man like Mark, even with a few glasses of wine in him, to ask for help, and I wanted to make sure that he didn't regret it. In addition, I don't like feeling that my colleagues and I are perceived as useless. While I knew I couldn't fix this man's son, I hoped that I might be able to give him some tools that would allow him to ride out his boy's troubled adolescence.

He called Simone the day after our meeting to book a time to see me.

TODAY, A WEEK LATER, courtesy of a cancellation, Mark walks into my office. He seems taller than he did at the fund-raiser, and better groomed, probably because he has not downed several glasses of wine before the appointment, definitely a good sign. I estimate that he must be about ten years younger than me. I'd thought he was younger at the fund-raiser, but in the daylight I can see that his abundant blond hair is gray at the temples. After thanking me for seeing him, Mark tells me he is not sure why he is here.

"When I told Jane I had talked to you and that you said I could come and see you, she jumped on it." He pauses. "I'm skeptical about this whole psychiatry thing, as you know. My father kicked me out of the house when I was seventeen, said if I wanted to put myself through university I was on my own. I worry that Sam's had it too easy, doesn't understand the value of things, that we've spoiled him."

I tell Mark that I appreciate his honesty. I remind him that his wariness about psychiatry is common. I explain that it can be difficult early on in a psychiatric illness to be entirely clear how it is going to develop and what it represents, and that my guess is that this uncertainty is part of why he and Jane have heard so many possibilities from doctors about what's led to Sam's difficulties.

He has relaxed back into his chair, so I seize the opportunity to see if I can ask him some questions about himself. I explain that my goal is to find out what he needs most urgently.

He laughs, and I see a glimpse of the warmth and self-deprecating humor that underlie his current distress. "Sure. Why not? In for a penny, in for a pound."

I begin the process of teasing out more details of Sam's troubles and their impact on Mark and his wife. I reflect on the fact that the guilt and self-doubt that characterize Mark's account are pretty much ubiquitous among parents of children with mental illness. There are very few medical illnesses that parents blame themselves for to the same extent. Purely genetic disorders or birth defects can be a source of guilt, as can childhood accidents and burns perhaps, and maybe a belief that a child with early onset diabetes was fed too much sugar, but these parents will soon be disabused of that idea by a treatment team. In contrast, parents of mentally ill children – and, sadly, many of their relatives, friends, colleagues, and even health-care professionals – assume that bad parenting is in large part to blame for the child's difficulties. My profession has done its fair share historically to contribute to this cruel and destructive perception, particularly early practitioners of Freudian psychoanalysis, who attributed the majority of psychic disturbances to unresolved conflicts in the parent-child relationship.

"Tell me about Sam as a kid," I say.

Mark tells me about his son's early years with an air of bafflement and loss. He was clearly an involved father – changing diapers, giving middle-of-the-night feeds when his son was an infant, and as Sam got older, coaching his soccer team and driving him to ice hockey practices.

"I think we were good parents, particularly Jane," he says. "She must have read hundreds of books about parenting. And she knew being a father was incredibly important to me. More important than my work."

As Mark pauses, I sense there's a contrast hanging in the air.

"I'd promised myself long before Sam was born that I wasn't going to be like my father, who left everything to my mother except the belt. I must have driven Sam to a thousand hockey games, all over the city, up until last year. I loved those drives. I miss them now that he won't play anymore. Says he can't be bothered, that it takes up too much of his time. Not that he's doing anything else, except endless video games. And smoking dope with his friends. He won't let me do anything for him except give him cash. And I won't do that anymore, knowing he'll spend it on drugs."

His wistful recollection of a lost relationship accentuates for me his current anger and frustration. He – and the whole family – need to be able to set expectations and limits and navigate through conflict. And to be relieved of guilt.

As though he can hear my thoughts, Mark starts to talk about his and his wife's experience of blame.

"One of the psychiatrists said that Sam seemed to have had a poor attachment to us when he was younger. Jane was devastated. After Jane gave me some articles to read about attachment, I told her that it was bullshit, that the doctor was going on a fishing expedition. Mostly it was because we'd told him that Sam was colicky as a baby and drove us crazy by not sleeping for the first year."

I grimace inwardly. My fellow residents and I learned about attachment theory during the mandatory child and adolescent rotation in our psychiatric residency training program, but its current usage has expanded far beyond its original conceptualization by the American-born (although raised and educated in Canada) psychologist Mary Ainsworth and the British psychoanalyst John Bowlby in the 1960s. Their theoretical model rooted personality development in the early relationships that infants have with their primary caregivers. The model's central conclusion – which was to have enormous influence on 1960s child-rearing practices – was that to grow up psychologically healthy, "the infant and young child should experience a warm, intimate, and continuous relationship with his mother (or permanent mother substitute) in which both find satisfaction and enjoyment."[1]

Previous child-rearing guides had been dominated by the influence of behaviorists, who advised that children developed according to environmental conditioning, a process that consisted of their learning to respond to positive and negative stimuli. The most famous of these guides was written by the behavioral psychologist John Watson, whose 1928 book *Psychological Care of Infant and Child* counseled parents, especially mothers, not to smother children with demonstrations of affection, as doing so would impair their developing self-reliance, both emotionally and practically.[2] One of its chapters even had the ominous title "The Danger of Too Much Mother Love."[3]

In Bowlby and Ainsworth's theoretical world, however, responsive, affectionate mothers provided children with the predictable availability that gave them the confidence to explore the wider world. What has been lost in translation over the decades since the pair's first publications is that Bowlby's emphasis was never solely on the parent-child relationship; he also emphasized the importance of social networks and economic and health factors as contributors to a healthy mother-child relationship. In a conclusion that anticipated Hillary Clinton, he wrote, "Just as children are absolutely dependent on their parents for sustenance, so in all but the most primitive communities are parents, especially their mothers, dependent on a greater society for economic provision. If a community values its children, it must cherish their parents."[4]

My mother, who had no time for theoretical models of parenting, nevertheless had an intuitive grasp of attachment theory. When she taught me to take the city bus, she did so by following me in her car for my first-ever ride when I was nine years old. She told me to sit near the driver and to tell him my stop, but she also told me if I was worried, to look out the back window of the bus and I would see her car there. I looked once; it was all the reassurance I needed. I think I realized at that point I was better off relying on the driver of the bus for guidance than the woman racing behind the bus in a powder-blue 1962 Hillman Minx convertible.

Decades after my first solitary bus ride, attachment theory has become the basis for a fascinating branch of neuroscientific research investigating how soothing or disruptive relationships shape our neurobiology. But those attachment theory proponents who see it as a reliable basis for assessment of parenting capacity or as an autonomous template for good parenting are taking it far beyond its authors' original claims. And for parents like Mark and Jane, who are already racked with guilt by the thought that Sam's problems lie with inadequate parenting, attachment theory becomes yet another whip that they can use to flog themselves.

"That first year with Sam's colic and no sleep must have been grim. How were things once it calmed down?" I ask.

"Sam's always been a challenge. Jane sometimes says that he just came out that way. He's always been more out there, acting without thinking first, needing to have his own way, whereas Rosie is more reserved and unflappable." Mark smiles as he describes their two children. "Jane and I used to say we each got a mini-me. I was just like Sam as a kid, always in trouble, always covered in scrapes and bruises. Jane's much calmer, thinks about things carefully, always does her research before she makes a decision. Rosie is turning out just like her."

It's interesting for me to hear Mark ponder his children's differences. It reflects my own experience as a parent: our two started with very different personalities and ways of being in the world that have continued through to adulthood. During my psychiatry residency, before I became a father, I had read and been impressed by the work of two American child psychiatrists working in the United States in the 1950s, Stella Chess and Alexander Thomas. They were the first researchers to study children's temperament in a systematic way, their work constituting a challenge to psychoanalysis' focus on the child-rearing environment as the primary determinant of a child's outcome. The New York Longitudinal Study of Child Temperament, begun in 1956, collected data on child-rearing practices and behaviors among 138 white middle-class children and 95 lower socioeconomic Puerto Rican children, from infancy to eight years of age. The children were interviewed by psychiatrists, and given sensory, neurological, psychological, and IQ testing.

Drawing on the data collected, Chess and Thomas described three temperamental patterns that were evident in approximately two-thirds of the children. Easy children, constituting 40 percent of the total, had regular biological rhythms (sleep, appetite, bowel movements, etc.), responded positively to new stimuli, and were highly adaptive in the face of changes. Difficult children, about 10 percent, were irregular in their biological rhythms, rejected new stimuli, were nonadaptive to change, and took a long time to adjust to new situations. These difficult children were easily frustrated, leading to tantrums. The third category, slow-to-warm-up children, about 15 percent, had mildly negative responses to new stimuli but slowly adapted with repeated exposure, coming to show positive interest and involvement. Unlike the difficult children, their reactions were milder, whether positive or negative, and their biological functions were less irregular. The remaining children in the study, about a third, showed a variety of behavioral styles, all appearing to be within normal limits.[5]

Chess and Thomas came to believe that psychiatric interventions should include a focus on the fit between parents' expectations and their child's temperament, and seek to modify conflict by providing parents with education and suggestions for how to recognize and adapt to their child's temperaments. For Mark and Jane's purposes in dealing with Sam, this might mean considering his daily rhythms – sleep, appetite, and bursts of energy – his comfort with strangers and new experiences, his ability to control impulses and to focus, and his relative needs for both personal space and physical contact in his relationships with his parents. Chess and Thomas' work challenged the idea of cookie-cutter parenting advice, pointing out that to be successful, different children require different responses from the adults in their lives. By pointing to how character traits present at birth might shape the relationship between parent and children, Chess and Thomas avoided the oversimplified dichotomy of nature versus nurture.

Mark pauses and pulls off his glasses as though tired of their weight before continuing. "I've wondered too about both kids suffering from how good we've had it economically. I've done well, no question. I've been lucky when some of my colleagues weren't. Even through 2008. So the kids have everything – private schools, camps, hockey, skiing, holidays in crazy places."

"I don't think for a second that your and Jane's generosity to your children has created Sam's struggles," I say. "In fact, the opposite is more likely true. Any studies that have looked at the relationship between a child's economic status at birth and developmental outcomes contradicts the belief – which is surprisingly common – that affluence automatically spoils children. A better way to think about this is that you and Jane have the financial resources to help Sam to get the treatment and education he needs." I understand Mark's guilt about affluence and the concern about its impact on values. But there is an equal problem in ennobling poverty as a moral classroom for children.

Professor Michael Rutter, an eminent British child psychiatry researcher, spent his career trying to understand how social and economic factors affect children's mental health. After training as a neurologist and pediatrician, Rutter elected to work with Chess and Thomas during a self-funded sabbatical year in New York, subsequently becoming the first professor in child psychiatry to be appointed in the United Kingdom. Until his retirement, he was head of the Department of Child and Adolescent Psychiatry at the Institute of Psychiatry, London.

Rutter led the largest long-term follow-up study of children's mental health of its time, the Isle of Wight Studies. The entire population of ten- to twelve-year-olds living on the Isle of Wight was surveyed initially in 1964 for evidence of psychiatric disorders and physical handicaps, and again in 1969. A follow-up study comparing Isle of Wight children with ten-year-olds living in an inner-city London borough found that the children living in London had a rate of psychiatric disorder twice that of the island children,[6] a finding that Rutter attributed – after rigorous statistical analysis of other possible contributing factors – to the higher proportion of poor families in London compared to the Isle of Wight.[7]

Inspired by Rutter, researchers in other countries have also used epidemiological surveys to shed light on the impact of social and economic factors on children's developmental outcomes. One of the largest, the Adverse Childhood Experiences (ACE) Study, sponsored by the Centers for Disease Control and Prevention in the United States, links a wide variety of adverse childhood experiences such as poverty, neglect and abuse, and family dysfunction to the risk of later health problems. Outcomes as diverse as alcoholism, depression, ischemic heart disease, unintended pregnancies, and liver disease, among others, have all been shown to be more likely in people who have experienced adverse childhood experiences.[8]

I don't have an easy answer for Mark about what has caused his son's difficulties. I see epidemiological studies such as Rutter's work and the ACE as providing a treasure map, with theoretical models based on attachment, temperament, socioeconomic and psychological adversity, and variations in brain development all providing possible routes. There are likely many more. The treasure itself, of course, is a credible research base that will provide us with a comprehensive scientific understanding of healthy personality development and its potential roadblocks.

A new field of science with which I have become fascinated in recent years – epigenetics – may be that treasure. The term was coined by the British developmental biologist Conrad Waddington in the early 1940s, who described epigenetics as "the branch of biology which studies the causal interactions between genes and their products which bring the phenotype [all of the organism's observable characteristics] into being."[9] My hospital is home to Art Petronis, one of the world's leading researchers in what has become a burgeoning field. A tall, enthusiastic Lithuanian immigrant, he and I have talked about our common heritage in that Baltic country – except for the fact that my family fled to Canada more than one hundred years before he moved here, and for reasons of persecution rather than research career advancement! Some years after Art introduced me to this field, my book club of grumpy middle-aged guys decided to read a book on epigenetics by the science writer and virologist Nessa Carey.

Carey describes this new area of science in real-world terms: "Whenever two genetically identical individuals are non-identical in some way we can measure, this is epigenetics. When a change in environment has biological consequences that last long after the event itself has vanished into distant memory, we are seeing epigenetic effect in action."[10] Our old ways of thinking about genes were that they were our immutable destiny. But except for relatively rare disorders, genes simply increase or decrease potential for disorders, and environmental factors can turn genes on and off. Both the uterine environment and early social experiences appear to have direct influence on the epigenome and thereby contribute to cognition and behavior. The rapid neuronal growth, organization, and plasticity seen in adolescent brains suggests that epigenetic processes may also play an active role during this developmental stage.[11] In my limited understanding, epigenetics may one day lead us to discover the physiological pathways by which adversity and environmental insults may destroy a child's opportunity to live the life he or she was initially offered by nature, and perhaps even facilitate our learning how to prevent such distortions from becoming permanent. If our DNA is the seed that defines our biological potential or nature, and if our environments and relationships are the landscape of nurture, then epigenetics holds hope for explaining their interaction in a way that moves us meaningfully beyond either/or. But we still have a long way to go.

Mark brings me back to the present with a question that exposes one of child psychiatry's current challenges, one that raises questions of fads, diagnostic legitimacy, and potentially toxic treatment.

"What do you think about Sam's psychiatrist's suggestion that he may have an underlying bipolar disorder? I gather there's no test, no brain scan that will tell you. I don't understand how such a serious diagnosis can depend on the docs talking to Sam and to us, and simply waiting to see what happens."

I pause, aware I am stepping onto very thin ice. Childhood bipolar disorder is arguably the psychiatric diagnosis over which mental health professionals currently disagree the most. The source of the disagreement is not what laypeople sometimes imagine: a misdiagnosis of ordinary adolescent Sturm und Drang. Rather it is an academic debate (one with significant real-world impact) over whether very young children with oppositional and explosive behaviors, frequently found together with attention problems, are experiencing an early form of bipolar disorder, a variant of ADHD, or simply significant moodiness and relational patterns that may require some kind of intervention but stop short of the sustained, wide and deep mood swings characteristic of adult bipolar disorder. These three diagnostic possibilities require very different treatments and have very different outcomes. Of the three, the diagnosis of bipolar disorder has been much in vogue in recent years, especially in the United States, where children as young as three to five years of age have been treated with antipsychotic medication for a putative diagnosis of mania.

I explain to Mark that the diagnosis of early childhood bipolar disorder is largely the brainchild of Dr. Joseph Biederman, a brilliant Harvard clinician and researcher. In a 1995 article written with his colleague Janet Wozniak, Biederman widely popularized the new concept of pediatric bipolar disorder, asserting that manic symptoms occurred in a significant number of children under the age of twelve who had previously been diagnosed with ADHD.[12] Skepticism about the validity of the diagnosis within and beyond the profession was amplified in 2008 when Biederman was reported to have failed to disclose funds amounting to $1.6 million given to him and his research institute between 2000 and 2007 by drug companies, including Johnson & Johnson, maker of risperidone, and Eli Lilly, maker of olanzapine – both medications that Biederman had proposed as mood stabilizers for childhood bipolar disorder.[13]

One of the thorniest issues related to the controversy is that the medications prescribed to adults with bipolar disorder have significant and potentially lethal side effects. Many child psychiatrists were troubled by the idea of medicating young children, especially without knowing the long-term impact on developing brains as well as metabolic concerns (weight gain, susceptibility to diabetes, and others).

Bipolar disorder is not the only illness where child psychiatry has danced intimately and dangerously with drug companies. My colleagues in that area describe a widespread sense of outrage at being sold a false bill of goods in the form of studies of what were, at that time, the new generation antidepressants, serotonin-specific reuptake inhibitors (SSRIs), published in prestigious academic journals that turned out to be ghostwritten for the eminent academics who put their names on what were essentially products of the pharmaceutical industry's marketing departments. They feel they were bamboozled into presenting this second generation of antidepressant medications to parents in a much more positive light than the studies merited, and this in turn led, in the wake of newer evidence, to public suspicion not just of the drug companies but also of child psychiatry's competence as a profession.

I explain to Mark that I am hesitant to add my opinion to all those he has already received on Sam's diagnoses and potential treatments.

"I think the psychiatrist, the one who knew about your brother-in-law's bipolar disorder but also worried about the impact of drug abuse, the one who told you it is a waiting game and recommended trying family therapy and CBT before rushing in with medications, was doing you and Sam a favor, frustrating as it must be to hear that perspective. I respect her honesty and her caution. None of the drugs used to treat bipolar disorder are straightforward or free from side effects, so unless the diagnosis is crystal clear, the risks of treatment likely outweigh any possible benefits."

Mark nods, telling me that Sam has responded well to the psychiatrist's message that nothing will work without his involvement and an effort to decrease his drug use. Mark has also noted that Sam never protests going to see her. Apparently Sam told Jane after the police call to the house that he and the psychiatrist are talking seriously about the possibility of his attending a substance abuse program.

"If Sam trusts her and is telling your wife about her suggestions, this psychiatrist is obviously doing something right. It's not easy keeping a boy Sam's age, and with his problems, in treatment. I'd hang on to her if you can. It sounds to me as though she's a keeper."

Mark nods. "Jane says the same thing about her. I do appreciate her honesty about not having all the answers; maybe I just can't accept the idea that there's no one out there who has them."

There's a long pause.

"Mark, you're struggling with the same questions that we all do – parents, teachers, psychiatrists. All of us want to know how much of teenage behavior – especially when it's risky and obnoxious – is attributable simply to their developmental stage and what crosses the line into mental illness. I do think you are getting some answers; the psychiatrists who have seen Sam are clearly telling you that they think there's more going on here than can be explained by adolescent angst and bad behavior that requires limit-setting.

"We have some good research that tells us most teenagers are pretty happy a lot of the time, and don't struggle with depression or drug abuse.[14] Those who do, really do have underlying issues or vulnerabilities that are anything but simple and require careful attention and treatment. I don't say that to scare you but rather to reinforce that I think the efforts that you and Jane are making to help Sam are important and necessary, and that he's lucky the two of you are so committed to helping him rather than writing him off as a bad kid."

Mark flushes and looks away from me. "I'm glad you think that. It helps, coming from you."

I genuinely believe that if Mark and Jane can keep at it with Sam, and work with him and his doctors to get him back on track developmentally and academically, the fact that his brain is still developing may work in their favor. But parenting a child with issues as severe as Sam's demands a huge commitment, and Mark is here today because both he and Jane feel he is not coping well with the pressure.

Remembering the quantity of wine I had observed Mark imbibe at the fund-raiser, I ask him about his current alcohol use. He acknowledges that he is using alcohol to deal with a number of stresses, while recognizing that it is hindering his ability to relate to his wife and children. He also admits that it provides Sam with some unfortunate role modeling.

I need to tread lightly here. I don't want Mark for a second to feel that I am blaming Sam's difficulties on Mark's drinking. It would be inaccurate and an oversimplification. If Mark is to be believed, and I think he is, his use of alcohol has increased as a result of the stress associated with dealing with his son's problems. More important, any hint of blame, as opposed to pointing out potential links, will signifi-cantly lower the likelihood that Mark will pursue treatment on his own behalf. Very few parents, in my experience, need any help blaming themselves for their child's problems; it is my job to suggest to Mark that by addressing his own mental health problems, he may indirectly assist his son, although there are obviously no guarantees.

"From what you tell me, I agree with your assessment that your drinking is a reaction to what's been happening at home. While it may not be affecting your health or ability to work at this point, it sounds as though it is contributing additional stress to your relationship with Jane, and may be dulling your reactions to what goes on at home. And that may be making it harder for the two of you to deal collaboratively with Sam. I hear what you are saying about it making you less likely to lose it with him, but it may also be making you less sensitive to his and Jane's cues. What do you think?"

Mark takes his time before responding. "You know, it's a good point. By the time I've had two or three beers, I stop caring as much about what's going on. It doesn't feel as life-and-death. Which on the one hand feels better, but on the other leaves Jane dealing with Sam. And I don't want him to think that beer is any more the answer to stress and conflict than pot is."

So far so good.

"Do you think it's something you're ready to address? It may be that if Sam sees you making an effort to cut down on alcohol, he'll be less able to normalize what he's doing. It doesn't necessarily mean quitting drinking entirely. I know of a few good local programs that focus on an approach called harm reduction, which means not abstaining completely if that's not something you feel you need to do, but working to make sure that your drinking stays within safe limits – medically and psychologically."

I'm relieved that Mark's drinking has not reached a level where I would have to switch gears from informal adviser to attending physician, making me responsible for reporting him to the authorities. I'm relieved too that he has told me very clearly that he never drinks and drives, and that Jane will corroborate this. Another set of answers would legally obligate me to notify the Ministry of Transportation that as a driver he was a potential danger.

"That's an interesting idea, Doctor. Another thing that has been suggested is family therapy. We've tried to get Sam to go a few times, but he refuses. How much of a priority do you think it is?"

Nate, my father-in-law, was a great proponent of family therapy's usefulness in caring for psychiatrically ill children. I would argue (unlike a significant proportion of my colleagues, trained to provide ongoing care to patients in one-to-one, confidential relationships) that all psychiatric treatment should involve families, and child psychiatry requires it, at least where parents are willing. Children cannot get better without the help of their families. Removing children from their families is a miserable fourth-best choice and needs to occur only where parents are incapable or flagrantly abusive. Family therapy, however, places a significant burden on families' time and money and is beyond the reach of, or poses major challenges for, many families. I had held off asking Mark more about their attempts to get Sam to go only because I didn't want to overwhelm him with suggestions and referrals.

I tell Mark that my guess is that family therapy will be offered as part of the adolescent substance abuse program and that it may be helpful to try again if Sam's psychiatrist is in agreement.

Mark looks at his watch. He's been with me almost an hour. My internal clock, conditioned over thirty years of clinical practice, has already told me I need to get on with my day.

He thanks me for seeing him. As he leaves, I know I am lucky that in serving as senior medical adviser to my hospital, my stipend covers not only some of the community talks I provide but also the kind of encounters that these outreach efforts inevitably engender, such as this one with Mark.

Parents like Mark need answers about the causes of their children's distress that we are decades away from being able to provide. They need help understanding the potential (and the limitations) of medication and psychotherapy for their children. They also need help in negotiating increasingly complex systems to access the treatments that their children require. For Mark, the many possible diagnoses and mental health treatments offered to Sam had become an impenetrable obstacle to getting a clear explanation of what had gone wrong for his son and suggestions to help him. But my hope is that Jane and Mark will be successful in finding effective help for Sam. Navigating the children's mental health system shouldn't be a matter of luck, geography, or privilege. But Mark and his family are among the fortunate; they live in a large Canadian city with treatment options. They have family and financial resources to support Sam's treatment, and the boy's psychiatrist can refer them to a program that I'm confident will provide them with an informed, balanced approach to Sam's psychiatric problems.

"BOSS, STAN SCHWARTZ LEFT a message on your inside line. It's important," Simone says.

Daryl Orzech's cousin Stan rarely calls except to ask whether some work he is moving Daryl's way is a good idea.

As I listen to Stan's message on my voice mail, I organize some stuff on my desk. Stan's recorded voice sounds uncharacteristically small and hesitant. He tells me that earlier this afternoon Daryl jumped to his death from his apartment balcony.

Everything is suddenly still.

I play the message several times, listening closely for something I may have missed, but my thoughts are inexorably drawn to my meeting with Daryl two days before, seeing his wrinkled, checkered shirt, his unshaved face, his slow smile.

I sit at my desk, staring out the window, trying to think of the orderly steps of notification and documentation dictated by our policy and procedures manual. Then, in the privacy and silence of my office, I hold my head in my hands and weep.

I don't cry easily or often. This is not my first encounter with suicide in thirty years of practice, but it is the first time with someone I have known so long and, I thought, so well. It is also the first time a patient has died by suicide such a short time after I characterized him as safe. I recall what I now realize were his last words to me, a hand on my shoulder as he turned to leave my office: *It's hard.*

Daryl had obviously had enough. Enough of feeling that life, in the form of technology, relationships, children, had passed him by. I call Sylvia, his mother. She tells me this was what she had feared most during the decades of Daryl's illness. We speak about his talents, his foibles, and the awful toll bipolar disorder took on his life. She asks me to thank everyone at the hospital for what they did for him. Even in her grief, she finds room for gratitude and generosity. She says she will email me details of the funeral and the shiva, and says I am welcome to come by her apartment anytime. I promise to drop by after work.

Daryl's words as he left my office intrude relentlessly on my thoughts. Why hadn't I stopped him? Made him sit down and asked him what he meant? I know I am grasping at straws. Though screening for suicidal thoughts and documenting the findings are part of clinical routine, a shorthand evolves that clinicians know well. It may be a facial expression, a way of walking, a pattern of speech – something that sets off alarm bells of familiarity. With Daryl, his typical "tell" when he was depressed was that he couldn't finish a sentence; he was slowed down, frustrated, and tearful. I saw none of that two days ago. I will never know if the thought of suicide was in his mind, undisclosed, then, or whether it seized him today and led him to an impulsive flight off the balcony.

I compulsively review Daryl's tumultuous course of treatment in my mind, ruminating over the choices toward which I steered him, wondering where I failed him. Our relationship involved my having an intimate knowledge of him and his depending on and trusting me. Week after week, month after month, his name appeared in my calendar. He accepted that the nature of my work commitments meant that no one had a regular, fixed appointment time, but he was mindful not to let the interval between appointments exceed what he thought was necessary. Each visit reflected a specific conversation, a joke, a plea for help.

I call Nancy to tell her what has happened. She is also a physician and knows of Daryl from the conversations we share over dinner about our patients. We don't know each other's patients by name, but have found that confiding in each other about patients has helped ease the burden of responsibility. Our dining room, in that regard, is a little like the doctors' lounge that used to exist in hospitals – where colleagues could talk candidly and privately about their clinical uncertainties and quandaries. At the same time, both Nancy and I have had the experience of meeting people who are surprised that we don't know that our spouse is that person's doctor.

Today, Nancy's comfort is instant and real, free of platitudes.

"Dave, I'm so sorry. I know how much you liked him. His poor family – what a blow. And for you. That's terrible."

Nancy knows that I don't want anyone to tell me it is "okay" or "to be expected," because neither is true in this moment. I simply need someone I trust and love to know the intensity of this loss and to relieve me of the sudden sense of being alone and of having failed a patient. Logic and grief are at best distant cousins. I am considered a good psychiatrist. What does Daryl's death say about my skills? Yes, people with bipolar disorder are at a significant risk of suicide. But that's *all* people with bipolar disorder, being treated or not treated by *all* mental health professionals. This is Daryl and this is me.

I have studied the small literature on the subject of psychiatrists' responses to patients' suicide, which has grown little over the years despite surveys that suggest that as many as half of all psychiatrists lose a patient to suicide and that about one-third of those endure the loss during their residency training.[15] Sadly, I often have occasion to provide support to trainees and colleagues whose patients have died by suicide. I remind them that what has occurred is in part a reflection of the fact that they chose to treat more severely ill people and that such tragic outcomes are painful but inevitable. I often ask them whether they would trust an oncologist who claimed he had never lost a patient to cancer. Today I feel the limits to the comfort of that perspective.

Every doctor lives with risk. We know from the first day we write a prescription for a medication or an order on a hospital chart that we have the power to harm or kill a patient. We joke about it, utilizing medicine's most ubiquitous and useful defense mechanism, but a doctor who is not awed by that knowledge, while resisting being paralyzed by it, is not a safe physician. Psychiatrists, however, live with a different kind of risk. Suicides and the rare homicide committed by psychiatric patients are seen as preventable in a way that deaths from pancreatic cancer or a stroke or a lifelong diagnosis of diabetes are not. While an oncologist may be criticized for telling a patient with end-stage cancer that medicine cannot accurately predict how long he or she has to live, a psychiatrist's failing to foresee a patient's decision to die or his or her likelihood of acting violently toward others is viewed more harshly.

Attempts to find more objective predictors of suicidality, both biological and behavioral, have met with mixed success. Although there is evidence for familial clustering of suicide (the Hemingway family being a notable example), no "suicide gene" has been identified. Neurobiological characteristics that have been associated with suicidality – disturbances in the serotonin system or of the hormones associated with the human stress response – are not specific and therefore have limited practical usefulness. In the case of the serotonin by-products we can measure, there is persuasive scientific evidence to link decreased levels of serotonin metabolites in cerebrospinal fluid with serious suicide attempts. But the feasibility of performing spinal taps on patients thought to be at risk of suicide – as well as the limits to the evidence itself – renders this a scientifically interesting finding but not yet one that can change practice or provide psychiatry with a suicide crystal ball. On Monday I had no diagnostic test other than my clinical experience and acumen. Both failed me, and therefore Daryl. And now he's gone, and Sylvia is waiting for me at her home.

Daryl had lived with a diagnosis of bipolar disorder for more than thirty years, and many of those years contained friendship, laughter, and romance. But in my own mind, and for most people who knew him, those thirty years of meaningful living now risk being completely overshadowed by how he died. By contrast, people who die of cancer are routinely valorized as "having fought a courageous battle" against their illness, and their funerals are a "celebration" of their lives.

All this ruminating is doing me no good. I tidy up my desk and drive to North Toronto, where Sylvia's apartment stands clustered among numerous condo developments. Her place is packed with friends and relatives, most of whom I don't recognize. But I know Sylvia and her daughters, and we embrace and cry. They offer me food. Sylvia introduces me to everyone as Daryl's doctor of many years, and these strangers warmly thank me. I appreciate their gratitude, though all I feel is loss and failure. But they want to tell me stories about him, to help me know him better than I already did. As we talk about Daryl, inevitably we laugh, because Daryl was funny and he loved to make other people laugh; maybe that was our bond, his and mine, across the boundaries that separate doctor and patient, health and illness, success and struggle. But today I don't feel as if I have any jokes left in me.

10

Doubt

I arrive at my office just after eight o'clock to find my resident from Monday morning, Josh, waiting outside the door. A lot has happened since I watched him earnestly assess a new outpatient at the beginning of the week.

"Good morning, Dr. Goldbloom. Did you play squash this morning?"

I must look surprised. My racquets are at the gym and the bag filled with my sweaty athletic clothes is in the car, so I am not sure what gave me away (apart from my beet-red face and heavy breathing).

Josh looks sheepish. "I forgot what time we were starting today so I asked Simone when I should get here. She explained that you always come straight from squash so you wouldn't get here much before eight. I didn't want to be late."

Clearly Josh has enough perceptiveness to have picked up that his assessment on Monday had not impressed me. I ask him if he plays and he says yes, that he started playing seriously at university and recently has joined a league downtown. I consider suggesting a game but decide to wait until I have had a chance to see how the morning goes. Squash may not be a good idea for all sorts of reasons, particularly given that Josh is more than thirty years younger than I am, fit, and from his own account, highly competitive. If I need to give him a negative evaluation based on our assessments together this week, our relationship may need some work before we are ready to play squash together.

This assessment starts off on a better note. Josh has made sure to read about the patient we are seeing together today. I ask him to summarize the main points.

"He's a physician, a pathologist at a community hospital. According to the GP, there's a problem with anxiety, and the GP wonders if the patient has PTSD [post-traumatic stress disorder]."

"Any other concerns?"

Josh smiles. "Yes, our patient isn't the only one who's anxious; I've never assessed a doctor before. I wonder if he knows he'll be seeing a resident."

I assure Josh that our clinic staff informs all patients they will be seen by a resident, but add that it's worth addressing in case it is a concern for this particular patient. I also tell him that he may be more anxious about this than the patient, since many physicians choose to seek care in a teaching hospital where the degree of subspecialization and innovation may be higher, knowing that they will also be seen by medical students and residents. This is exactly what happened when I had surgery for a torn meniscus in my knee. There were so many students and residents evaluating me that just before the anesthetic knocked me out, I asked the surgeon if I qualified for continuing education credits. But that was my knee, not my mind.

I tell Josh about the anxiety I felt as a junior resident when my first assigned case for long-term individual psychotherapy was a recently qualified social worker.

At our first meeting, she asked me, "What year resident are you?"

"First year," I answered in a barely audible voice.

"I can't believe it. Every colleague I know who's in therapy is seeing a real psychiatrist."

Luckily, my acute anxiety and her acute disappointment abated over time, and I ended up treating her for three years. But in the immediate wake of her lament, I remember feeling like Fred Flintstone, who when criticized by his wife, Wilma, immediately shrank to a tenth of his normal size – the perfect representation of the experience of shame and humiliation.

"Have you seen many patients with PTSD?" I ask Josh.

"A bunch of times. I've seen women in the ER dealing with the impact of sexual abuse that occurred years earlier, and refugees who were tortured. Most of them had horrendous nightmares, really compromised functioning, and bad anxiety. Their lives were devastated by their experiences. It bugs me now when I hear the diagnosis misused. What I saw wasn't the trivial stuff where you hear people throw the diagnosis around, like a fender bender or a hockey concussion. I'm lucky to have seen the real thing."

I bristle. "'Lucky' seems an unfortunate word to use. I get that those clinical experiences helped you understand PTSD and made you feel lucky in that regard, but those people were anything but. It's important our patients know we see them as more than just a good teaching case."

Josh reddens.

I move on. "I agree though that PTSD is in danger of becoming a diluted buzzword. I try to talk to people about its history. That tends to give more context than explaining the *DSM* criteria."

War has taught us that exposure to overwhelming events can produce harrowing symptoms – flashbacks, nightmares, avoidance of triggers of recollection, depression, anxiety, and substance abuse. And then there's the impact on people's functioning – problems in relationships and trouble keeping a job. Movies often romanticize war, but soldiers who have been through it don't.

In the aftermath of the First World War, the symptoms were known as "shell shock." The term was later banned by the British Army and replaced in the Second World War with "combat stress reaction." "Post-traumatic stress disorder" became the dominant diagnostic label for the same symptoms among American veterans of Vietnam, the first and second Gulf wars, and Afghanistan. In Canada, more recently PTSD has been relabeled "operational stress injury," defined by Veterans Affairs Canada as "any persistent psychological difficulty resulting from operational duties . . . It is used to describe a broad range of problems which include diagnosed medical conditions such as anxiety disorders, depression, and post-traumatic stress disorder (PTSD) . . . as well as other conditions that may be less severe, but still interfere with daily functioning. The symptoms and the injuries themselves vary according to the individual and nature of their experience."[1]

The labels operational stress injury and post-traumatic stress disorder are an attempt to explain and legitimize the injury and symptoms, relating them to the traumatic event rather than blaming and stigmatizing the person. At a pragmatic level, it's also about ensuring access to the same supports and services that someone with a war-related physical injury would receive. But the fact that the name keeps having to change to describe the same phenomenon suggests to me that these repeated attempts to remove stigma from the illness are not entirely successful.

I ask Josh if he's ready for the patient.

He nods. "Thanks. I'm good to go."

Josh opens the door leading to Simone's office, where our patient is seated, scanning my bookshelf.

"Dr. Zeigler? I'm Dr. Joshua Leitner, working with Dr. Goldbloom. Please come in."

Josh shows a tall, lanky man with a receding hairline and graying beard into the room. He is dressed in black jeans, a checkered shirt, and a light-brown leather jacket that looks left over from a previous life. Josh points him to a comfortable chair. The patient acknowledges me silently as I sit off to the side at the conference table, and Josh begins.

"Dr. Zeigler, welcome to the Assessment Clinic. Before we get started, let me tell you a bit about who we are and what's going to happen today. I'm a fifth-year resident in psychiatry and Dr. Goldbloom is my supervisor. I'm going to be doing the interview today with you, although Dr. Goldbloom is going to be here the whole time and will probably have some questions for you at the end. We're going to meet for about an hour and I'll be asking lots of questions. You'll have a chance to ask questions of us at the end. We want to do our best to figure out what's going on and how we can help you. To begin with, what would you like me to call you?"

"Philip. That would be fine. I'm not here as a doctor." He speaks quietly.

"Okay, Philip it is. But I need to be honest with you, I am not going to be able to ignore that you're a doctor. It will either make it easier or harder – for both of us!"

This is a different Josh from the one I saw at the beginning of the week – more natural, less rote, more ready to use humor appropriately to acknowledge sources of difficulty for both the patient and the interviewer. As I make note of these changes, I wonder what has made the difference.

Josh expresses genuine curiosity about the nature of Philip's work. The doctor's expertise is in cancer diagnosis. He works full-time in the pathology lab and has had no direct clinical contact with patients since completing his internship almost twenty years earlier. It's a reminder of the career spectrum within medicine, the thousands of paths beyond the entry door to medical school.

Josh adds that because Philip is a physician, Josh may learn things about him that would require him to report them to the College of Physicians and Surgeons of Ontario (CPSO), the regulatory body for all physicians in the province. In Ontario, mandatory reporting by individual physicians of colleagues is currently limited to the sexual abuse of a patient. This may change in the near future to resemble the legal frameworks that exist in other provinces and countries, such as the UK and Australia and many US states, which have wider mandates for mandatory reporting of physicians. But for now, there is "permissive reporting," where it is not mandatory but nevertheless recommended and permissible for physicians to report other physicians when there is evidence of physician incapacity or incompetence.[2]

Philip nods. I notice he is picking at the skin around his nails, apparently unconsciously.

"I'm already terrified of making a mistake in my line of work. Go ahead and ask."

I note that Josh has done his duty in informing Philip about reporting obligations but has also set the stage for Philip to feel comfortable to talk. It's not an easy balance, but he's done it.

Josh soon learns that Philip has been divorced for the last decade, with joint custody of two teenage sons. He lives alone in a condo not far from his hospital. He describes his problem as "overwhelming anxiety for the past year."

Briskly, Josh gets him to describe the contours of this otherwise amorphous experience. In the moment, they are both pathologists, discussing the findings under a single microscope with two viewing scopes. I feel relatively invisible, a sure sign that there is strong engagement between them.

"Is it continuous or episodic? Physical, emotional, or both?"

"It comes in waves – sometimes every day, sometimes every few days. It's intensely physical. The first time I had it was a year ago. I was alone in my condo at night, I was sure it was an MI [myocardial infarction; a heart attack]. I could barely catch my breath. My cardiac rhythm was all over the place and my chest felt tight. I felt woozy and my fingers went numb. I thought, 'This is it. I'm forty-eight, divorced, and alone, and my cleaning lady is going to find my corpse in two days.' I called 911 and begged them to take me to a hospital other than my own. That hospital kept me overnight and I got the full nine yards of assessment, including a cardiologist who came into the ER in the middle of the night to make sure I was okay. I'm sure they went the extra distance because I'm a doc. It was humiliating when all the results of the labs were negative. 'It's just a panic attack,' the ER doc said. I felt like a fool. It was as though I had disappointed them by not having a 'real' diagnosis."

Josh carefully gauges the frequency of subsequent attacks, which usually occur once or twice per week but sometimes almost daily, their symptom profile (similar to the first one, but less likely to be associated with fear of a heart attack), and their duration (usually about twenty to thirty minutes). But he also notes that the first forty-seven years of Philip's life had been free of panic attacks, and he digs a little deeper into the context of the very first attack a year ago.

Good. He is mindful of gathering the evidence to support a diagnosis, but he is also paying due attention to context. It's not a cookbook interview.

"I've thought a lot about it myself. The first time it happened was the evening after a particularly busy workday where I'd been covering for a colleague who was off. Early in the afternoon, a surgeon – deep in the belly of a patient – had sent a frozen section of a biopsy down to the lab from the OR for rapid interpretation to figure out how extensive a surgical resection was needed. I interpreted the biopsy as benign and called the OR. But something was gnawing at me. As I said, it was a really busy day in the lab and we were overwhelmed with specimens to interpret. I suddenly realized I had looked at the wrong slide. I triple-checked the ID on the specimen, started over, and then asked a colleague to take a look as well. It was an aggressive cancer. I called the OR back. The surgeon hadn't started the closure yet, so they were able to proceed with the resection. He thanked me for double-checking, but all I could think about were all those cases across the country of incorrectly interpreted pathology specimens, of people dying of incorrectly undiagnosed malignancies or having perfectly healthy tissue removed, of the pathologists who made the mistakes written up in the newspapers and disciplined by their colleges."

"Do you find yourself thinking about the events of that day a lot? Brooding, flashbacks, dreams, or even nightmares?"

Josh pursues the question of PTSD, raised by Philip's GP, weaving his specific inquiry into the interview without disrupting the rhythm.

"No. It's not so much being stuck on what actually happened. It's worrying about the next possible mistake, imagining getting sued, losing my spot at the hospital, being unable to support my kids."

It might be argued that Philip's belief that he was experiencing a heart attack immediately following the lab error met the initial necessary but not sufficient criterion for a diagnosis of PTSD – that a patient has been exposed to actual or threatened death, serious injury, or sexual violence. However, Josh has effectively ruled out the diagnosis, eliciting Philip's denial of any of the disorder's defining symptoms: recurrent, involuntary, intrusive memories, and dreams of the traumatic event (or events); flashbacks where the patient feels or acts as if the event is actually happening in the present; intense or prolonged distress, intense physical reactions, and avoidance if confronted with cues that recall or resemble details of the event; increased irritability and anger, pessimism, insomnia, distrust of others, hypervigilance, and reckless or self-destructive behaviors.[3]

"How's your sleep? Any trouble falling asleep or staying asleep?" Josh asks.

"Apart from getting up to pee, I seem to be okay."

"Having you been missing work or dodging particular cases?"

"I can't afford to. I've seen that surgeon a number of times since and done cases with him, but now I triple-check my findings and it slows me down."

Satisfied he has enough information from Philip's description of the lab error and his response to it to answer the GP's question, Josh moves on to explore other areas of Philip's psychiatric history.

Josh asks about the course of Philip's career over the fifteen years since completing his pathology residency. He has never experienced professional difficulty and has never been in trouble. He found the intellectual intrigue and rigor of pathology preferable to the muddier world of clinical care. But he made an uncharacteristic visit to the bedside of the surgical patient the day after the near miss had happened – "I needed to be sure he was still alive. I see lots of slides of cancer in the lab every day. My job is to tell the surgeon it's there or it isn't there, not the patient. But that day I almost blew it."

"Are there thoughts or events that trigger the panic attacks for you now?"

"Not that I know of. They seem to have a life of their own. So far, it hasn't happened at work. Just at the condo, when I'm alone. Maybe it's when there's nothing else going on and I'm just thinking about things, but honestly I don't know anything specific."

"What helps?"

"Sometimes before it gets too intense I'll make a phone call to my kids, my brother, or a friend, and that works. But I can't keep just calling people. Sometimes a bolt of vodka does the trick."

I'm aware of sitting up straighter now, an unintended bodily cue to Josh that something of note has just been said.

Philip has opened an important door, and Josh enters. In seamless transition, he explores Philip's alcohol use – frequency, amount, context, and consequences. Thoroughly but naturally, Josh determines that the alcohol use is not escalating or compromising Philip's ability to work. Philip is fastidious about never getting behind the wheel of his car after drinking, and he doesn't drink at work or when on call. But nothing is left implicit as Josh asks systematically about other behaviors that would put Philip or others at risk.

Reporting clinical conditions that you believe interfere with a patient's car-handling ability to the Ministry of Transportation in Ontario is mandatory – although discretionary in other jurisdictions – but it can also create an angry patient and a damaged therapeutic relationship. As an ophthalmologist, Nancy has had to deal with this in older patients with failing vision more than I have in my practice. People can be devastated by this loss of autonomy, especially if it affects their livelihood.

"What about drugs?"

Silence. Philip looks away.

"This is where it gets difficult. I'm not proud of what I need to tell you. I am probably addicted to Ativan. I feel like such an idiot to have got here. It's not like I don't know the risks, and I am forty-nine, for God's sake, not fourteen. When I was younger, from about fifteen to thirty, I smoked pot nearly every day. Never more than a joint, or at most two. It was the only thing I ever found that really relaxed me, turned my head off. It never got in the way of my studies. My ex-wife was okay with it, even smoked with me until our kids were born. Then she started to nag me to stop, said it made me stupid, emotionally unavailable, whatever that meant. It was one of the things that split us up, although one of many. She'd want to talk about what was wrong with the marriage, always after a long day at work, and all I would want to do was light up. Funnily enough, after we split up, I finally gave it up. Figured she was right, and I didn't want the boys seeing me smoke up and think it was okay. I didn't really miss it until the panic attacks started."

While Philip's story of anxiety ostensibly started in the wake of a near miss at work, I wonder whether some subclinical level of anxiety both drove and was contained by his use of marijuana. Many patients have told me, sometimes sheepishly, that it worked better than any pill or psychotherapy for this problem.

"And then on that trip to the ER with this, they gave me some Ativan. It was a relief like I'd never experienced before, better than pot. They gave me a couple of pills to take home, but pretty soon I was out of them. My GP's a good guy, and he gave me a refill. Then another. Eventually, I didn't want to wait for the anxiety train to leave the station before taking one, so I started popping an Ativan each morning when I got to work. Just half a milligram under my tongue. It helped me get through the day. I take a second pill, sometimes two, when I get home and want to put my feet up. You have to understand, it's me alone at night in the condo, rewinding the events of the day, second-guessing myself, worrying about my future."

"How are you on the days you don't take it?"

Philip pauses.

"Those days don't exist anymore. Last time I went in, my GP called the prescription in to the pharmacy for a month's supply with three repeats. I don't want to face him, and I think it's easier for him not to see me, but I know he'll insist on my coming in to see him before he gives me another renewal."

"What's the most you've taken in a day?"

"It's rare, but a couple of times I've taken four or five pills on a Saturday or Sunday if I don't have the boys. And I'm not just telling you I only take those amounts on weekends because I'm scared you will report me; I am here because I don't want it to get to the point that I take those doses when I am at work, and I am starting to see that it could happen if I don't take a stand now. Having said that, right now four or five pills would be a really bad day for panic, but I worry about those days happening more and more often. I think the days when I have no structure, like weekends, with nothing to distract me, are the hardest. I've tried going to movies by myself but that actually makes it worse. Something about being in a crowd of people I don't know. I've also thought about going to a gym, but it's been difficult to get motivated."

"It seems pretty clear you think the Ativan is a problem."

"The real problem is that it really works for me. I'm at a point where I can't function without it – and I don't know what I'll do if my GP doesn't renew the prescription. I wouldn't have the first clue how to buy this stuff on the street or anything like that. But I need it. That's why I said that I think I may be addicted to it. So the short answer is yes. I'm really in a tough spot."

His tough spot is very different from that of Sofia, the woman I saw in ER two days ago who couldn't get on a plane. Although they are both struggling with anxiety, Sofia has, over the course of her life, learned to live with and adapt to her anxiety. She has found "work-arounds" such as travel by car instead of by plane so she and her family can enjoy holidays together, and she has a supportive husband. She has also managed to keep her anxiety confined to one area, largely success-fully, until the crisis point triggered by her recognition that there was no alternative to airplane travel to see her aging parents. By contrast, Philip is experiencing his first sustained period of significant anxiety, and his work-around – Ativan – is likely to prove more destructive to his psyche than the anxiety symptoms themselves.

Ativan, or lorazepam in its generic form, is a powerful antianxiety drug from the benzodiazepine family. It can be very useful in the short term over a period of days to weeks for management of overwhelming anxiety and insomnia, but it can also be highly addictive for vulnerable patients with a personal or family history of addiction or with no other resources for addressing their problems. It is from the same family as Valium, infamously known in the 1960s as "mother's little helper," the pill given by usually well-meaning but socially traditional physicians to unhappy housewives cursed with what the feminist Betty Friedan called the "problem that has no name."

Josh responds to Philip's disclosure with surprising empathy and lack of judgment. He finishes his interview with a survey of Philip's early life, medical and family history, and current social functioning. It is here that he hits another bull's-eye.

"What about sex?" Josh asks after learning that Philip has had only a few dates since his divorce.

"I've shied away from dating. I can't imagine doing the online dat-ing thing that everyone seems to do these days, and what with work and the boys, there doesn't seem time to meet anyone. At work I mainly meet residents, who are obviously off-limits. Most of my colleagues and the lab staff are either married or involved in a relationship."

He pauses. "So no sex. I have used some porn sites, which also doesn't feel great. I think Jake, our oldest, busted me recently after using my laptop for homework. He didn't say anything, but I noticed the history was erased and he seemed embarrassed. I hate porn really; it doesn't fit with who I am, but it's like the Ativan. I just find when I get home and I am really tired, it's easier than picking up a phone and calling a friend, or asking someone out. And once I start, I can't seem to stop. Often I am on for hours without realizing. It will be three or four in the morning before I realize it. Which doesn't help with work the next day."

Philip seems relieved after sharing his shame about this behavior. I am pleased by how comfortable he and Josh seem with each other. It bodes well for Josh's future work as a clinician. I wonder, though, if Philip would have been as open with a female resident. I find generally that the residents are reluctant to ask about sexual thoughts and behavior, despite the centrality of sexuality to the lives of most adults. Dorothy Horn, a talented and tough family therapist who worked with my father-in-law, said the first rule of seeing couples in treatment was to "think dirty."

My own questions at the end of the interview are a series of minor grace notes, mostly to convey to Philip that he should not attribute my silence over the preceding hour to inattention. I indicate to Philip that Josh has covered all the areas that I thought needed to be addressed. I see a slight smile at the corner of Josh's mouth on hearing this. I take the lead, as previously discussed with Josh, on providing Philip with our assessment. Unlike Josh's Monday assessment with Anya, this one does not require a debrief before the feedback. Today Josh and I are in sync.

"Philip, your openness with us today, which can't have been easy, has been very helpful. You've provided us with a good sense of what it feels like inside your head these days and the challenges you experience living your life. It's clearly been a tough road for you the last several months."

I go on to explain that in answer to his GP's primary question about possible PTSD, we don't think that diagnosis applies to him. Bad things happen all the time to people, and the most common response is resilience. Philip kept working, rather than avoiding the place where the error happened, and while his near miss was clearly incredibly stressful, it wasn't something outside the realm of experience for most physicians. A preceding traumatic or stressful event doesn't necessarily explain why someone becomes depressed or anxious, but it might tap into someone's vulnerability. In Philip's case, there was clearly something about the near miss that triggered significant anxiety that has subsequently seeped into the rest of his life.

I tell him that part of his recovery may well involve looking at what it was about that experience that was a trigger.

Philip nods and answers no when I ask if he has any questions so far, so I continue.

"We agree with your self-assessment that your use of both Ativan and pornography, which you describe as addictive, are getting in the way of your pursuing other activities that might help you to feel better. You probably know better than us that it will be hard to stop them because they help to calm you down when you're anxious, tired, or lonely. Both Dr. Leitner and I think that you would benefit from professional help tackling them."

Together, we offer Philip a series of recommendations, including referral to the Physician Health Program of the Ontario Medical Association to get help with his benzodiazepine abuse as well as the anxiety that fuels it. Although the program has the same reporting obligations as any clinician, it exists independently from regulatory agencies like the College of Physicians and Surgeons of Ontario. The program's case managers are available to assist physicians, veterinarians, and pharmacists experiencing mental illness or substance abuse to connect with specialized treatment. We don't think Philip meets reporting requirements to his college at this point but tell him that, like him, we worry he may get there if he doesn't address his prescription drug use immediately. We also tell him that the fact that he came for help is a good sign.

We tell Philip we will also advise his GP of our findings and the plans for treatment to keep him in the loop. We will explain to the GP that while Philip has some problems that need addressing, he doesn't have PTSD. And as I do with most patients, I recommend some self-help books on panic that help people achieve better understanding of and mastery over their problem as a complement to professional help.

I also suggest some reading material on compulsive Internet pornography use and give him the name of a private mental health program in the city that runs groups for patients struggling with this problem, the numbers of whom have burgeoned over the last decade as technology has created opportunities for dopamine-stimulating experiences online that were never possible before the Internet. From Philip's account, he craves real-life relationships, a desire that will never be satisfied by virtual ones.

Beyond his problems with anxiety and Ativan use, there are elements of an existential crisis as Philip hits his midcentury mark alone. I wonder what challenges he will still face if he is successful in addressing his more immediate problems.

"Philip, once you feel you have a grip on these issues, you may want to look at how you got here. My sense is that you are a guy who has always worked hard at your job, raising your boys. Now you are turning fifty and your kids are getting older. Maybe it's time to start turning your mind to what might make you enjoy life more. We've given you lots of recommendations, and you need to get these things in order first, but later, when you are off the Ativan and feeling less anxious and more like yourself, feel free to come back and talk to me. If you're interested and in need, we can look at potential therapy referrals. I'll leave that option open in our letter to your GP."

Philip's sense of disconnection from other people, apart from his sons, seems to me to underlie his vulnerability to addiction going back to his teens, both to drugs and compulsive online behavior. I wonder if Josh is looking for psychotherapy patients, as he and Philip clearly made a good connection. To my mind, Philip would be a great candidate for interpersonal therapy (IPT), which focuses on how people's perceptions of their relationships based on early experience determine their behavior in their current relationships, frequently to the detriment of the latter. IPT is a time-limited, focused therapy, supported by scientific evidence, which echoes themes of the more meandering psychotherapies of an earlier era. I like its practicality and efficiency.

After Philip has left, Josh and I debrief. "Apart from your being four days older, why do you think it went so much better today?"

"I felt like I got him right from the beginning. Not just the fact we've both been to med school. It was the dread of making a mistake; I know what that's like."

Josh is less guarded than usual as he goes on to tell me that Philip's account of his devaluing dismissal from the ER, after being told his pain was psychological in origin, had enraged him.

"It reminded me of how some of my instructors in internal medicine reacted to my decision to go into psychiatry. It pissed me off. This guy needs help as much as any patient with a cardiac condition."

I decide to use his identification with Philip to push home a teaching point.

"Josh, I generally hate to use technical lingo, but in this instance it's fair to say that your identification with the patient facilitated empathy. Now your challenge is to figure out how to make that connection when the patient's world and experiences are so far removed from your own, the way they were on Monday with Anya. You did a great interview today, partly because you connected with Philip's experience. Studying your reactions to different patients will teach you an enormous amount, not just about them but also about your strengths and weaknesses as a psychiatrist."

He nods. "You're right. Sometimes it seems like psychobabble to me when my psychotherapy supervisors want to talk about my transferences to the patients, but what you're saying today makes sense to me."

He pauses for a moment.

"I have an easier time connecting with male patients."

I want Josh to feel good about this disclosure. I tell him that it's not uncommon to find interviews with your own gender easier.

"It's as though you both speak the same language, although the risk of course is that can sometimes lead to mistakes based on false assumptions."

I tell him that when I first worked with women with eating disorders, it was a whole new world for me. It took me many months to feel I had a true understanding of my patients' experiences. My female colleagues seemed to have a much easier time connecting with the patients' worries about weight and shape as rooted in a cultural reality, even if they were distorted and dangerously extreme.

"Keep talking about this with your psychotherapy supervisor. Exploring your reactions with different patients will help you to adjust your interviewing style in ways that may surprise you."

AFTER SENDING JOSH ON his way with a reminder to get back to me with some dates for squash, I check to see whom I am seeing next. I haven't seen Kirsten Halpin recently, but for eight years she made an appearance every other week in my calendar of outpatient appointments. Kirsten had contacted me a few months ago. After an exchange of emails, we agreed to meet to catch up and to discuss some treatment options about which she wanted my opinion. In a coincidence of timing, Kirsten was one of the patients whom I had just confessed to Josh that I had struggled to understand early in my career.

I first met Kirsten in the late 1980s when I was an eager young psychiatrist starting my career with a research fellowship in eating disorders. When she arrived in my office for the first time, I was struck simultaneously by her dangerous emaciation and her obvious intelligence and charm. Her youth and her life-threatening illness evoked an immediate rescue response in me.

I had no intention of working in eating disorders when I started psychiatry. In 1984 I was in my final year of residency in psychiatry at McGill. I had spent much of the previous year in the Clinical Psychopharmacology Unit and the Schizophrenia Follow-Up Clinic. I had published a couple of minor papers, participated in a number of drug treatment studies, and learned how to gauge the therapeutic and toxic effects of antipsychotic medications. Extensive exposure to people with schizophrenia and their families led me to want to do further academic training in that area.

Then in November, I went to a day-long symposium at the Jewish General Hospital. The speaker was someone I had never met, and his topic was something I knew absolutely nothing about: eating disorders. The speaker, Paul Garfinkel, a tall, lean man with a close-cropped beard and a thoughtful, contemplative style, was the psychiatrist-in-chief of Toronto General Hospital. What I heard over the course of an hour was the most influential and engaging talk of my entire residency. Eating disorders were entirely unfamiliar to me, and his view of them integrated biology, psychology, culture, family, and normal development – all subjects that appealed to me because of their inherent complexity and the need for multiple perspectives.

Anorexia nervosa has been well described for more than 150 years. Primarily but not exclusively a disorder of girls and women, typically with onset between ages fourteen and eighteen, it is one of the few psychiatric disorders that has multiple physical manifestations – including striking thinness – that can cause numerous health problems and premature death. The profound weight loss that occurs comes from severe dietary restriction, sometimes punctuated by episodes of binge eating and then frantic efforts to purge the ingested calories. For people with this disorder, the body becomes a metaphor for self-appraisal, self-definition, and control taken to an extreme that ultimately renders the person a slave to her own weight.

Dieting is common in Western societies, but anorexia nervosa is rare. It is much more than a diet, which is usually a transient exercise to lose a modest amount of weight (and one associated with a very low success rate over time). While dieting is often the first step in the journey for people with anorexia, the disease leaves normal dieting in the rearview mirror as it hurtles down a highway of severe caloric restriction and the tyranny of body weight and shape as the primary expression of personal identity.

At the end of his lecture, I went up to Paul and introduced myself. I had a question (which I no longer recall), and he answered it genuinely and with interest. The formality of his answer gave way to curiosity, and he asked about my plans. I made vague noises about going to the United States to one of the hotbeds of research into schizophrenia. He must have sensed that I was either ambivalent about that possibility or intrigued about this terra incognita known as eating disorders. He mentioned that he was having an eating disorders conference in Toronto in several weeks and that I should consider attending. Flattered to be invited and curious as to whether his lecture was reflective of work by others, I impulsively agreed.

Weeks later, I found myself in Toronto, meeting Garfinkel's colleagues and students. The 1980s was a period of intense academic productivity and clinical innovation in eating disorders, and Toronto General Hospital was one of the epicenters. I met a highly collaborative group of people from a variety of disciplines – psychiatry, psychology, social work, nursing, occupational therapy – who were fired up about what they were doing. And, in contrast to McGill at that time, Toronto seemed a land of resources and opportunity. At McGill, budgets were tight, the hospitals were crumbling, and the government had placed severe restrictions on the recruitment of new psychiatrists.

Looking back, during my four years of residency, before meeting Paul, I must have encountered people with eating disorders. But I didn't think to ask, and I didn't know to ask. My ignorance is a reminder of why training is so critical in shaping awareness and sensitivity.

After the conference in Toronto, I changed my plans. I applied for a research fellowship funded by the Medical Research Council of Canada to work under Paul's supervision. When I received it, Nancy and I made plans to move to Toronto with our infant son, Daniel. We had completed our residencies simultaneously, with Nancy literally giving birth in the final weeks of her training. I soon found myself both a research fellow and a staff psychiatrist at Toronto General Hospital.

My new position required me to talk with women about their bodies and how they perceived them. It was not something my medical or psychiatric training had prepared me for. I was soon no longer surprised by a world dominated by scales, mirror checking, and elaborate rules about food. As an unrestrained omnivore, I was amazed to learn about foods being categorized as "good" and "bad," from bran muffins to potato chips. I entered a world of ritual around weighing and the goal of being in "double digits" (below one hundred pounds). Asking, "Where do you feel fat?" revealed detailed self-scrutiny, judgment, and self-loathing. I worried at first that my questions would be perceived as prurient interest, but most commonly they were greeted with a sense of relief that even though I was a guy, I had some professional sense of how, to their humiliation, these distorted perceptions and beliefs permeated people's lives. Surprisingly for me – and in contrast to some political dogma in the 1980s that only women can help women – for some of my patients, my gender was an asset. They told me they found it easier to trust my statements about their weight and extreme thinness than similar comments from a female therapist, with whom they might feel competitive.

Between 1985 and 1993, the five hundred women with eating disorders whom I saw in psychiatric consultation and treatment influenced my perceptions of female beauty as well as my own body image. If I had ever wanted to be thinner, this in-depth exposure to their struggles with the tyranny of caloric restriction relieved me of that desire. I witnessed at close range the horrendous psychological and physical impact of low body weight, and body image preoccupation and distortion, and the vicious cycle of disordered eating and dieting. Suddenly, when flipping through magazines, I became acutely aware of the fashion models, with their impossibly tubular bodies punctuated by pneumatic breasts. As I learned more about what women went through to achieve such thinness by semistarvation, purging, and joyless exercise, the look lost whatever allure it might have had for me.

Learning to treat those with eating disorders involved first building a trusting relationship with people who often had difficulty trusting themselves, let alone others. Establishing this trust was crucial to engaging with them in the highly threatening work of gradual weight restoration. It meant regular weighing, talking about meal plans, but also uncoupling their sense of identity from the numbers on the scales. It meant challenging beliefs that had taken root in an all-or-nothing thinking style – "I'm thin or I'm fat, the best or the worst" – and helping them to explore the threatening gray zone in which most of us live. It meant vigilance about the many medical complications of the disorder and even the threat of death. For patients, it meant relinquishing absolute control to a treating clinician, even though too often a sense of being out of control in various aspects of life was the problem for which the eating disorder was the maladaptive cure – a "cure" that often proved worse than the "disease" of perfectionism, dysfunctional thinking patterns, overwhelming life changes, and, frequently, trauma.

During my early years in Toronto, I became fascinated by the medical and cultural history of eating disorders, perhaps hoping to find answers there that would help me understand my patients such as Kirsten and their vulnerability to this life-threatening disease. Contrary to popular perception that these disorders developed only recently and are related to our cultural preoccupation with thinness, historians of the subject have pointed out that extreme fasting, ostensibly for specific religious purposes, was widely recorded in ancient Greek and Egyptian culture, as well as in early Eastern religions.[4]

In the Middle Ages, following the example of St. Catherine of Siena, who died in 1380 from self-imposed malnutrition at the age of thirty-two, self-proclaimed virgins starved themselves. The so-called miraculous maids committed to neither eating nor drinking, and disavowed the usual bodily excretory functions. The implication inherent in these extreme behaviors, defying human survival, was that some supernatural force permitted the young women's extraordinary state, perhaps angels who dropped heavenly ambrosia into their mouths. The motivation of these women was generally understood to be fame seeking; this indeed was the result for many of them, with various members of the medical, clerical, and political establishments visiting them to verify their claims.

Not until the end of the seventeenth century was the possibility entertained that there was a psychological underlay for self-starvation. In 1694, Sir Richard Morton described two patients who in his view suffered from a "nervous consumption" caused by "sadness and anxious cares."[5]

Sarah Jacobs was one of the most famous of the nineteenth-century cohort of fasting girls, young women who rose to fame through fasting in the United Kingdom and the United States in the 1860s. Sarah, who stopped eating as she entered puberty, also claimed to need no form of nourishment and became a tourist attraction, bringing her family money and fame. A medical team was sent to observe this apparent miracle, providing nurses to watch Sarah around the clock and ensure that she wasn't surreptitiously given any food or water. After six days of this, Sarah was clearly failing, and the nurses appealed to the doctors on the team and to Sarah's father to feed the girl. Mr. Jacobs refused, presumably determined that the family's golden goose not be slaughtered, and after ten days of observation, Sarah died.[6]

Sarah Jacobs' case would likely have been known to Sir William Withey Gull, the preeminent British physician who coined the term "anorexia nervosa." He had previously thought that the disease, which affected predominantly young women who became emaciated, pale, and listless, had a physical cause. By 1873, Gull concluded that "the want of appetite is, I believe, due to a morbid mental state."[7]

One of Gull's contemporaries, Dr. Charles Lasègue, worked initially for the Parisian police force, where he wrote detailed forensic reports on the criminals he examined and grew increasingly fascinated by psychiatry. He published his paper on hysterical anorexia in 1873, the same year that Gull gave his address to the Clinical Society of London. He, too, described his patients with anorexia in details astonishingly evocative of patients described in clinical teaching rounds today:

> A young girl, between fifteen and twenty years of age, suffers from some emotions which she avows or conceals. Generally it relates to some real or imaginary marriage project, to a violence done to some sympathy, or to some more or less conscient desire . . . at first, she feels uneasiness after food, vague sensations of fullness, suffering, and gastralgia [stomach ache] post-prandium, or rather coming on from the commencement of the repast . . . the patient thinks to herself that the best remedy for this indefinite and painful uneasiness will be to diminish her food.

Lasègue described the progression of the disease from these early stages to increasing abstention from all sources of nourishment. He also described the physical signs and symptoms that characterize anorexia today, including constipation, loss of menstrual periods, dry skin, vertigo, pallor, anemia, cardiovascular abnormalities, among others. He pointed to the hyperactivity demonstrated by these patients, describing them as pursuing "a fatiguing life in the world."[8]

The twentieth century, particularly its second half, saw an explosion of medical interest in eating disorders. Clinicians were educated by Ancel Keys, a physiology professor and consultant to the US War Department, who cast light on the medical complications that such patients shared with starvation victims: endocrine abnormalities such as low basal metabolic rates; decreases in reproductive hormones; loss of protein, leading to fluid buildup, called edema, in patients' limbs; electrolyte imbalances (particularly in the context of vomiting) and their potential for cardiac injuries; and the risk of life-threatening medical complications if patients were provided too quickly with normal amounts of nutrition rather than starting with small amounts of food and gradually increasing these.[9] A slow process of improved nutrition and weight restoration, therefore, came to be recognized as essential medical and psychological treatments for these patients.

In addition, the late twentieth century saw the emergence of "new" eating disorders, characterized as specific to the era. In 1979, the distinguished British psychiatrist and eating disorders expert Gerald Russell described what he termed "bulimia nervosa." It featured people eating thousands of calories of food in an uncontrolled and rapid manner at one sitting, often followed by deliberate attempts to rid themselves of the food through vomiting, laxatives, extreme exercise, and other forms of violent purging. It was seen among people with anorexia nervosa but also among those who were at statistically normal body weights.

The question for scholars looking at the historical origins of eating disorders is whether the older accounts of voluntary self-starvation, erratic swings between over- and undereating, and self-induced vomiting are prototypes – wearing different costumes depending on the culture of the time – for our modern eating disorders, anorexia nervosa and bulimia nervosa. Or do they describe separate and distinct disorders where only the symptom – whether voluntary starvation or self-induced vomiting – is the same but the underlying mechanisms, including sociocultural pressures, are entirely different? An analogy to the latter possibility would be headache. Headache is a symptom seen historically, frequently, and globally, but there are any number of possible causes.

I lean toward the explanation most frequently endorsed by physicians: that anorexia's core symptoms of voluntary self-starvation and bodily self-disgust in the face of eating and weight gain in obsessional, perfectionistic, and psychologically vulnerable patients are influenced by cultural context. For example, only in the last century, and even then only within certain cultural groups until recently, has the perception of an unnaturally thin female body as aesthetically attractive been widespread. Previously women with eating disorders did not refer to a desire to be thin in aesthetic terms but rather explained their starvation as related to religious devoutness or medical symptoms. Today, a majority (but not all) of sufferers refer to an extremely thin appearance as an aspiration.

Within psychiatry, psychosis lends itself to a similar paradigm with its key symptoms (delusions, hallucinations, and loss of touch with reality) consistent through historical eras, but the contextual content of the psychosis – whether medieval fears of demonic possession, postwar delusions regarding CIA surveillance, 1960s psychotic experiences of extraterrestrial mind control, and current delusions regarding terrorist activities and Internet conspiracies – varies from era to era.

SIMONE CALLS THROUGH TO tell me that Kirsten has arrived. When she enters my office – twenty-three years after our first meeting – my initial response is that she has not changed at all. This is because one's involuntary first response to Kirsten is shock at how painfully underweight she is. When I move beyond this first response, I realize that of course she has aged, as have I. Not wanting my response to her appearance to be visible, I move forward to shake her hand.

"Kirsten. It's good to see you. It's been a long time. I think the last time we met I was still a brunette."

For most of her adult life, Kirsten Halpin has been the thinnest person she – or anyone who knows her – knows. At five foot six, for the last twenty-five years she has weighed between sixty-five and a hundred pounds. At forty-seven years old, she has had anorexia nervosa far longer than she hasn't, and it has affected her physical health ruinously. She has had extensive dental problems and has the bones of an eighty-year-old woman. She has not been able to have children as a result of her emaciation and recently discovered that she has early signs of kidney failure. A fiercely intelligent and capable woman, she has not had a paid job since her mid-twenties.

Even after knowing many women with anorexia at various states of emaciation, I find that the sight of Kirsten's skeletal frame cuts through my defenses. I am confronted visibly by my failure to help her, and I feel, in the moment, useless.

"How you have been since I saw you last?" I ask her as she sits down.

Kirsten tells me about her activities, her husband, their travels together. She mentions proudly that she has maintained sobriety for fifteen years, following a decade-long struggle with alcoholism. She now acts as a mentor and sponsor to other alcoholics seeking recovery.

"It still amazes me I was able to stop drinking but have never been able to get over my eating disorder. I've thought a lot over the years about why not. Maybe I am one of those people who can do things only in an all-or-nothing way? The abstinence model makes perfect sense for alcoholics, but it doesn't really work for anorexia nervosa. I can't abstain from food. I think, too, by throwing myself into supporting other people who are struggling with their recovery and my volunteer work I can ignore the risk of my eating disorder and persuade myself I am okay. Sometimes I think that my eating disorder is the only way I can have fun. I can't drink anymore, I can't steal food for binges anymore – I've promised myself that. I'm committed to helping and providing for other recovering alcoholics and to being a good wife. Bingeing and purging is one of the only things I can still do where I can have fun."

I tell Kirsten, "I remember our talking years ago about how this illness perpetuates itself, how people get locked into an endless cycle of food restriction, bingeing, and purging. I could see you understood the cycle but couldn't break out. I wish I could have helped you more."

Rigidly straight until now, Kirsten relaxes back into her chair.

"You know, I remember the times I came to see you incredibly clearly. I liked you. I liked our meetings. I only missed appointments when I was drinking. I remember liking the fact that we talked about the books in your office. And that you had a photograph of your sons on your desk."

Kirsten pauses, fiddling with her wedding ring, heavy on her bony finger. "I hope you won't take this the wrong way, but I wish you had been more aggressive. That anyone had been more aggressive. Pushed me into treatment. I know this illness now, and I know that if you can get it early, you have a chance of escaping its clutches. Why didn't you or my parents – anybody – step in more forcefully?"

It's a good question. Why I didn't step in? I realize I don't have an answer to give her. It's unusual for me to feel at such a loss for words. Why wasn't I more intrusive and directive twenty-five years ago when her illness was less entrenched? What held me back? I tried on a number of occasions to persuade her to enter more intensive treatment, and at times when she dropped weight like sweat I struggled with whether I should hospitalize her without her permission to prevent imminent death.

"Kirsten, to be honest, I am not entirely sure why I never forced treatment on you. There were certainly times when I thought about it. I think I was worried about losing you as a patient. When I first met you, you had just left home and your independence was incredibly important to you. I suspect I was afraid that you might never see another doctor if I did something that you felt betrayed your trust."

The balancing act of winning someone's trust, a particular challenge with anorexia nervosa, and taking charge in a way that undermines the patient's sense of autonomy is the high-wire act of psychiatry. Around the same time that I was treating Kirsten, I detained another patient with anorexia, Elise Francoeur, under the powers of the Mental Health Act. At the time, she weighed seventy pounds (a terrifying weight to which Kirsten also dropped at times), and I feared she would die, even though she didn't want to. Although Elise is alive today, she is chronically and severely underweight – and my act of taking away her choice did end the therapeutic relationship. Perhaps I hadn't wanted to fail twice in the same way. I will never know whether Elise would have died without involuntary hospitalization, but I definitely know she refused to see me afterward. Would Kirsten have come around over time to seeing the value of the psychiatrist temporarily taking control? Knowing that Kirsten liked me, did I not want to jeopardize that? Many other patients of mine, particularly those with bipolar disorder or psychosis, have made that journey of involuntary hospitalization to voluntary inpatient and outpatient care. They have talked with me about "how crazy" they were when their fundamental freedoms of movement and choice were taken away, but later they thanked me for stepping in.

Perhaps the difference between my treatment of Kirsten and my treatment of patients with overt psychosis stems from the fact that more than any other psychiatric illness, except perhaps substance abuse, eating disorders raise questions of free will and the appropriateness of involuntary treatment. The image of a fragile young woman held down by psychiatric staff to insert a feeding tube into her nose does not fit with our notions of empathic mental health treatment. What's more, unlike someone whose perception of reality and normative behavior can be eroded by psychosis, many patients with anorexia, apart from being very thin, can seem more "like you and me." Despite the severity of her illness, Kirsten was working as a lawyer when I met her; she was as driven to be productive professionally as she was to be at a perilously low body weight.

And yet is not the belief that one is fat at 50 percent of one's healthy body weight as much a delusion as the patient with schizophrenia's belief that she has been implanted with monitoring devices by the CIA? A delusion is defined as a fixed false belief despite evidence to the contrary, but we don't consider people with eating disorders to be psychotic (although some clinicians and researchers argue this point[10]), and there is no evidence that the antipsychotic medications that relieve delusions in schizophrenia have any impact on the thinking disturbances characteristic of patients with eating disorders. If the patient with schizophrenia is convinced that she needs to cut open her skull to remove the implant, most of us believe that the health-care system is justified in restricting her ability to harm herself irrevocably, even if that means temporary involuntary treatment and, as a last resort, physical and chemical restraint. For complex reasons, the notion that a patient with anorexia nervosa whose disease has already inflicted irrevocable physiological damage should be forced to accept treatment is far more controversial.

Part of the discomfort with the idea of involuntary treatment is that society as a whole tends to deny or not to realize how lethal these disorders can be. Anorexia nervosa has one of the highest mortality rates in psychiatry, a fact that those who see it as a frivolous phase of female development seem unaware. Even when it does not kill its victim, anorexia shortens life spans by close to twenty years.[11] One in five of the patients with anorexia who die does so by suicide, while the majority who die suffer fatal physical complications.[12] During the eight years I spent in clinical and research work in this field, a number of women in our eating disorders program died of medical complications of their illnesses, including electrolyte imbalances and cardiac rhythm disturbances. Some clinicians leave the field because of the high risk that the illness poses to patients, and those who stay acquire a certain resilience and resolve in the face of repeated patient deaths. A colleague who headed the eating disorders program where I used to work tells patients considering intensive treatment and their families, "I have been to too many funerals for my patients," before encouraging them to take on their disease with all the resources at their disposal.

"Do you think it would have made a difference, Kirsten?" I ask her. "I remember you telling me that it helped if someone else told you that you had to eat. I remember you saying that during one of your worst periods you could allow yourself to eat only if your husband ordered food for you in a restaurant."

She nods. "That was a crazy time. The food rules were all wrapped up with my OCD [obsessive-compulsive disorder]. Do you remember when I couldn't leave my house without vacuuming the carpet in the hall all the way to the door? I had so many rules; only some of them were about eating. I remember feeling safe only in restaurants, where my husband would order food for me off the menu. For some reason I could eat it, knowing he was saying it was all right. Those meals were among the few times that I remember enjoying food, feeling able to relax and to savor it. It worked for a while, and then suddenly it didn't anymore.

"Maybe it would have helped to be in the hospital and to be forced to eat, to know if I didn't, I wouldn't be able to leave the hospital, and that I would be given a nasogastric tube if I refused to eat or drink for long enough. But I also know I'd have hated it and fought you. I don't know the answer."

Kirsten would likely not have needed tube feeding. Involuntary treatment for patients with eating disorders rarely involves its use. Most patients respond to the insistent and empathic pressure of skilled mental health staff and, where appropriate, the support of copatients, and they begin taking food by mouth voluntarily. In cases where a patient feels she cannot take the food by mouth, she will frequently accept a feeding tube. Patients have explained to me over the years that one of the few ways they can resist the relentless dictates of their eating disorder is to have others make it impossible for them not to do so. Or as Kirsten says, using the language of the twelve-step programs, to give themselves over to a higher power.

Kirsten now tells me about the positive things in her life, as if to let me know that my failure is less than I think. I suspect she has sensed my unease. I remember her gift for empathy, her double-edged ability to put another's needs above her own.

"It's not so bad these days, my life. I have come to terms with what's happened to me. I have my husband, my house, my friends, my work in the fellowship. And I love my nephews and nieces; they have given me great joy over the years."

There is a pause during which we both confront the obvious. Kirsten breaks it. She has reached a stage in her life where she has decided there is no longer a point to pretending.

"I think I would have liked children of my own. But that wasn't in the cards for me. I hope I would have been a good mother. Maybe it would have helped me to put my eating disorder aside. I'll never know."

Why Kirsten? Why not any of her contemporaries in Toronto in the 1970s and 1980s who were exposed to the same destructive cultural thin ideal for women, one that is physiologically impossible and undesirable for 95 percent of women? The randomness of disease incidence in families feels cruel to me. When she was my patient, Kirsten used to talk to me at length about her feelings of competitiveness toward other women, including those close to her. She incessantly compared their clothes sizes and weights.

"Kirsten, do you remember how it all started?"

She sighs. "I do. It's sad that is so clear after all these years. It's tragic, really. I'd always been thin, but no one had ever explained to me about puberty and how your body changes. I was fourteen and I hit 125 pounds at five foot six. I didn't realize it was natural to gain weight and become rounder at that age; I panicked and assumed I was getting fat. Then one day I decided I was too big and that I was going to go on a diet. And I've never stopped. I also got into long-distance running. I remember that my mother always seemed to be on a diet. Most women were in those days."

I nod. "I've learned from my pediatric colleagues and seen for myself how confusing the bodily changes that girls experience in early adolescence can be. If a girl is vulnerable — as you were, given the cumulative impact of your anxiety, obsessive-compulsive tendencies, perfectionism, and your parents' breakup — and she doesn't feel support and approval for those physical changes from the people around her, her body image can be damaged, sometimes irreparably. As yours was . . ."

We share a short silence. Perhaps we are both imagining the life that might have been if her environment had not squeezed the trigger on fourteen-year-old Kirsten's eating disorder, to use an analogy coined by US researcher Cynthia Bulik.

"David, I want to get your opinion of Ann Kerr." Kirsten's use of my first name catches me off guard. It's new for her to use it, a sign she has known me for a long time but no longer sees me as her doctor. She has mentioned a therapist I know well and admire. "Apparently Ann has developed a practice focusing on women who have had anorexia for a really long time. I'm thinking of going to see her. What do you think?"

I tell her that I think it would be wonderful for her to see Ann, and that she seems to be at a point in her life where she has achieved a degree of insight into the costs of her eating disorder that was not possible before. I suggest that working toward some realistic goals with Ann holds out real hope for change.

I am genuinely delighted to hear Kirsten has not given up on feeling better, although I am concerned about her ability to make meaningful gains after so many years of illness. Given Kirsten's insight, I know she is too. I admire her tenacity. Perhaps even after all this time, her survivor instinct can overpower her eating disorder. It is not beyond the realm of possibility. And the gains won't necessarily be measured in pounds. But meeting Kirsten again and encountering the reality of her chronic struggle with her disorder is difficult today, when Daryl's death has made me unusually vulnerable professionally. It shakes my ability to compartmentalize past mistakes and regrets, a denial necessary for my day-to-day work treating and giving hope to my patients. Still, I have learned, painfully, that authenticity inevitably requires us to look back at those memories in order to learn from them. I know that Kirsten's words to me today – "I wish you had done more" – will haunt me.

The field of eating disorders has, of course, moved on since I left it, although any apparent easy cures remain mirages. Our early hope in fluoxetine (Prozac) in the 1980s and 1990s as a possible protector for patients who achieved the incredible feat of weight restoration was undermined by a study in 2006 demonstrating no difference in rates of relapse between patients on the medication and those not.[13] There was initial excitement at the possibility that the so-called new generation of antipsychotics might help dangerously low-weight women, but that has given way to a realization that so far, research looking at the effectiveness of these drugs has produced equivocal results at best. To date, food itself remains the drug of choice in reversing the dangerous starvation of anorexia nervosa. The only relative bright light derives from studies demonstrating that children and adolescents with anorexia tend to do better, particularly with family therapy, which supports the theory – and Kirsten's regret – that if the disease is caught early and treated aggressively, intervention may support better outcomes.[14]

"I've lived with this illness more than I've lived without it," says Kirsten. "Most of the time, I can't imagine life without it. It's cost me so much, but it's also always there for me. In a strange way it's come to define me to myself. I am not even sure who I am without an eating disorder. That isn't to say that I don't wonder sometimes what my life would have been without it. It took up so much time, so much energy, so much mental space."

"Kirsten, maybe when you see Ann, you can talk to her about this. It seems very important to me that you give yourself the chance to imagine your life, the time you have left, without an eating disorder."

I've learned in my work that an inexhaustible capacity for hope is essential – for me and for my patients. There is a controversial literature on a palliative-care approach for patients who have struggled with eating disorders for decades and have reached a point when any chance at recovery appears long gone.[15] For those who support such an approach, the only sensible path seems to be to prepare the patient and her family for the fact that the patient will die a cruelly early death.

I am more drawn to a small group of authors who have written about the importance of continuing to work therapeutically with patients with chronic illnesses. Predictably, these clinicians tend to draw on a vast experience in treating patients with eating disorders and have been sufficiently humbled in doing so that they no longer see it as their job to coerce patients to try yet another treatment. Rather, they ally with them to understand their experience of treatment and consider with the patient how to build a life worth living.[16] And who knows – if a patient who has been ill for decades can build a life, maybe she will decide she can tolerate some minimal weight gain that will allow her to enjoy it that much more. This is indeed the broader definition of recovery that is now the zeitgeist in mental health – that recovery means not a narrow definition of "cure" but rather a broader concept of a journey toward a meaningful life, an adaptation, an acceptance, and a focus on strengths despite limitations.

Today, Kirsten tells me, "It must have been so frustrating to you when you couldn't find a way to shift the needle on the weight scale in the nurse's office, but it wasn't nothing that you saw me whenever I asked to see you, and that you made it clear I mattered to you."

I hope that Kirsten will follow up with Ann Kerr, but I also ask if she would ever consider another try at more intensive treatment, such as a hospital-based refeeding program. She takes a long time to answer. I see tears in her penetrating blue eyes. She blinks them away before they can fall.

"I still have hope that God has a plan for me to recover from this. I haven't closed the door."

AFTER ESCORTING KIRSTEN TO the door and saying good-bye, I experience a compulsive urge to open my email even though I have only a few minutes before I am due to see Frederick and his wife, Colleen, for a debrief of his ECT experience earlier this week. I recognize the urge for what it is – a means to avoid the sadness and helplessness that I feel for Daryl, Kirsten, and countless others whom I have not helped to achieve a significant and sustained period of remission from their illness, let alone a cure.

Answering my email would be the Goldbloom way. Getting on with things, staying active, not wallowing, not mourning spilt milk – all worthy principles and ones that have served my family well. But I stop myself. I have learned various lessons from my decades in psychiatry: the importance of stillness, waiting, doing nothing, taking time and space to pay appropriate attention to my own feelings and those of others. Not doing so risks missing important clues lying beneath the surface of everyday behavior and consciousness as to what needs attention, what needs to be done. These lessons still don't come easily to me; they are counter to my temperament and natural (and familial) inclinations, but I have learned to be more process-oriented, less goal-focused than I likely would have become in a different vocation.

I take a moment to recognize my sadness at Kirsten's predicament and Daryl's death. Underlying this is a wider, deeper emotion that threatens to overwhelm me. My psyche, despite all the defense mechanisms at my disposal, can't keep at bay this new idea, this grappling with the possibility of the world without my mother – my funny, energized, no-holds-barred, loving mother. I acknowledge for a moment that such a world will be a much less joyful, less lively, less driven place for me and my family.

Frederick and Colleen will arrive any moment. I bookmark the feeling, turning my mind instead toward what the couple will need from me to make sense of Frederick's experience of ECT and to buttress their hope that after so many false starts, this treatment will finally alleviate his symptoms. I marshal my resources by structuring in my mind a brief, reasoned account of the research behind the use of ECT in patients like him, together with potential explanations regarding any side effects that he may be experiencing.

When Simone tells me they have arrived, I am ready. They enter together and sit at the circular conference table in my office.

"Well, you've had two ECTs so far this week. How have they gone for you?"

"Better than I expected," Frederick replies.

"Especially since you thought you'd end up as a turnip," Colleen adds, smiling slightly.

"How have you tolerated them?"

"My jaw was really sore after the first one, but not the second. I felt pretty groggy for much of the day. And I forgot we had seen my in-laws last week for supper until Colleen reminded me – but then it all came galloping back to me. More than I actually wanted to remember."

He smiles, a small miracle, given the depths of depression in which he has been submerged. I glance over to Colleen to make sure she has seen it. As she leans over and takes her husband's hand in hers, it is clear that she has.

I explain that for reasons we don't understand, the jaw pain he described – likely from clenching during the muscle contraction phase of the seizure – is more common with the first treatment than with subsequent ones.

"Have you noticed any changes for the better?"

"Not really. I can't say I'm less depressed or anything."

"I can," Colleen interjects. "The day after the first treatment he just seemed a little quicker off the draw, more responsive to me. Even more so yesterday. I could see a change in his face. This morning, as we got ready to drive here, he was perkier, taking more initiative to do things. I'm beginning to see flickers of old Freddy." She starts to cry. Frederick moves his chair closer to her and puts his arm around her.

"This is really good news. In my experience, people who get better with ECT often respond early to it, but they have a sawtooth pattern of response, feeling better for a few hours and then feeling low again, but all the time arcing upward to sustained relief of depression. People around you often notice the improvement before you do, because you're stewing in your own juice twenty-four/seven. So it's no surprise that Colleen is picking up changes first. And it sounds as if you're tolerating it pretty well. I suggest you continue, and we'll meet again after another four treatments to see how it's going."

Their fear of the treatment itself has subsided, modest but significant changes are emerging, and they can move forward now with some hope – not based on my word but on their experience, the most persuasive evidence.

AS I HEAD DOWN to get lunch, my thoughts wander back to the three patients seen this morning. All have had their lives thrown off course by psychiatric disorders – Philip crippled by anxiety that, left untreated, has the potential to grow into a destructive typhoon of addiction that could blow away his career and residual relationships; Kirsten's intelligence and capacity for relationships limited by the ravages of an eating disorder that robbed her of her physical health, and the career and children that she might otherwise have chosen; and Frederick, whose depressions have threatened the equilibrium of the happy and successful life he worked hard to build. I am hopeful that both Philip and Frederick can be helped to keep their lives on track by their encounters with Josh and me and our recommendations for treatment, but it remains to be seen. The life that Kirsten might have had if freed from her anorexia – despite her generosity today in telling me that our years of appointments and medication trials helped her – has not been salvaged, despite her strength in carving out and maintaining long-term relationships, and the contribution to others' lives that she has made in her volunteerism and in her family.

Inevitably, given my psychological state today, I think back to the mistakes I have made in my career and that I hope to help Josh avoid: missed opportunities to act as well as rushes to judgment; consultations provided to other physicians where I did not follow up assiduously enough with helpful telephone calls or offers to check in with the patients at a future date; Code Whites that potentially could have been avoided by more strategic use of verbal de-escalation or medication; not following up on Daryl's final words to me: *It's hard.* There are too many.

But perhaps in dwelling on my perceived mistakes, I am guilty of therapeutic omnipotence, believing I have far more influence on my patients' decisions and outcomes than is the case. And arrogance, in believing that I could make it through thirty years of practice without error and reasons for self-recrimination.

Psychiatry has few easy answers for either its patients or its doctors. Even when immediate responses to medication or ECT or psychotherapeutic interventions occur, they can be maintained only through hard work and usually repetition. What it does have is the potential for connections between two people built on trust, whether based on interactions lasting no more than fifty minutes or on interactions over months or years. Those connections at their best facilitate good responses to treatment and mitigate the collateral damage of psychiatric disorders by preventing the loss of work, housing, and relationships, and perhaps most of all by reducing patients' isolation and suffering.

11

Public and Private

FRIDAY AFTERNOON AND EVENING

I run from the parking lot to the anonymous ballroom, arriving ten minutes before my scheduled presentation, clutching the speaking notes I will likely not use. My last task of the day is a talk to a union group of telecommunications workers who are holding their annual national meeting at a midtown hotel. Participants are just returning from their late buffet lunch in the hallway, and I take my place at a circular table near the podium marked RESERVED FOR SPEAKERS. An attractive woman with a short, spiky haircut who I think is about my age (in other words, she is probably younger than me) introduces herself as one of the union representatives and organizers of the event.

We chat about the locale and the salad she's finishing, and then – just as I think we are about to run out of topics – she asks me, "What do you think of my new haircut?"

I am taken aback by what seems like an odd question for two people meeting for the first time, but perhaps she is simply trying to keep the conversation going. I am nevertheless hesitant; in my experience there are few minefields riskier than commenting on a woman's appearance.

After a moment I throw out, "Well, it's kind of . . . punky." As I say it, I kick myself for not coming up with an adjective that is more complimentary than descriptive.

"Thanks – I think," she says. "I used to have shoulder-length hair, but a year ago I was diagnosed with breast cancer. I had surgery, then chemo and radiation. My hair fell out – they told me it would – but now it's grown back to this length and I'm kind of liking it. I step out of the shower and it's done!"

"You're right; it looks great," I offer weakly, but now I'm emboldened and decide to plunge in. "You and I met less than two minutes ago, and you obviously feel comfortable enough to tell me about your cancer, the treatment and the side effects. I'm here to give a talk about mental illness. Do you think you would have disclosed a mental illness to me so quickly?"

She smiles. "Nope. Not in a million years. And I know mental illness. My husband was hospitalized for depression two years ago. One of my biggest fears when I was diagnosed with cancer was that he wouldn't be able to cope. In my dark moments I worried that if I ended up dying, he wouldn't be okay psychologically and wouldn't be able to be there for our kids. I think I was more worried about the impact of my diagnosis on him than on how things would turn out for me. I know it was crazy. He's been fine, better than fine. I don't know how I would have managed without him."

I ask for her permission to use the first half of this story to make a point, and she agrees – another departure from my speaking notes.

After the moderator of the session introduces me, I step up to the podium.

I begin my talk by recounting the conversation I just had with my tablemate. Then I ask the audience to do a shout-out exercise with me. The only prop I have requested is a flip chart. I tell them to park their political correctness at the door and to shout out adjectives that describe someone who is mentally ill.

It starts slowly, with one person saying "nuts." I write it on the chart, then goad them, challenging them to say something I haven't heard before. The wave of adjectives swells: "Whack job . . . psycho . . . loony tunes . . . dangerous . . . weird . . . scary . . . out to lunch . . . an enchilada short of a combo plate."

In less than a minute, writing as fast as I can, twenty adjectives fill the page. I flip it over and ask them now to think of someone they know personally who has had cancer and shout out the adjectives that would describe that person. This time there is no delay: "brave . . . scared . . . sick . . . courageous . . . inspiring . . . alone."

The final thing I ask them to do is raise their hand if in the course of their lives they have known anyone who died by suicide. There are two hundred people in the room. All but a few raise a hand.

I tell them that this is why they are having this talk, because mental illness affects every Canadian family and every workplace. And I point out what they have already realized – that every one of the adjectives they use to describe a person with cancer is relevant to a person facing mental illness, and yet there is no shortage of words to denigrate, lampoon, and ultimately distance the latter. I tell them that the plethora of pejorative terms reflects the greatest disability that patients with mental illness face: stigma. I explain that stigma is a sociological concept that has its linguistic origin in the ancient Greek word describing the skin markings that branded someone as a slave or criminal. Research focusing on psychiatric stigma has looked backward to the myriad historical, cultural, religious, and ethnic contributions to perceptions of the mentally ill as outside mainstream society and therefore undeserving of the respect and rights owed to more desirable citizens. A 2001 *British Journal of Psychiatry* article that reviewed the vast literature on the topic summarized the impacts of psychiatric stigma as threefold: social exclusion, financial hardship, and discrimination.[1]

The mood in the room is more somber now, and I wonder if people are thinking about their friends and relatives who have mental illness. But it would be physically impossible for me to sustain an hour at the podium without jokes, so I oscillate between surefire punch lines and take away messages.

"One in five. That's the number of Canadians each year who will experience some form of mental illness. That's not just one in five over the course of a lifetime. It's every year. And it's not the same one in five each year. These numbers can be confusing. It's like that statistic about traffic accidents in Manhattan – that a man is hit by a car there every twenty-three seconds. Some people think, 'Wow, that guy should get out of town.'

"Unlike the diseases that people jog along highways and climb skyscrapers to raise money for, which are usually diseases of middle age and old age, mental illnesses typically hit people in mid- to late adolescence and young adulthood, just as they are coming into their own identities personally and professionally. The thirty-six hundred Canadians who die tragically by suicide each year, most commonly in the grip of mental illness, represent a small percentage of Canadians who live with these disorders year in, year out. In Ontario, where a third of the entire Canadian population lives, the most comprehensive study of illness burden – which is defined and measured as the combination of lives lost prematurely and lives lived with diminished function – has shown that mental illnesses and addictions represent one and a half times the burden of all cancers combined."

I pause to take a question from the audience.

A South Asian woman who looks about fifty says, "Did you say one and a half times of all cancers? That sounds high to me."

"Yes, that's right. They looked at data for all adults in this province and examined the illness burden of just six psychiatric disorders – depression, bipolar disorder, schizophrenia, social phobia, panic disorder, and agoraphobia – as well as three substance use disorders – alcohol, cocaine, and prescription painkiller abuse. And when they compared that burden with the burden of all cancers combined in adults, it was one and a half times greater. But if you look at the resources available, the public and private support provided, there are nowhere near one and half times the resources for mental illness compared to cancer.

"If these statistics seem shocking, I would argue that one of the main reasons is that mental illnesses tend to be hidden. People don't talk about mental illnesses the way they do these days about cancer or heart disease. Which leaves us with the illusion that mental illness is much less common than it really is. Which in turn leaves patients feeling isolated and strange, rather than having the experience that other types of patients do – of knowing that many of their friends, neighbors, and colleagues have shared something similar."

I see people in the audience nodding. My interrogator sits down after thanking me for my response and whispers something to the person sitting next to her.

"There's more. In terms of the Canadian workplace, where estimates are that each day there are five hundred thousand people off from work due to mental illness, we know that mental illnesses are the leading cause of disability requiring a leave of absence in the private and public sectors. Forget the incalculable human cost to individuals and their families; there is also a measurable cost for organizations and for countries. It's said that mental illnesses cost the Canadian economy $51 billion a year in lost productivity as well as health-care costs."

Now that the devastating consequences of mental illness on the economy have caught their attention, I turn to some specific findings on the impact of mental illness on the workplace. While I refer primarily to Canadian studies (which I know the best), it's the same story in the United States, Australia, and Europe. In addition to the obvious consequences of absenteeism, there is the more subtle "presenteeism," when ill workers dutifully show up but are prone to lower productivity and error. The reasons for presenteeism are many – a person may not even be aware that she is ill, or she may not be able to find treatment or accept it if it is offered, or she might not want to admit she is ill because of the stigma or shame.

I describe what someone in the workplace who is mentally ill might look like. There might be changes in his demeanor – he might seem less responsive verbally and emotionally, or seem less engaged with his work, or make uncharacteristic mistakes; he might appear unusually irritable or even explosive. He may seem more isolated, making excuses not to take part in the kind of office socializing that was previously routine for him. Emails and voice mail messages may uncharacteristically be left unanswered. There may be vague health complaints as well as increased sick days. I had one patient who told me that her boss had called her in for a meeting to let her know that colleagues had noticed a deterioration in her grooming and hygiene and had complained. My patient knew it was true but felt unable to talk about the real reason: she was so depressed that she was barely making it to work at all, let alone managing to shower, do laundry, or style her hair.

I move on to discuss the climate in the workplace. I ask the audience what their organization's response is when a colleague is struck by a bus and hospitalized on an orthopedic unit of the local hospital. They describe delegations of visitors, flowers, cards, and gifts. Then when she is at home recovering, they send over casseroles, and later, when she is up to it, work that she can do at home. When she is ready to return to work, albeit in a wheelchair with her legs in casts, they raise her desk and build a ramp.

"And what if she had thrown herself under the bus, escaped physical injury, but was admitted to the psychiatric ward of the local hospital?"

Silence.

In the remainder of the hour, I review the initiatives of the Mental Health Commission of Canada around workplace mental health in an effort to promote psychological health and safety in the workplace. "Our occupational health and safety standards seem a bit stuck on steel toes and protective eyewear, but in our postmodern economy it is what is between our ears that is our greatest work asset. That's why the Mental Health Commission has led the creation of the world's first standards for psychological health and safety in the workplace. They address everything from organizational culture and leadership to the known factors associated with good employee mental health and the need for resources when people are mentally ill."

An audience member asks me to elaborate.

"Let me start with what we know about healthy workplaces: these are environments that support procedural justice in the resolution of issues, fairness, and respect toward all employees, give employees a sense of control over their work, and reward them appropriately. As for necessary resources for employees with mental illness, the commission has identified the need for employee and family assistance programs that provide counseling, appropriate disability leaves, and tailored return-to-work strategies."

I am interrupted by a burst of applause. As it subsides, I suspect that beyond the technical elements of my talk, the applause stems from the audience's emotional reaction as they think about themselves, their families, and their colleagues.

A woman raises her hand and says that she sometimes would like to express concern about a colleague but worries about confidentiality. In reply I tell them the story of a speech I gave at a major bank. At the end of my talk, a woman stood up and announced that she had had bipolar disorder for the last decade. Three times in the preceding ten years, she had needed to take a medical leave for her illness. And each time when she returned, no one said anything to her about her absence. "It would have meant so much to me if you had simply asked, 'How are you? What happened?' It wasn't a matter of confidentiality. I would have told you; I figured you already knew anyway, you had seen the signs." As tears rolled down her cheeks, she sat down. Then, quietly, one by one, other managers stood up and divulged their family histories – a brother with schizophrenia, a mother who drank herself to death, a niece with anorexia nervosa, a son with depression. As a group, they realized this common experience was unspoken. I left that group hopeful that now that the door had been opened, it would not be allowed to shut again. But I also tell today's audience something they already know: that such disclosures, however courageous, don't always elicit such positive responses. I have learned the hard way from my patients that we have a long way to go before employees can safely disclose mental illness in their . workplaces without fear of repercussion, however subtle. There are now tools – such as decision aids that help people to articulate pros and cons of disclosure, whom to tell, and when to tell – to help people work through whether to disclose in the workplace, and there is good research evidence that such aids reduce uncertainty and dissatisfaction with making these difficult choices.[2]

I see that the speaker scheduled to follow me, who is listed in the program as the chief negotiator for their collective agreement, is in the bullpen, waiting to stride to the podium. I have no idea how long I've been speaking and, in these circumstances, often fall back on a one-liner I stole from my parents, both loquacious public speakers.

"Sorry that I've lost track of time. A few minutes ago I saw the fellow in the blue suit checking his watch, and a moment ago I saw him checking his calendar." This gets the exit laugh that allows me to leave the stage comfortably and head to my car.

I DELIBERATELY TAKE A circuitous route home, one of my favorites, along a one-way road that curves along the bottom of the wooded ravine that is our backyard. There is little or no pedestrian traffic, and in the middle of a busy city, the valley provides a brief stretch of quiet and natural beauty. My car stereo is blasting Robert Schumann's piano quartet, its third movement one of the most meltingly beautiful and simple melodies I've ever heard. Schumann's life included recurrent episodes of depression and mania, suicide attempts, and an ignominious death in an asylum, his creativity silenced by the ravages of illness. Glenn Gould made this recording half a century ago with members of the Juilliard String Quartet, one of the rare chamber recordings by an artist who was a soloist in music and in life. Gould was the object of endless postmortem psychological speculation, an activity I have become more cautious about over the years, given its risks of inaccuracy, presumption, and even exploitation. I allow myself to be drawn back into the recurring cello theme of the movement. I drive more slowly than usual, and the world outside my car seems suspended. There is a melancholy to the music that ushers me back to Daryl.

I believe that Daryl's mother was sincere when she thanked me on Thursday night for all I had done for Daryl. My father and brother, both pediatricians, have attended patients' funerals, never questioning whether their presence was desired by the family and taking their welcome for granted. Psychiatrists who lose patients don't have that confidence, and before attending they check carefully to ascertain whether the family is comfortable with this customary sign of respect.

I am forced to remember at times like this that psychiatrists remain outliers in medicine. Our field's relative lack of diagnostic certainty, together with our focus on intangible and nonquantifiable signs and symptoms in our patients such as mood, consciousness, identity, cognition, and awareness of reality, singles us out.

This lack is almost as frustrating for psychiatrists as it is for patients. Many of my colleagues working in clinics, hospitals, and private offices talk about the current gap between the neuroscience research that dominates our academic journals and preoccupies the popular media, and their day-to-day hopes and disappointments for their patients. Some of them study and advocate loudly for essential services and treatment supports for patients with mental illness: the need for accessible and affordable housing to prevent relapse and revolving-door hospitalizations, the impact of health-care professionals' and the public's negative beliefs regarding mentally ill patients on their medical care and employment opportunities, and the need for more mental health services for prison populations. Unfortunately, the work of these clinicians and researchers tends not to come to the public's attention until there is some sort of disaster – a death of a homeless person, or an assault. Their studies are much less sexy than cover articles in *Time* magazine showing a brain lit up like a lightbulb and a headline that promises that the mysteries of consciousness will be revealed inside.

As a result, the public's perception of psychiatry is ambivalent at best. It is seen – accurately – as a divided profession that cannot get its clinical, academic, or public relations acts together. Patients are often baffled and disappointed by our explanations that they are suffering from what is likely to prove a chronic illness that may have recurrences, and that they will require ongoing treatment and possibly medication. After all, if we now have machines that can look inside your head and describe which areas of your brain are activated when you see a picture of an attractive person, or a piece of chocolate cake, or a zombie, how is it that we do not have treatments that provide a 100 percent cure for psychosis or depression?

I don't see the limits to psychiatric knowledge as a failure, but rather as an acceptance that not everything is knowable in the empirical language of medical science. The myth of certainty is alive and well in areas of medicine beyond psychiatry, despite the reality that the precise causes of most noninfectious diseases remain unknown.

Psychiatry has made its greatest mistakes when its practitioners claimed miracle-cure status for new treatments without adequately testing their hypotheses, or without recognizing that some hypotheses are unprovable with current knowledge and tools. The example of psychoanalysis – whose proponents expanded its original Freudian mandate based on treating the Viennese bourgeoisie to treating patients with schizophrenia, bipolar disorder, and suicidal depression – leaps to mind. So too do lobotomies, originally conceived by the Portuguese neurologist Egas Moniz in 1935 as a treatment for obsessive-compulsive disorder (for which a less invasive version of neurosurgery is still used today) but which fast spread as a treatment – in many cases catastrophic – for a range of psychiatric illnesses. Arguably, psychiatrists' fervent desire to prove themselves scientists, and equal to those medical colleagues with more robust evidence for their practice, has led some of them to postulate certainty where none can exist. And in their overzealous efforts, these few have rendered psychiatric practice vulnerable to excesses and unethical treatments that have tainted the entire profession.

A less sinister outcome of psychiatry's blind faith in scientific progress has been a blinkered approach to knowledge that has undermined what I believe could be psychiatry's unique contribution to modern medicine. Neuroscientific advances are not sufficient to lessen the stigma, desperation, and suffering associated with major mental illness. Research in the humanities and social sciences that focuses on individual psychological development and what binds and divides human communities is essential to our understanding of how to alleviate the burden of mental illness. At least in the short term it is likely to outperform our current brain science discoveries. I am happy to have supported in my work for the Mental Health Commission of Canada examples of immediately useful research such as At Home/Chez Soi and the initiatives produced by the National Standards for Psychological Health and Safety in the workplace.[3]

If psychiatry pursues diverse research paths that lead to concrete help for our patients and direction for our policy makers, it will offer the rest of medicine a uniquely modern way forward. There is an urgent need for physicians to grapple with the oppressively quantitative and technological model of medicine that dominates in developed countries struggling with aging patient populations and ballooning health-care costs without correspondingly increased budgets. The current model in these countries focuses on numbers and efficiency instead of looking at less obvious contributors to patients' outcomes, such as their relationships with their doctors and health-care providers, the aesthetic design of clinical settings, and the role of psychosocial and economic life stressors in disease, including unemployment, poverty, abuse, ethnicity, and immigration.

One of the most interesting series of studies I have come across in recent years describes how patients who trust and have a good relationship with their doctors have better diabetes outcomes.[4] We are a long way from understanding the biological and psychological mechanisms that link feeling good in a medical appointment to having better glucose control, but to my mind it is an eminently worthwhile pursuit. Good physician-patient relationships may be the cheapest possible treatment intervention yet discovered.

Doctors don't like to admit their own biases. They especially do not like to admit in front of a patient that they don't know what is wrong or how to help. Physicians are taught to present ourselves as rational, objective professionals with answers for every human ailment or dilemma. And yet my own experience has taught me not to see uncertainty as a failure. In fact, I have found that patients can tolerate a much greater degree of humility on our part than we think (or perhaps than we are comfortable with) as long as it is matched with a commitment to see them through whatever treatment trials and retrials and advocacy their disease requires.

Psychiatry's intellectual eclecticism – historically a source of controversy and characterized as a weakness – allows it to offer this new medical paradigm, which emphasizes the importance of providing both physicians and patients with relationships within which science, technology, and humanism come together to ameliorate the suffering imposed by mental illness.

TURNING ONTO OUR DEAD-END street, I see small children running up and down the sidewalk, laughing and chasing each other as our boys did when we moved here twenty years ago. I need to pay attention and slow down. A week of thinking about uncomfortable things – my failures with patients, psychiatry's stigmatized status within medicine, and my emotions, things that are usually stored far in the back of my brain – is now affecting my driving, and the finale of the piano quartet has led me to accelerate without noticing. I have inherited my liking for speed from my mother, who has a long history of speeding tickets and traffic court appearances in both Quebec and Nova Scotia. Like me, she is impatient. She finds it frustrating to wait for my father to take another practice swing before he tees off at golf, preferring what she calls "ready steady golf."

Daniel and Will are already at the house when I get home. Daniel, our older son, is articling at a downtown law firm this year. I don't see him as much as I would like as a result of his hectic work schedule and full social life with his girlfriend. It's good to see him tonight. Will, our younger son, is going to start law school in the fall, though he is not sure if it fits with his commitment to social justice and challenging orthodoxy and wonders if it signifies too great a degree of conformity to a Goldbloom worldview where the professions are held sacrosanct. Neither son has evinced any interest in medicine as a career, although once when Daniel was young and was asked about his future, he said he'd like to be "either a doctor or an actor who plays a doctor." This comment has always stayed with me. It's funny, but also it contains the truth that draws me to both theater and medicine: we seek out roles for ourselves before fully understanding them, emulating those who have most profoundly inspired us. Neither Nancy nor I regret that our sons won't follow in our career footsteps. It seems to me a good sign that the boys are finding their own ways in the world.

Nancy has spoken to both boys about my mother's possible (I still cannot say *probable* to myself) diagnosis. Knowing Nancy, I suspect she may also have told them that I lost a patient this week as a way of explaining why I may seem distracted or aloof. Daniel asks me right away how I am doing. The honest answer is that I don't know, but that doesn't seem a particularly helpful response.

"This week's been no walk in the park. It's the waiting that's the hardest part. I keep reminding myself that even if the news is bad, it's hardly unexpected, or even tragic. Your grandmother is eighty-seven; she has lived almost every minute of that time in perfect health. It doesn't get much better."

I think I am comforting them, repeating phrases about my mother and the long, rich life she has led. Deep down I already know that I will repeat them many, many times over coming weeks. And even I know how ridiculous it sounds, because what Will and Dan are concerned about is not the logic of mortality but the emotional impact on me of losing my mother. Our sons are young men in their twenties now, and they want to comfort me. Losing a grandmother seems more in the natural order of things to them than losing a parent does to me.

Daniel is dressed in his work clothes, a suit and tie, a sight that still sometimes catches me off guard. He gives me a hug. "True, Dad. But that doesn't mean you don't get to feel sad."

My eyes are suddenly hot. I wonder if I am about to cry. I see Will watching me. I can feel his compassion, and I pull myself together. "I know, Dan, I know, and I will. But it's premature still. We need to wait for the MRI."

Nancy comes in from the kitchen.

"Dave, don't forget to call your parents. They called earlier; they're leaving shortly for dinner with Laura and Jim. Boys, why don't you help me set the table, dress the salad. Can one of you open the wine? Dan, will you light the candles?"

I take the phone into our family room and look out over the fir trees towering in the ravine. I take a breath and dial my parents' number. It is my mother who picks up.

"David? How are you, darling? Nanner said she thought you'd be back in time to call. She said you're having the boys for dinner. I had such a good time with them at the law school graduation. They're terrific." Her descriptions are rarely less than superlative, like a television infomercial with products for sale and operators standing by. "I hope they're planning on coming to the cottage this summer. Mind you, your father and I have so much scheduled it's ridiculous. I haven't even told him half the things we're going to. You know, he doesn't have the energy he used to. He takes a nap *every afternoon* like clockwork." She is astounded that someone in his late eighties requires this and clearly views it as both a moral failing and a problem she will fix. She barely stops for a breath. When she does, I manage to tell her that I am well. She resumes immediately.

"Your father and I are having dinner with Laura and Jim at a new restaurant on Hollis Street. They called to see if we wanted to try it this weekend, and when your father asked if I was up to it, I told him not to be ridiculous. What else are we going to do? Sit around all weekend and worry about what may or may not be in my brain? I feel fine."

My mother chatters on, with my offering intermittent "uh-huhs." It's oddly comforting, as though nothing has changed, as though nothing ever will change. Then she stops for a moment.

"You sound tired, David. I hope you're going to get some rest this weekend. I hear from Nanner that you've been working like crazy."

It is unlike my mother to comment on my sounding anything less than my usual ebullient self, even less like her to advise slowing down. I know Nancy will not have burdened her with the fact that a patient of mine killed himself this week. I realize her unusual sensitivity to the fatigue she hears in my voice reflects the dance that she and I have begun as we face the dark probabilities of her diagnosis. I tell her that I am glad it is the end of the week and promise to follow her advice. We say good-bye and she hands over the phone to my father. I have a brief conversation with him about arrangements for the following week when I'll meet him in Montreal for the annual Alton Goldbloom lecture at the Montreal Children's Hospital.

He ends quietly, saying, "We should have the MRI results by then." He doesn't want to say more, and neither do I.

I say good-bye and ask him to pass on my best to Laura and Jim.

Dinner feels charmed. Nancy, the boys, and I talk about Daniel's work and colleagues, Will's summer plans, and politics. I contribute less to the conversation than usual, but no one seems to mind. Both boys are engaged and informed; I am proud of them and couldn't feel more comforted than sitting at our dining table with them and Nancy.

As we start on dessert – flourless chocolate cake in honor of the boys – I can see through the windows behind us that the sun is setting and the light outside is that pinky blue that says summer's long nights are coming. I watch Nancy as she scoops ice cream onto the boys' plates, and Dan and Will as they tuck into their food and talk about their circles of friends. I am pierced by an overwhelming sense of how lucky I am. Lucky to be facing the potentially imminent (and eventually inevitable) loss of my mother with the support of these three people.

I think back to my university squash partner, Andrew Balkos, and wonder what happened to him and whether he is still alive. I think of Sylvia, surrounded by her family and friends tonight as she mourns her son's death; of Richard, who has likely taken advantage of the good weather to get in a late tennis game with a friend before the light fails; of Frederick and Colleen, wary but starting to see a response to ECT, and heading into the weekend with tentative hope; of Josh, who is on call, no doubt chatting and joking with the ER team in between seeing patients; of Kirsten, struggling to eat some supper to reassure her husband; of Georges, whom the team hopes to transfer out of ACU on Monday to the general psychiatry unit on the fifth floor, where he knows the nurses and psych assistants well and will stay until he is ready for discharge to his boardinghouse; and of each of the ER patients whom I sent home to their families and friends on Wednesday. I wonder how each of them is managing. Our lives have intersected and then spun off into a dozen directions.

It has been a long week; its events in my head are a cacophony of people and relationships, diseases, investigations, diagnoses, and hoped-for treatments. Coming from a family of doctors, I know better than most that much of modern medicine remains shrouded in darkness. There is no treatment that can reverse the march of my mother's cancer if it has indeed entered her brain, nor decelerate her aging.

Of all the medical specialties, mine remains the darkest – complex and filled with residual mysteries. This is not an easy thought but a true one. Almost simultaneously, I recognize another true thought, one that got me and all but one of my patients through the week: human relationships and their support are our best medicine. I hope I have served my patients well this week, even – especially – Daryl.

Epilogue

As I walk quickly to the restaurant, I regret not bringing a jacket. The September sun is bright but doesn't give much warmth, and there's a brisk breeze. Pier arrives just after me and joins me at our usual table. She gives me a hug.

"Nice to see you."

We chat about our summer holidays, our children, our relative busyness at work, the recent change in weather. After we order our food, I surprise myself.

"It's hard to believe it's been over a year since my mother's funeral."

Pier pauses almost imperceptibly before responding. She is as taken aback as I am that I have raised this subject unprompted.

"So it is. I had forgotten it was at the end of August. I wish I could have gone. I remember your telling me the funeral was packed. Half of Halifax there . . . How are you? Anniversaries can be hard."

"Okay, I think. I miss her, of course. I did a funny thing last night, though. I reread the eulogy I gave at the service. It's not like me to look back, but for some reason I wanted to remember that day. I don't think I ever showed it to you at the time. Here, I brought you a copy."

I pull it out from my pants pocket and hand it to her. The eulogy began as a letter I wrote to my mother when we both knew she was dying. It listed the top ten gifts and life lessons she had given me and chronicled the things about her – mainly funny but also value-laden – I would most miss. She loved the letter and read it over and over. Later she told me she wanted me to read it at her funeral, which I did.

As I watch Pier read it now, I think back to the signal events of the past eighteen months: the day in Montreal when, at a lecture in honor of my grandfather, my father told me that my mother's MRI confirmed brain metastases and described it as "a setback, a definite setback"; the summer weekend at my parents' cottage when I cried with my mother for the first time in decades and she told me that I had been "easy" for her; the two memorials I attended, my mother's and Daryl's, both full of humor and warmth; and the monthly meetings with Pier to review our progress on the book.

The pale autumn sunshine suddenly lights up the window next to us. As Pier reads, I recognize that through the act of writing our book, I have come to a new appreciation of how much my view of psychiatry has changed over the course of my career. The brash, privileged, overconfident twenty-six-year-old who chose psychiatry would have predicted a career spent researching biological cures for severe mental illness and a clinical practice in which he would single-handedly bring patients back from the brink of madness and restore them to their former selves.

But in the intervening years, my training, my clinical experience, and the important relationships in my life took me in a different direction. I learned the essential value of trust in relationships: between doctors and patients, between doctors and patients' families, and between colleagues who necessarily work together to support one another in providing the best possible care for patients. I learned other things, of course, things that might have deterred me from my choice of psychiatry had I known them at twenty-six. I also learned, with the help of my wife – the psychiatrist's daughter – how to understand and express my feelings, so that I can now receive comfort even while providing consolation to others.

Writing also forced me to recognize some hard lessons about my chosen field. Despite psychiatry's therapeutic advances and greater public education, mental illness remains a hard path to walk. Its travelers need a community that looks beyond the strangeness of madness to those things all its members share: a need for symptom relief, relationships, shelter, employment, respect, and caregivers whom we can trust. In psychiatry we provide some of those things some of the time, but not consistently or sufficiently.

At sixty, I am not done yet. I will continue to talk and write about psychiatry in order to demystify and destigmatize the work we do. By doing so, I hope to make psychiatrists' work more transparent so that people suffering from mental illnesses and their families may face one less barrier to seeking our help and trusting our ability to steer them toward the best treatments, however imperfect. I will also continue to teach psychiatry's newcomers what I have learned until I am no longer able to do so: that we prove ourselves worthy of our patients' trust by giving them our respect and care; by pursuing self-knowledge in order that we not harm them by our blind spots, biases, arrogance, or greed; by painstakingly accumulating and understanding the best evidence for what works and what doesn't; and, always, by acknowledging our responsibility toward those trapped in the darkness of madness. For they are not only our patients; they also are our friends, our family, ourselves.

Authors' Note

Significant issues of trust arise for physicians who write books that include their patients. Neither of us can forget the criticism thrown at the late neurologist and author Oliver Sacks by Tom Shakespeare, a geneticist and disability activist offended by Sacks' portrayals of neurologically impaired individuals. Shakespeare characterized Sacks harshly as the "man who mistook his patients for a literary career."[1] The ethics of physicians writing about patients have been written about in many forums, testifying to the unease that both physicians and patients experience when the extraordinary access offered to physicians in the course of their work is used for a literary purpose.

Arguably the ethical risks are greatest for psychiatrists and our patients, given the vulnerability and stigma associated with those who experience mental illness. We have identified "real" patients only with explicit permission. All others are fictitiously described, most representing composites we have created from our shared experiences of meeting thousands of patients over several decades.

We greatly respect our working environments and have also

identified "real" colleagues only with their agreement. We are grateful to those who provided feedback on their experiences and perspectives. All others are fictitious, again drawn compositely from our experience.

Someone who has lived through a psychiatric disorder and its treatment – whether the person directly affected by it or a family member or intimate – brings an essential understanding and point of view to the public discourse. On the other hand, our years of caring for patients, often during their most acute periods of illness, and of working within a mental health system that can only be characterized as fragmented and difficult to access, has given us a particular perspective. We have seen not only the barriers to receiving treatment faced by patients both within and outside the mental health system, but also the larger societal barriers that prevent desperately needed mental health research and treatments from receiving the funding and attention they require.

While we have attempted to write about psychiatry as a medical specialty that is international in scope, our experience as physicians working in Canada has inevitably shaped our descriptions. It is also true that in an attempt to avoid a book that extends to six volumes, we have left out fascinating chunks of psychiatric history and scientific discovery, and provided limited accounts of the sociological and philosophical critiques of how societies approach mental illness. We have therefore included a section on further reading for those who wish to know more about the subjects that we have only touched upon.

We should also note that we have compressed particular patient events that in fact took place over several months into a one-week period – although the variety of professional activities that occurs in one of David's weeks is realistic. We did so in the interest of meeting our publisher's requirement of not putting readers to sleep, as well as to emphasize the intersect between David's clinical and personal lives.

Of course, all mistakes, inaccuracies, and inevitable omissions are our own, as are passages where we have been inadvertently insensitive, cavalier, or simplistic. For these we apologize.

We want to offer our thanks to those without whom this book would never have come about. First, Malcolm Lester, who provided input and encouragement on a much different conception of a book, which nonetheless was the seed from which this book was born. Next, to colleagues Drs. Vivian Rakoff, Shitij Kapur, and Patricia Cavanagh, who patiently allowed themselves to be interviewed on their careers and ideas about psychiatry, again for a version that anticipated but was not included in this book. Michael Levine, our literary agent, tirelessly advocated for us with publishers that this was a book that mattered, and insisted that despite the gravity of its content, a book that would find an audience.

To Kevin Hanson, Alison Clarke, Phyllis Bruce, Patricia Ocampo, and the team at Simon & Schuster, thank you for believing we could learn to write a book and for treating us gently when we delivered our first draft.

To Jennifer Glossop, our literary editor, who patiently, kindly, and rigorously taught us how to write a readable book – without her eagle eye, insistence on clear, nontechnical language, and extraordinary understanding of what makes a book engaging, we would not have been able to deliver a manuscript.

Thank you to Judith Kwok for her invaluable assistance researching bibliographic resources on psychiatric history and science.

Pier wishes in addition to thank her colleagues in the Department of Psychiatry at the Hospital for Sick Children, who supported her in a part-time sabbatical to write the book, and who covered her on-call duties during that time. She thanks too her colleagues at the University of Toronto Undergraduate Medical Program, who supported her to reduce her workload there during the same time period. And David is grateful for all the opportunities that the Centre for Addiction and Mental Health has provided him to be a clinician, a teacher, a researcher, and a writer.

We both thank our families, who put up with our endless phone calls, weekend meetings, papers strewn over tables, and general abdication from much of family life while the book was being written.

Thank you, Nancy, Daniel, and Will.

Thank you, Micheil, Diana, Callum, and Euan.

Finally, we thank our colleagues and patients, both those who agreed to be in the book and those who inspired different parts of our composites of patients, residents, and colleagues. Our colleagues share the work and challenge of trying to do their best for patients with resources that are often limited and imperfect. Our medical students and residents come to psychiatry with fresh eyes and ask us why we can't do more for our patients, demanding that we respond to their questions with real solutions and with hope, rather than becoming jaded or resigned to the status quo.

Our patients teach us daily what it means to struggle with psychiatric disorders, and about the challenges they face in trusting mental health professionals after what is too often an illness history characterized by rejection, lack of collaboration, and failure to understand the breadth of damage that these disorders create across all domains of someone's life. They are amazingly generous in giving us chances to do better, and we owe them our best. We are extraordinarily grateful to Kirsten Halpin, Richard Braudo, and Sylvia Orzech (Daryl's mother), whose courage, honesty, and determination to battle the stigma associated with mental illness by sharing their stories have been an inspiration.

It has been a privilege to write this book. We hope that in doing so we have made psychiatry and psychiatrists less frightening, because as long as psychiatric disorders exist, we need to help one another to safety.

Notes

INTRODUCTION: "THEY" ARE "US"

1. Graham Thornicroft, Diana Rose, and Aliya Kassam, "Discrimination in Health Care Against People with Mental Illness," *International Review of Psychiatry* 19 (Jan. 2007): 113–122, doi: 10.1080 /09540260701278937; C. Lauber, C. Nordt, C. Braunschweig, and W. Rössler, "Do Mental Health Professionals Stigmatize Their Patients?" *Acta Psychiatrica Scandinavica* 113 (Jan. 2006): 51–59, doi: 10.1111/j.1600-0447.2005.00718.x.

1. FAMILY MEDICINE: SUNDAY

1. Ian F. Brockington and David B. Mumford, "Recruitment into Psychiatry," *British Journal of Psychiatry* 180 (2002): 307–12, doi: 10.1192/bjp.180.4.307.
2. Ivan W. Miller, Christine E. Ryan, Gabor I. Keitner, Duane S. Bishop, and Nathan B. Epstein, "The McMaster Approach to Families: Theory, Assessment, Treatment, and Research," *Journal of Family Therapy*

22 (2000): 168–89; see also Christine E. Ryan, Nathan B. Epstein, Gabor I. Keitner, Ivan W. Miller, and Duane S. Bishop, *Evaluating and Treating Families: The McMaster Approach* (New York: Routledge, 2005).

3. Edward Shorter, *A History of Psychiatry: From the Era of the Asylum to the Age of Prozac* (New York: John Wiley, 1997), 26.

4. Leon Eisenberg, "Mindlessness and Brainlessness in Psychiatry," *British Journal of Psychiatry* 148 (1986): 497–508, doi: 10.1192 /bjp.14.5.497.

2. LISTENING FOR A DIAGNOSIS: MONDAY MORNING

1. www.cambridgeshire.gov.uk/NR/ . . . /O/AHistoryofCounty Asylums.pdf. "A History of County Asylums," https://web .archive.org/web/20140414130409/http://www.cambridgeshire .gov.uk/NR/rdonlyres/DEF85AEC-CCCB-429D-8328 -BB802A2E77EC/0/AHistoryofCountyAsylums.pdf.

2. "Mental Health Services," *Te Ara – The Encyclopedia of New Zealand*, www.teara.govt.nz/en/mental-health-services/page-2.

3. Susan Piddock, "Convicts and the Free: Nineteenth-Century Lunatic Asylums in South Australia and Tasmania (1830–1883)," *Australasian Historical Archaeology* 19 (2001): 84–96.

4. Stefan Priebe, Claudia Palumbo, Sajjad Ahmed, Nadia Strappelli, Jelena Gavrilovic, and Stephen Bremner, "How Psychiatrists Should Introduce Themselves in the First Consultation: An Experimental Study," *British Journal of Psychiatry* 202 (June 2013): 459–62, doi: 10.1192/bjp.bp.112.123877.

5. Canadian Institute for Health Information, report, November 18, 2014.

6. Robert Lindner, *The Fifty-Minute Hour: A Collection of True Psychoanalytic Tales* (New York: Rinehart, 1955).

7. Abraham M. Nussbaum, *The Pocket Guide to the DSM-5 Diagnostic Exam* (Arlington, VA: American Psychiatric Publishing, 2013).

8. David S. Goldbloom, "General Principles of Interviewing," in

Goldbloom, ed., *Psychiatric Clinical Skills*, rev. 1st ed. (Toronto: Centre for Addiction and Mental Health, 2010), 6.

9. American Psychiatric Association, *Diagnostic and Statistical Manual of Mental Disorders*, 5th ed. (Arlington, VA: American Psychiatric Publishing, 2013).

10. American Psychiatric Association, "Homosexuality and Sexual Orientation Disturbance: Proposed Change in DSM-II, 6th Printing, Page 44," APA Document Reference No. 730008 (Arlington, VA: American Psychiatric Publishing, 1973).

11. Allen Frances, *Saving Normal: An Insider's Revolt Against Out-of-Control Psychiatric Diagnosis, DSM-5, Big Pharma, and the Medicalization of Ordinary Life* (New York: William Morrow, 2013).

12. British Psychological Society, "British Psychological Society Statement on the Open Letter to the DSM-5 Taskforce," http://www .bps.org.uk/sites/default/files/documents/pr1923_attachment _-_final_bps_statement_on_dsm-5_12-12-2011.pdf.

13. Heinz E. Lehmann, "Clinical Evaluation and Natural Course of Depression," *Journal of Clinical Psychiatry* 44, sect. 2 (May 1983): 5–10.

14. Ronald C. Kessler, Katherine A. McGonagle, Shanyang Zhao, Christopher B. Nelson, Michael Hughes, Suzann Eshleman, Hans-Ulrich Wittchen, and Kenneth S. Kendler, "Lifetime and 12-Month Prevalence of DSM-III-R Psychiatric Disorders in the United States. Results from the National Comorbidity Survey," *Archives of General Psychiatry* 51 (Jan. 1994): 8–19, doi: 0.1001/arch psyc.1994.03950010008002.

15. Ellen Frank, Barbara Anderson, Charles F. Reynolds III, Angela Ritenour, and David J. Kupfer, "Life Events and the Research Diagnostic Criteria Endogenous Subtype: A Confirmation of the Distinction Using the Bedford College Methods," *Archives of General Psychiatry* 51 (July 1994): 519–24, doi: 10.1001/arch psyc.1994.03950070011005.

16. American Psychiatric Association, *Desk Reference to the Diagnostic*

Criteria from DSM-5 (Arlington, VA: American Psychiatric Publishing, 2013).

17. Karen Amner, "The Effect of DBT Provision in Reducing the Cost of Adults Displaying the Symptoms of BPD," *British Journal of Psychotherapy* 28 (Aug. 2012): 336–52, doi: 10.1111/j.1752 -0118.2012.01286.x.

18. Goldbloom, "General Principles of Interviewing," 9.

19. Richard B. Goldbloom, "Interviewing: The Most Sophisticated of Diagnostic Technologies," *Annals of the Royal College of Physicians and Surgeons of Canada* 26 (1993): 224–28.

20. Eric Kandel, *The Age of Insight: The Quest to Understand the Unconscious in Art, Mind, and Brain, from Vienna 1900 to the Present* (New York: Random House, 2012).

3. COPING BUT NOT CURED: MONDAY AFTERNOON

1. Joanna S. Bromley and Sara J. Cunningham, "'You Don't Bring Me Flowers Any More': An Investigation into the Experience of Stigma by Psychiatric In-Patients," *The Psychiatrist* 28 (Sept. 2004): 371–74, doi: 10.1192/pb.28.10.371.

2. Michael Serby, "Psychiatric Resident Conceptualizations of Mood and Affect Within the Mental Status Examination," *American Journal of Psychiatry* 160 (Aug. 2003): 1527–29, doi: 10.1176/appi.ajp.160.8.1527.

3. Joel Paris, *The Bipolar Spectrum: Diagnosis or Fad?* (New York: Routledge, 2012).

4. Kay Redfield Jamison, *An Unquiet Mind: A Memoir of Moods and Madness* (New York: Alfred A. Knopf, 1995).

5. Kenneth I. Shulman and Ivan L. Silver, "Assessment of Older Adults," in Goldbloom, *Psychiatric Clinical Skills.*

6. World Health Organization, *Adherence to Long-Term Therapies: Evidence for Action* (Geneva: World Health Organization, 2003).

7. American Psychiatric Association, *Diagnostic and Statistical Manual*

of Mental Disorders, 4th ed., Text Revision (Arlington, VA: American Psychiatric Publishing, 2000).

8. American Psychiatric Association, *DSM-5.*

9. Cited in Roy Porter, "Mood Disorders: Social Section," in German Berrios and Roy Porter, eds., *A History of Clinical Psychiatry: The Origin and History of Psychiatric Disorders* (New York: NYU Press, 1995).

10. Philip B. Mitchell and Dusan Hadzi-Pavlovic, "Lithium Treatment for Bipolar Disorder," *Bulletin of the World Health Organization* 78 (2000): 515–17.

11. Andrea Cipriani, Keith Hawton, Sarah Stockton, and John R. Geddes, "Lithium in the Prevention of Suicide in Mood Disorders: Updated Systematic Review and Meta-Analysis," *BMJ* 346 (June 2013): 136–46, doi: 10.1136/bmj.f3646.

12. Martin Zinkler and Stefan Priebe, "Detention of the Mentally Ill in Europe – A Review," *Acta Psychiatrica Scandinavica* 106 (July 2002): 3–8, doi: 10.1034/j.1600-0447.2002.02268.x.

4. SHOCKED: TUESDAY MORNING

1. David S. Goldbloom and Dennis J. Kussin, "Electroconvulsive Therapy Training in Canada: A Survey of Senior Residents in Psychiatry," *Canadian Journal of Psychiatry* 36 (March 1991): 126–28; Edward Yuzda, Kathryn Parker, Vivien Parker, Justin Geagea, and David Goldbloom, "Electroconvulsive Therapy Training in Canada: A Call for Greater Regulation," *Canadian Journal of Psychiatry* 47 (Dec. 2002): 938–44.

2. Maurizio Pompili, David Lester, Giovanni Dominici, Lucia Longo, Giulia Marconi, Alberto Forte, Gianluca Serrafini, Mario Amore, and Paolo Girardi, "Indications for Electroconvulsive Treatment in Schizophrenia: A Systematic Review," *Schizophrenia Research* 146 (2013): 1–9, doi: 10.1016/j.schres.2013.02.005.

3. Cynthia J. Tsay, "Julius Wagner-Jauregg and the Legacy of Malarial Therapy for the Treatment of General Paresis of the Insane," *Yale*

Journal of Biological Medicine 86 (June 2013): 245–54, doi: 10.1176/appi.ajp.2014.13060787.

4. Edward M. Brown, "Why Wagner-Jauregg Won the Nobel Prize for Discovering Malaria Therapy for General Paresis of the Insane," *History of Psychiatry* xi (October 2000): 371–82.

5. "Notes and Comment," *American Journal of Psychiatry* 79 (April 1923): 721–23.

6. Joel T. Braslow, "Effect of Therapeutic Innovation on Perception of Disease and the Doctor-Patient Relationship: A History of General Paralysis of the Insane and Malaria Fever Therapy, 1910–1950," *American Journal of Psychiatry* 152 (May 1995): 660–65, doi: 10.1176/ajp.152.5.660; Tsay, "Julius Wagner-Jauregg," 251.

7. Edward Shorter and David Healy, *Shock Therapy: A History of Electroconvulsive Treatment in Mental Illness* (New Brunswick, NJ: Rutgers University Press, 2007), 9–10.

8. Jean Michel Barbier, Gérard Serra, and Gwenolé Loas, "Constance Pascal: Pioneer of French Psychiatry," *History of Psychiatry* 10 (1999): 425–37, doi: 10.1177/0957154X9901004002.

9. Shorter and Healy, *Shock Therapy*, 11.

10. "Insulin Coma Therapy," *The American Experience*, PBS, www.pbs.org/wgbh/amex/nash/filmmore/ps_ict.html.

11. Robert M. Kaplan, "A History of Insulin Coma Therapy in Australia," *Australasian Psychiatry* 21 (Dec. 2013): 587–91, doi: 10.1177/1039856213500361; Joan Acocella, "Secrets of Nijinsky," *New York Review of Books*, January 14, 1999, www.nybooks.com/articles/archives/1999/jan/14/secrets-of-nijinsky/.

12. Shorter and Healy, *Shock Therapy*, 11–13.

13. Shorter, *A History of Psychiatry*, 215.

14. Richard Abrams, *Electroconvulsive Therapy*, 4th ed. (New York: Oxford University Press, 2002), 526–27.

15. Ferdinando Accornero, "An Eyewitness Account of the Discovery of Electroshock," *Convulsive Therapies* 4 (1988): 47.

16. Shorter and Healy, *Shock Therapy*, 43.

17. Jennifer S. Perrin, Susanne Merz, Daniel M. Bennett, James Currie, Douglas J. Steele, Ian C. Reid, and Christian Schwarzbauer, "Electroconvulsive Therapy Reduces Frontal Cortical Connectivity in Severe Depressive Disorder," *Proceedings of the National Academies of Sciences* 109 (April 2012): 5464–68, doi:10.1073/pnas.1117206109.

18. Ion Anghelescu, Christoph Jürgen Klawe, Peter Bartenstein, and Armin Szegedi, "Normal PET After Long-Term ECT," letter to the editor, *American Journal of Psychiatry* 158 (Sept. 2001): 1527, doi: 10.1176/appi.ajp.158.9.1527.

19. Jennifer Hughes, B. M. Barraclough, and W. Reeve, "Are Patients Shocked by ECT?" *Journal of the Royal Society of Medicine* 74 (April 1981): 283–85.

20. Kitty Dukakis and Larry Tye, *Shock: The Healing Power of Electroconvulsive Therapy* (New York: Penguin, 2006); Sherwin Nuland, "How Electroshock Therapy Changed Me," lecture, TED Talks, February 2001, www.ted.com/talks/sherwin_nuland_on_electroshock_therapy .html; André Picard, "In Praise of 'Electroshock,'" *The Globe and Mail*, October 16, 2009, www.theglobeandmail.com/life/health-and-fitness /health/conditions/in-praise-of-electroshock/article597040/.

21. Nuland, "How Electroshock Therapy Changed Me."

22. Richard's final course of ECT was administered in 2009. His last episode of major depression requiring hospitalization was during the fall of 2011. After forty years of learning to live and repeatedly thrive with familial treatment-resistant bipolar disorder (Type II), including some fifty-five episodes of major depression (1972–2011), a psychotropic medication regimen proved to be the first drugs to bring Richard's major depression into remission without triggering hypomania. The combination of a typical dosage of 30 mg of tranylcypromine (available for the treatment of depression since the 1950s) and an atypically low dosage of 2 mg of aripiprazole (a second-generation antipsychotic medication) has proven to be effective not only in bringing his major depression into remission but also in preventing recurrence of severe episodes and need for ECT

or hospitalization. Since January 2012, Richard has experienced stable wellness sufficient to establish and maintain a productive law practice, including corporate/commercial transactions and litigation; wills and estates; family, mental health, and criminal matters. He works with unique expertise in mental health law and tireless passion to advise clients on how to best resolve civil or criminal legal problems associated with mental disorder. Richard's unprecedented stable wellness since January 2012 has facilitated his happy marriage to Pam in spring 2014 and his joy in parenting their daughter born in June 2015.

5. BRIDGING DISTANCES: TUESDAY AFTERNOON

1. World Health Organization, *Telemedicine: Opportunities and Developments in Member States* (Geneva: World Health Organization, 2010), www.who.int/goe/publications/goe_telemedicine_2010.pdf.

2. Azhar Rafiq, James A. Moore, Xiaoming Zhao, Charles R. Doarn, and Ronald C. Merrrell, "Digital Video Capture and Synchronous Consultation in Open Surgery," *Annals of Surgery* 239 (April 2004): 567–73, doi: 10.1097/01.sla.0000118749.24645.45.

3. Liron Pantanowitz, Clayton Wiley, Anthony Demetris, Andrew Lesniak, Ishtiaque Ahmed, William Cable, Lydia Contis, and Anil V. Parwani, "Experience with Multimodality Telepathology at the University of Pittsburgh Medical Center," *Journal of Pathology Informatics* 3 (2012): 45–53, doi: 10.4103/2153-3539.104907.

4. Christopher Lau, Sean Churchill, Janice Kim, Frederick A. Matsen III, and Yongmin Kim, "Asynchronous Web-Based Patient-Centered Home Telemedicine System," *IEEE Transactions on Biomedical Engineering* 49 (Dec. 2002): 1452–62, doi: 10.1109/TBME.2002.805456.

5. Sally Gainsbury and Alex Blaszczynski, "A Systematic Review of Internet-Based Therapy for the Treatment of Addictions," *Clinical Psychology Review* 31 (April 2011): 490–98, doi: 10.1016/j.cpr.2010.11.007.

6. Evan Osnos, "Meet Dr. Freud: Does Psychoanalysis Have a Future

in an Authoritarian State?," *The New Yorker*, January 10, 2011, www .newyorker.com/magazine/2011/01/10/meet-dr-freud.

7. Laura Eggertson, "High Rates of Childhood Abuse, Depression in Inuit Suicides," *Canadian Medical Association Journal* 185 (July 2013): E433–E434, doi: 10.1503/cmaj.109-4518.

8. Slavash Jafari, Ray Copes, Souzan Baharlou, Mahyar Etminan, and Jane Buxton, "Tattooing and the Risk of Transmission of Hepatitis C: A Systematic Review and Meta-Analysis," *International Journal of Infectious Diseases* 14 (Nov. 2010): e928–e940, doi: 10.1016 /j.ijid.2010.03.019.

9. National Institute of Neurological Disorders and Stroke, "Asperger Syndrome Fact Sheet,"www.ninds.nih.gov/disorders/asperger/detail _asperger.htm.

10. J.M.S. Pearce, "Kanner's Infantile Autism and Asperger's Syndrome," *Journal of Neurology, Neurosurgery & Psychiatry* 76 (2005): 205, doi: 10.1136/jnnp.2004.042820.

11. Steve Silberman, *NeuroTribes: The Legacy of Autism and the Future of Neurodiversity* (New York: Avery, 2015).

12. Ami Klin and Fred R. Volkmar, "History of Asperger's Disorder," psychcentral.com/lib/history-of-aspergers-disorder/000879.

13. Giulia Rhodes, "Autism: A Mother's Labour of Love," *The Guardian*, May 24, 2011, www.theguardian.com/lifeandstyle/2011/may /24/autistic-spectrum-disorder-lorna-wing.

14. "Asperger Syndrome Fact Sheet."

15. Hilary Stace, "Mother Blaming; or Autism, Gender and Science," *Women's Studies Journal* 24 (Dec. 2010): 66–70.

6. EMERGENCIES I: WEDNESDAY MORNING

1. Craig Morgan, Rosemarie Mallett, Gerard Hutchinson, Hemant Bagalkote, Kevin Morgan, Paul Fearon, Paola Dazzan, Jane Boydell, Kwame Mckenzie, Glynn Harrison, Robin Murray, Peter Jones, Tom Craig, and Julian Leff, "Pathways to Care and Ethnicity: 1.

Sample Characteristics and Compulsory Admission," *British Journal of Psychiatry* 186 (2005): 281–89, doi: 10.1192/bjp.186.4.281.

2. Since the time of this clinical experience, the emergency room has been completely renovated and doubled in size, opening in 2015 and named for donors. It is safer, more respectful of the needs of patients and families, and more hopeful. And the fact that prominent citizens were willing to give not only their money but their names to it heralds a welcome change in the stigma about mental illness and its treatment.

3. Malcolm Gladwell, *Blink: The Power of Thinking Without Thinking* (New York: Little, Brown, 2005).

4. M. Alvarez-Jimenez, J. F. Gleeson, L. P. Henry, S. M. Harrigan, M. G. Harris, G. P. Amminger, E. Killackey, A. R. Yung, H. Herrman, H. J. Jackson, and P. D. McGorry, "Prediction of a Single Psychotic Episode: A 7.5-Year, Prospective Study in First-Episode Psychosis," *Schizophrenia Research* 125 (Feb. 2011): 236–46, doi: 10.1016/j.schres.2010.10.020.

5. Emil Kraepelin, *Lebenserinnerungen*, cited in Shorter, *A History of Psychiatry*, 66–67.

6. Roy Porter, *Madness: A Brief History* (New York: Oxford University Press, 2005), 184.

7. Eric J. Engstrom, "Kraepelin: Social Section," in Berrios and Porter, *A History of Clinical Psychiatry*, chap. 10.

8. Shorter, *A History of Psychiatry*, 102.

9. Ibid., 107–108.

10. Shitij Kapur, "Psychosis as a State of Aberrant Salience: A Framework Linking Biology, Phenomenology, and Pharmacology in Schizophrenia," *American Journal of Psychiatry* 160 (Jan. 2003): 15.

11. Harvey A. Whiteford, Louisa Degenhardt, Jürgen Rehm, Amanda J. Baxter, Alize J. Ferrari, Holly E. Erskine, Fiona J. Charlson, Rosana E. Norman, Abraham D. Flaxman, Nicole Johns, Roy Burstein, Christopher J. L. Murray, and Theo Vos, "Global Burden of Disease Attributable to Mental and Substance Use Disorders:

Findings from the Global Burden of Disease Study 2010," *Lancet* 382 (Nov. 2013): 1575–86, doi: 10.1016/S0140-6736(13)61611-6.

12. Kapur, "Psychosis as a State of Aberrant Salience," 13–23.

13. Bernard A. Fischer and Robert W. Buchanan, "Schizophrenia: Epidemiology and Pathogenesis," UpToDate, updated October 9, 2015, http://www.uptodate.com/contents/schizophrenia -epidemiology-and-pathogenesis.

14. World Health Organization, *Mental Health Atlas 2011* (Geneva: World Health Organization, 2011), p. 22, hwhqlibdoc.who.int /publications/2011/9799241564359_eng.pdf.

7. EMERGENCIES II: WEDNESDAY AFTERNOON

1. Herbert Y. Meltzer, Larry Alphs, Alan I. Green, A. Carlo Altamura, Ravi Anand, Alberto Bertoldi, Marc Bourgeois, Guy Chouinard, M. Zahur Islam, John Kane, Ranga Krishnan, J.-P. Lindenmayer, and Steve Potkin, "Clozapine Treatment for Suicidality in Schizophrenia International Suicide Prevention Trial (InterSePT)," *Archives of General Psychiatry* 60 (2003): 82–91, doi: 10.1001/archpsyc.60.1.82.

2. Cornelius L. Mulder, Gerrit T. Koopmans, and Jean-Paul Selten, "Emergency Psychiatry, Compulsory Admissions and the Clinical Presentation Among Immigrants to The Netherlands," *British Journal of Psychiatry* 188 (April 2006): 386–91, doi: 10.1192 /bjp.188.4.386.

3. Ibid.

4. Peter P. Roy-Byrne, "Postpartum Blues and Unipolar Depression: Epidemiology, Clinical Features, Assessment, and Diagnosis," UpToDate, updated November 24, 2014, http://www.uptodate .com/contents/postpartum-blues-and-unipolar-depression -epidemiology-clinical-features-assessment-and-diagnosis.

5. Meir Steiner, "Postpartum Psychiatric Disorders," *Canadian Journal of Psychiatry* 35 (1990): 89.

6 Michael W. O'Hara and Annette M. Swain, "Rates and Risk of Postpartum Depression – A Meta-Analysis," *International Review of Psychiatry* 8 (1996): 37–54, doi: 10.3109/09540269609037816.

7. Postpartum Support International, "Postpartum Psychosis," www .postpartum.net/learn-more/postpartum-psychosis.

8. James F. Paulson and Sharnail D. Bazemore, "Prenatal and Postpartum Depression in Fathers and Its Association with Maternal Depression: A Meta-Analysis," *JAMA* 303 (2010): 1961, doi: 10.1001 /jama.2010.605.

8. RESTRAINT: THURSDAY MORNING

1. Thomas Bewley, *Madness to Mental Illness: A History of the Royal College of Psychiatrists* (London: RCPsych Publications, 2008), chap. 1.

2. Shorter, *A History of Psychiatry*.

3. Ibid., 3.

4. Ibid., 4.

5. Ibid.

6. Richard Warner, "The Roots of Hospital Alternative Care," *British Journal of Psychiatry* 197, supp. 53 (Aug. 2010): s4–s5, doi: 10.1192 /bjp.bp.110.080036.

7. Philippe Pinel, *A Treatise on Insanity*, trans. D. D. Davis (New York: Hafner, 1962), 63–64, 67.

8. Ibid., 67.

9. Bridget M. Kuehn, "Criminal Justice Becomes Front Line for Mental Health Care," *JAMA* 311 (May 2014): 1953–54, doi: 10.1001 /jama.2014.4578.

10. World Health Organization, *Mental Health Legislation & Human Rights* (Geneva: World Health Organization, 2003), www.who.int /mental_health/resources/en/Legislation.pdf.

11. Mark Moran, "New Law to Transform MH Services in China," *Psychiatric News*, June 7, 2013, psychnews.psychiatryonline.org/doi/full /10.1176%Fappi.pn.2013.6a9.

12. Janet S. Richmond, Jon S. Berlin, Avrim B. Fishkind, Garland H. Holloman Jr., Scott L. Zeller, Michael P. Wilson, Muhamad Aly Rifal, and Anthony T. Ng, "Verbal De-escalation of the Agitated Patient: Consensus Statement of the American Association for Emergency Psychiatry Project BETA De-escalation Workgroup," *Western Journal of Emergency Medicine* 13 (2012): 17–25, doi: 10.5811/westjem.2011.9.6864.

13. Paula Goering, George Tolomiczenko, Tess Sheldon, Katherine Boydell, and Donald Wasylenki, "Characteristics of Persons Who Are Homeless for the First Time," *Psychiatric Services* 53 (2002): 1472–74, doi: 10.1176/appi.ps.53.11.1472.

14. Paula Goering, Scott Veldhuizen, Aimee Watson, Carol Adair, Brianna Kopp, Eric Latimer, Tim Aubry, Geoff Nelson, Eric MacNaughton, David Streiner, Daniel Rabouin, Angela Ly, and Guido Powell, *National at Home/Chez Soi Final Report* (Calgary, Alberta: Mental Health Commission of Canada, 2014), mhcc _at_home_report_national_cross-site_eng_2.pdf.

9. OFF THE PATH: THURSDAY AFTERNOON

1. Inge Bretherton, "The Origins of Attachment Theory: John Bowlby and Mary Ainsworth," *Developmental Psychology* 28 (1992): 759–75.

2. Kathryn M. Bigelow and Edward K. Morris, "John B. Watson's Advice on Child Rearing," *Behavioral Development Bulletin* 1 (Fall 2001): 26–30, doi: 10.1037/h0100479.

3. Ann Hulbert, "He Was an Author Only a Mother Could Love," *Los Angeles Times*, May 11, 2003, http://articles.latimes.com/2003/may /11/opinion/oe-hulbert11.

4. Bretherton, "Origins of Attachment Theory," 762.

5. Harriet P. Lefley, review of Stella Chess and Alexander Thomas, *Temperament: Theory and Practice*, *American Journal of Psychiatry* 155 (1998): 144.

6. Michael Rutter, Anthony Cox, Celia Tupling, Michael Berger, and William Yule, "Attainment and Adjustment in Two Geographical

Areas I – The Prevalence of Psychiatric Disorder," *British Journal of Psychiatry* 126 (June 1975): 493–509, doi: 10.1192/bjp.126.6.493.

7. Michael Rutter, Jack Tizard, William Yule, Philip Graham, and Kingsley Whitmore, "Research Report: Isle of Wight Studies, 1944–1974," *Psychological Medicine* 6 (May 1976): 313–32, doi: 10.1017/S003329170001388X.

8. Centers for Disease Control, Injury Prevention & Control: Division of Violence Prevention, ACE Study, www.cdc.gov/violencepreven tion/acestudy/.

9. Cathérine Dupont, D. Randall Armant, and Carol A. Brenner, "Epigenetics: Definition, Mechanisms, and Clinical Perspective," *Seminars in Reproductive Medicine* 27 (Sept. 2009): 351–57, doi: 10.1055 /s-0029-1237423.

10. Nessa Carey, *The Epigenetics Revolution: How Modern Biology Is Rewriting Our Understanding of Genetics, Disease, and Inheritance* (New York: Columbia University Press, 2012), 6.

11. Michelle S. Horner, "Epigenetics and Child and Adolescent Psychiatry," *Journal of the American Academy of Child & Adolescent Psychiatry* 48 (Nov. 2009): 1048, doi: http://dx.doi.org/10.1097/CHI.0b013e3181bb8d56.

12. Janet Wozniak, Joseph Biederman, Kathleen Kiely, J. Stuart Ablon, Stephen V. Faraone, Elizabeth Mundy, and Douglas Mennin, "Mania-Like Symptoms Suggestive of Childhood-Onset Bipolar Disorder in Clinically Referred Children," *Journal of the American Academy of Adolescent Psychiatry* 34 (July 1995): 867–76.

13. Scott Allen, "Backlash on Bipolar Diagnoses in Children," *Boston Globe*, June 17, 2007, www.boston.com/yourlife/health/diseases /articles/2007/06/17/backlash_on_bipolar_diagnoses_in_children/; Gardiner Harris and Benedict Carey, "Researchers Fail to Reveal Full Drug Pay," *New York Times*, June 8, 2008, www.nytimes.com/2008/06 /08/us/08conflict.html?_r=0; Alan Schwarz, "The Selling of Attention Deficit Disorder," *New York Times*, December 14, 2013, www.nytimes .com/2013/12/15/health/the-selling-of-attention-deficit-disorder.html.

14. Daniel Offer, Eric Ostrov, and Kenneth I. Howard, "The Mental

Health Professional's Concept of the Normal Adolescent," *Archives of General Psychiatry* 38 (Feb. 1981): 149–52, doi: 10.1001 /archpsyc.1981.01780270035003; Angela Boak, Hayley A. Hamilton, Edward M. Adlaf, Joe Beitchman, David Wolfe, and Robert E. Mann, "The Mental Health and Well-Being of Ontario Students, 1991–2013," OSDUHS highlights (Toronto, ON: Centre for Addiction and Mental Health, 2014); Rutter, "Research Report: Isle of Wight Studies."

15. Thomas E. Ellis, Thomas O. Dickey, and Eric C. Jones, "Patient Suicide in Psychiatry Residency Programs: A National Survey of Training and Postvention Practices," *Academic Psychiatry* 22 (September 1998): 181–88, doi: 10.1007/BF03341922.

10. DOUBT: FRIDAY MORNING

1. Veterans Affairs Canada, "Understanding Mental Health," www .veterans.gc.ca/eng/mental-health/osi.

2. College of Physicians and Surgeons of Ontario, "Mandatory and Permissive Reporting," policy statement 6-12, 2012, www.cpso.on.ca /uploadedFiles/policies/policies/policyitems/mandatoryreporting .pdf.

3. American Psychiatric Association, *DSM-5*.

4. Jules R. Bemporad, "Self-Starvation Through the Ages: Reflections on the Pre-History of Anorexia Nervosa," *International Journal of Eating Disorders* 19 (April 1996): 217–37, doi: 10.1002/(SICI)1098 -108X(199604)19:3<217::AID-EAT1>3.0.CO;2-P.

5. Joseph A. Silverman, "Richard Morton's Second Case of Anorexia Nervosa: Reverend Minister Steele and His Son – An Historical Vignette," *International Journal of Eating Disorders* 7 (May 1988): 439–41, doi: 10.1002/1098-108X(198805)7:3<439::AID -EAT2260070319>3.0.CO;2-N.

6. Bemporad, "Self-Starvation Through the Ages," 228.

7. William Withey Gull, "Anorexia Nervosa (Apepsia Hysterica,

Anorexia Hysterica)," October 24, 1873, *Obesity Research* 5 (Sept. 1997): 498–502, doi: 10.1002/j.1550-8528.1997.tb00677.x.

8. Walter Vandereycken and Ron van Deth, "A Tribute to Lasègue's Description of Anorexia Nervosa (1873), with Completion of Its English Translation," *British Journal of Psychiatry* 157 (Dec. 1990): 902–8, doi: 10.1192/bjp.157.6.902.

9. Eugene L. Bliss and Charles Henry Hardin Branch, "The Biology of Anorexia Nervosa," in *Anorexia Nervosa: Its History, Psychology, and Biology* (New York: Paul B. Hoeber, 1960), 74–105.

10. Joss Bray, "Is Anorexia Nervosa a Psychotic Illness?" letter to the editor, *BMJ* 334 (May 7, 2007): 894, doi: 0.1136/bmj.39171.616840.BE.

11. J. Harbottle, C. L. Birmingham, and F. Sayani, "Anorexia Nervosa: A Survival Analysis," *Journal of Eating and Weight Disorders* 13 (June 2008): e32–e34.

12. Jon Arcelus, Alex J. Mitchell, Jackie Wales, and Søren Nielsen, "Mortality Rates in Patients with Anorexia Nervosa and Other Eating Disorders: A Meta-Analysis of 36 Studies," *Archives of General Psychiatry* 68 (July 2011): 724–31, doi: 10.1001/archgenpsychiatry.2011.74.

13. B. Timothy Walsh, Allan S. Kaplan, Evelyn Attia, Marion Olmsted, Michael Parides, Jacqueline C. Carter, Kathleen M. Pike, Michael J. Devlin, Blake Woodside, Christina A. Roberto, and Wendi Rockert, "Fluoxetine After Weight Restoration in Anorexia Nervosa: A Randomized Control Trial," *JAMA* 295 (June 14, 2006): 2605–12, doi: 10.1001/jama.295.22.2605.

14. Seena S. K. Grewal, "A Comparison of the Presentation and Outcome of Anorexia Nervosa in Early and Late Adolescence" (master's thesis, Graduate Department of Medical Science, University of Toronto, 2011).

15. Małgorzata Starzomska, "Controversial Issues Concerning the Concept of Palliative Care of Anorexic Patients," *Archives of Psychiatry and Psychotherapy* 4 (2010): 49–59.

16. Michael Strober, "Managing the Chronic, Treatment-Resistant Patient with Anorexia Nervosa," *International Journal of Eating*

Disorders 36 (Nov. 2004): 245–55, doi: 10.1002/eat.20054; Josie Geller, Kim D. Williams, and Suja Srikameswaran, "Clinician Stance in the Treatment of Chronic Eating Disorders," *European Eating Disorders Review* 9 (Nov./Dec. 2001): 365–73, doi: 10.1002 /erv.443.

11. PUBLIC AND PRIVATE: FRIDAY AFTERNOON AND EVENING

1. Peter Byrne, "Psychiatric Stigma," *British Journal of Psychiatry* 178 (March 2001): 281–84, doi: 10.1192/bjp.178.3.281.
2. Claire Henderson, Elaine Brohan, Sarah Clement, Paul Williams, Francesca Lassman, Oliver Schauman, Lisa Dockery, Simone Farrelly, Joanna Murray, Caroline Murphy, Mike Slade, and Graham Thornicroft, "Decision Aid on Disclosure of Mental Health Status to an Employer: Feasibility and Outcomes of a Randomized Controlled Trial," *British Journal of Psychiatry* 203 (Nov. 2013): 350–57, doi: 10.1192/bjp.bp.113.128470.
3. Goering, et al. *National at Home/Chez Soi Final Report.*
4. Yin-Yang Lee and Julia L. Lin, "The Effects of Trust in Physician on Self-Efficacy, Adherence and Diabetes Outcomes," *Social Science & Medicine* 68 (March 2006): 1060–68, doi: 10.1016 /j.socscimed.2008.12.033.

AUTHORS' NOTE

1. Tom Shakespeare, review of Oliver Sacks, *An Anthropologist on Mars, Disability and Society* 11 (March 1996): 137–39.

Further Reading

In choosing books for this section, we tried to mingle the voices of people and family members of people who have lived with psychiatric disorders with works by writers, including mental health professionals, scientists, and the simply curious, who offer suggestions, strategies, information, and hope. The list is by no means exhaustive, but all the books have been read by one or both of us.

HISTORY OF PSYCHIATRY AND SOME CURRENT THEMES

Appignanesi, Lisa. *Mad, Bad, and Sad: Women and the Mind Doctors.* New York: W. W. Norton, 2008.

Bolton, Derek. *What Is Mental Disorder? An Essay in Philosophy, Science, and Values.* New York: Oxford University Press, 2008.

Foucault, Michel. *Madness and Civilization: A History of Insanity in the Age of Reason.* New York: Random House, 1965.

Gabbard, Glen O., Laura Weiss Roberts, Holly Crisp-Han, Valdesha

Ball, Gabrielle Hobday, and Funmilayo Rachal. *Professionalism in Psychiatry.* Arlington, VA: American Psychiatric Publishing, 2012.

Kallert, Thomas W., Juan E. Mezzich, and John Monahan, eds. *Coercive Treatment in Psychiatry: Clinical, Legal and Ethical Aspects.* Chichester, UK: Wiley-Blackwell, 2011.

Luhrmann, T. M. *Of Two Minds: The Growing Disorder in American Psychiatry.* New York: Alfred A. Knopf, 2000.

Porter, Roy. *Madness: A Brief History.* New York: Oxford University Press, 2002.

Sadler, John Z. *Values and Psychiatric Diagnosis.* New York: Oxford University Press, 2005.

Shorter, Edward. *A History of Psychiatry: From the Era of the Asylum to the Age of Prozac.* New York: John Wiley, 1997.

Watters, Ethan. *Crazy Like Us: The Globalization of the American Psyche.* New York: Free Press, 2010.

Weissman, Sidney, Melvin Sabshin, and Harold Eist, eds. *Psychiatry in the New Millennium.* Washington, D.C.: American Psychiatric Press, 1999.

ADDICTION

Carr, David. *The Night of the Gun: A Reporter Investigates the Darkest Story of His Life, His Own.* New York: Simon & Schuster, 2008.

Carroll, Jim. *The Basketball Diaries.* New York: Penguin, 1987.

Johnston, Ann Dowsett. *Drink: The Intimate Relationship Between Women and Alcohol.* New York: Harper, 2013.

Knapp, Caroline. *Drinking: A Love Story.* New York: Dial Press, 1996.

ANXIETY

Bourne, Edmund J. *The Anxiety & Phobia Workbook.* 5th ed. Oakland, CA: New Harbinger, 2010.

Pearson, Patricia. *A Brief History of Anxiety – Yours and Mine.* New York: Bloomsbury, 2008.

Smith, Daniel B. *Monkey Mind: A Memoir of Anxiety.* New York: Simon & Schuster, 2012.

Stossel, Scott. *My Age of Anxiety: Fear, Hope, Dread, and the Search for Peace of Mind.* New York: Alfred A. Knopf, 2013.

BIPOLAR DISORDER

Berger, Diane, and Lisa Berger. *We Heard the Angels of Madness: A Family Guide to Coping with Manic Depression.* New York: Harper, 1992.

Jamison, Kay Redfield. *An Unquiet Mind: A Memoir of Moods and Madness.* New York: Alfred A. Knopf, 1995.

Vonnegut, Mark. *Just Like Someone Without a Mental Illness Only More So.* New York: Delacorte, 2010.

BORDERLINE PERSONALITY DISORDER

Kaysen, Susanna. *Girl, Interrupted.* New York: Turtle Bay Books, 1993.

Linehan, Marsha M. *Skills Training Manual for Treating Borderline Personality Disorder.* New York: Guilford Press, 1993.

Mason, Paul T., and Randi Kreger. *Stop Walking on Eggshells: Taking Back Your Life When Someone You Care About Has Borderline Personality Disorder.* 2nd ed. Oakland, CA: New Harbinger, 2010.

CHILD PSYCHIATRY

Karen, Robert. *Becoming Attached: First Relationships and How They Impact Our Capacity to Love.* New York: Oxford University Press, 1994. First published 1994 by Warner Books.

Stern, Daniel N. *The Interpersonal World of the Infant: A View from Psychoanalysis and Developmental Psychology.* New York: Basic Books, 1985.

Warner, Judith. *We've Got Issues: Children and Parents in the Age of Medication.* New York: Riverhead Books, 2010.

COGNITIVE BEHAVIOR THERAPY

Beck, Judith S. *Cognitive Behavior Therapy: Basics and Beyond.* 2nd ed. New York: Guilford Press, 2011.

Burns, David D. *The Feeling Good Handbook: Using the New Mood Therapy in Everyday Life.* New York: Morrow, 1989.

Greenberger, Dennis, and Christine A. Padesky. *Mind Over Mood: Change How You Feel by Changing the Way You Think.* New York: Guilford Press, 1995.

DEPRESSION

Manning, Martha. *Undercurrents: A Therapist's Reckoning with Her Own Depression.* New York: Harper, 1994.

Solomon, Andrew. *The Noonday Demon: An Atlas of Depression.* New York: Scribner, 2001.

Styron, William. *Darkness Visible: A Memoir of Madness.* New York: Random House, 1990.

EATING DISORDERS

de Rossi, Portia. *Unbearable Lightness: A Story of Loss and Gain.* New York: Atria Books, 2010.

Fairburn, Christopher G., and Kelly D. Brownell, eds. *Eating Disorders and Obesity: A Comprehensive Handbook.* New York: Guilford Press, 2002.

Hornbacher, Marya. *Wasted: A Memoir of Anorexia and Bulimia.* New York: Harper, 1998.

Orbach, Susie. *Hunger Strike: The Anorectic's Struggle as a Metaphor for Our Age.* New York: W. W. Norton, 1986.

ELECTROCONVULSIVE THERAPY

Dukakis, Kitty, and Larry Tye. *Shock: The Healing Power of Electroconvulsive Therapy.* New York: Avery, 2006.

Fink, Max. *Electroconvulsive Therapy: A Guide for Professionals and Their Patients.* New York: Oxford University Press, 2009.

EPIGENETICS

Carey, Nessa. *The Epigenetics Revolution: How Modern Biology Is Rewriting Our Understanding of Genetics, Disease, and Inheritance.* New York: Columbia University Press, 2012.

MINDFULNESS

Kabat-Zinn, Jon. *Full Catastrophe Living: Using the Wisdom of Your Body and Mind to Face Stress, Pain, and Illness.* New York: Delacorte, 1990.

Teasdale, John, Mark Williams, and Zindel Segal. *The Mindful Way Workbook: An 8-Week Program to Free Yourself from Depression and Emotional Distress.* New York: Guilford Press, 2014.

PSYCHOTHERAPY

Grosz, Stephen. *The Examined Life: How We Lose and Find Ourselves.* New York: W. W. Norton, 2013.

Yalom, Irvin D. *Love's Executioner, and Other Tales of Psychotherapy.* New York: Basic Books, 1989.

PSYCHOPHARMACOLOGY AND PSYCHIATRY'S RELATIONSHIP WITH DRUG COMPANIES

Angell, Marcia. *The Truth About Drug Companies: How They Deceive Us and What to Do About It.* New York: Random House, 2004.

Carlat, Daniel. *Unhinged: The Trouble with Psychiatry – A Doctor's Revelations About a Profession in Crisis.* New York: Free Press, 2010.

POST-TRAUMATIC STRESS DISORDER

Barker, Pat. *Regeneration.* New York: Viking, 1991.

Feinstein, Anthony. *Journalists Under Fire: The Psychological Hazards of Covering War.* Baltimore: Johns Hopkins University Press, 2006.

Sebold, Alice. *Lucky.* New York: Scribner, 1999.

SCHIZOPHRENIA

Cockburn, Patrick, and Henry Cockburn. *Henry's Demons: Living with Schizophrenia, A Father and Son's Story.* New York: Scribner, 2011.

Saks, Elyn R. *The Center Cannot Hold: My Journey Through Madness.* New York: Hyperion, 2007.

Torrey, E. Fuller. *Surviving Schizophrenia: A Manual for Families, Patients, and Providers.* 6th ed. New York: Harper, 2013.

SUICIDE

Colt, George Howe. *November of the Soul: The Enigma of Suicide.* New York: Scribner, 2006.

Durkheim, Émile. *Suicide: A Study in Sociology.* Trans. John A. Spaulding and George Simpson. Glencoe, IL: Free Press, 1951.

Jamison, Kay Redfield. *Night Falls Fast: Understanding Suicide.* New York: Alfred A. Knopf, 1999.

Index